I0890399

THE HEALTHY COUNTRY?

We know much about how personal behaviours, choices and genes influence individual health. This enterprising, well-written and timely book asks a bigger question: What cultural, political, commercial and socioeconomic influences explain the trends over several centuries in New Zealand's population health and life expectancy? The authors' exploration of major differences in health trends between Māori and Europeans (Pākehā) provides further valuable insights – and just when the need for sustainable and healthier ways of living is pressing on us all.

– Professor Emeritus Tony McMichael, Australian National University

The history of life and death in New Zealand is of wide interest, both because New Zealand held the record for life expectancy over a long period and because of the experience of the indigenous population. Written in a lively style by internationally renowned scholars, this book provides a convincing synthesis of life expectancy from pre-European times to the present and it will be welcomed by readers around the world.

– Professor Dr Johan P. Mackenbach, Erasmus MC, University Medical Center Rotterdam

THE HEALTHY COUNTRY?

A History of Life & Death in New Zealand

Alistair Woodward & Tony Blakely

AUCKLAND
UNIVERSITY
PRESS

First published 2014

Auckland University Press
University of Auckland
Private Bag 92019
Auckland 1142
New Zealand
www.press.auckland.ac.nz

© Alistair Woodward and Tony Blakely, 2014

ISBN 978 1 86940 813 8

A catalogue record for this book is available from the
National Library of New Zealand

This book is copyright. Apart from fair dealing for the purpose of private study, research, criticism or review, as permitted under the Copyright Act, no part may be reproduced by any process without prior permission of the publisher. The moral rights of the authors have been asserted.

Cover design: Keely O'Shannessy

Printed by Printlink Ltd, Wellington

Contents

LIST OF FIGURES

LIST OF TABLES

PREFACE

New Zealand offers unexpected insights into human longevity and, especially, helps to explain the astounding mortality reductions that have occurred in most countries, most of the time, in the last 150 years. For New Zealanders this book is about who we were, who we are now and how we might live in the future. Further afield, we hope our story will attract readers who are curious about the links between location, history, social circumstances, physical environments and health. Stephen Kunitz notes that it is 'particular realities' as much as generalities that matter when trying to decipher trends in longevity;[1] and as a small island nation remote from the mainstream of biological history and human settlement, New Zealand certainly does have its own particularities. We are writing also for students in public health and epidemiology, be they formally enrolled students or (like us) just wanting to learn more. Don't mistake this for a comprehensive textbook. It roams the borders and neglects disciplinary heartlands, but we hope our book adds to the standard treatments with detail, colour, connections and, perhaps, surprise.

ACKNOWLEDGEMENTS

Sam Elworthy of Auckland University Press prompted the idea for this book over coffee some years ago, and then shepherded us through the process.

The University of Auckland and the University of Otago have generously granted sabbatical time for us to research and write the majority of this book.

The Health Research Council of New Zealand and the Ministry of Health funded the New Zealand Census-Mortality Study and the CancerTrends Study that together contributed many of the data we present in chapter 6.

We have been fortunate to receive enthusiastic and wise comment on drafts of this book from many of our colleagues and friends: Robert Beaglehole, Ruth Bonita, Linda Bryder, Hera Cook, Caroline Daley, Tahu Kukutai, Richard McKenzie, Tony McMichael, Alison O'Connell, Papaarangi Reid, Anthony Rodgers, Diana Sarfati, Richard Taylor, Martin Tobias and Nick Wilson. We also appreciate the comments of two anonymous Auckland University Press reviewers.

We thank Kate Sloane, who helped with the preparation of the figures and numerous other editing tasks; Ginny Sullivan, for copyediting and indexing; and Igor Drecki for the redrawn map of New Zealand.

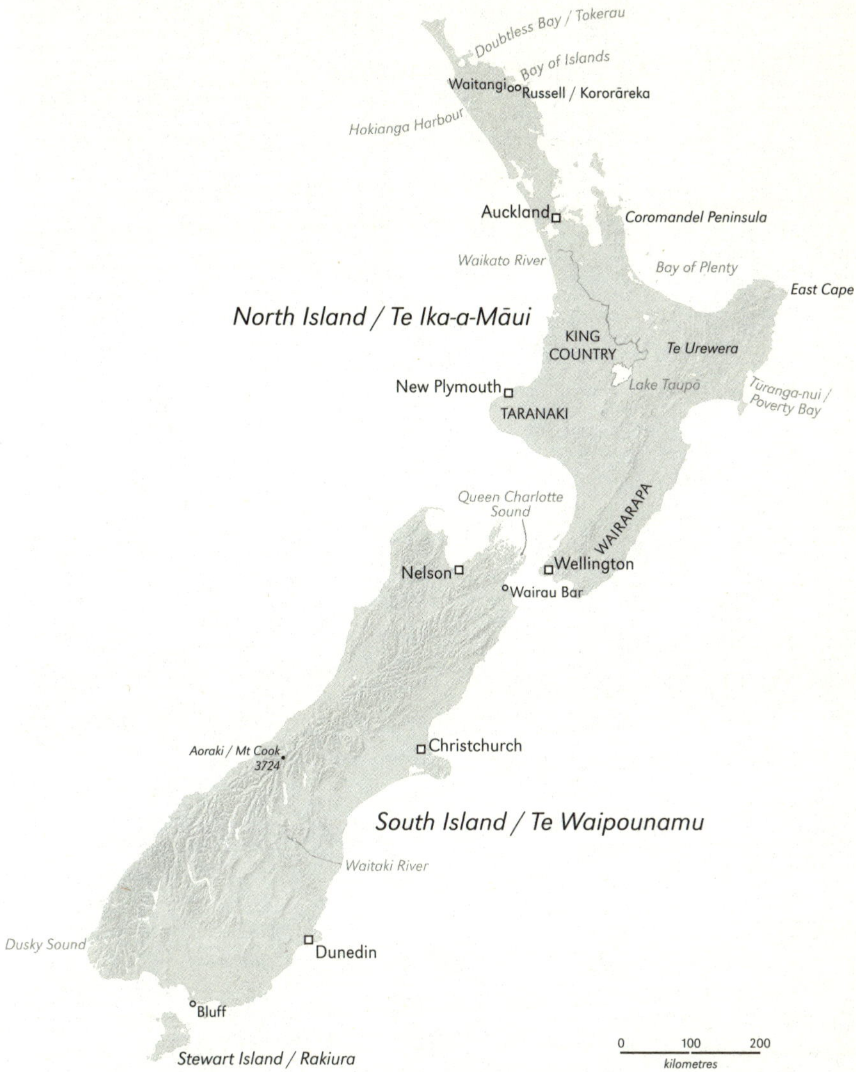

Doubtless Bay / Tokerau
Bay of Islands
Waitangi
Russell / Kororāreka
Hokianga Harbour
Auckland
Coromandel Peninsula
Waikato River
Bay of Plenty
East Cape
North Island / Te Ika-a-Māui
KING COUNTRY
Te Urewera
New Plymouth
Lake Taupō
Tūranga-nui / Poverty Bay
TARANAKI
Queen Charlotte Sound
WAIRARAPA
Nelson
Wellington
Wairau Bar
Christchurch
Aoraki / Mt Cook 3724
South Island / Te Waipounamu
Waitaki River
Dusky Sound
Dunedin
Bluff
Stewart Island / Rakiura
0
100
200
kilometres

Introduction

Was born, is dead.
Let this be said
on stone over my head
or graven on urn
when it is my turn.
— DENIS GLOVER, 'EPITAPH'

We live in an age of speed and transformation. Since 1965, computer-processing power has doubled roughly every two years. If you were born before 1970, the world's population has doubled in your lifetime. The press of human activity has overwhelmed the natural environment. If current trends continue, carbon dioxide (CO_2) levels in the atmosphere will double by the end of the century, and the acidity of the oceans will increase by 150 per cent. These changes are remarkable. But for a species to double – actually soon triple – its life expectancy over a period of less than ten generations is, simply, astounding. There is no singular and uncontested explanation. Rather, each country achieved its incredible mortality decline at different times, at different speeds and with (somewhat) differing determinants.

Measuring life expectancy is one way of capturing the mortality experience of a population. It also acts as a proxy measure for 'health' more generally. Life expectancy is a sentinel measure of the social, political and environmental undercurrents in a society; it summarises the causes of disease and injury in a single number. Life expectancy takes account of the credits as well as the debits: it embodies all the behaviours, circumstances and interventions that promote health, or detract from it, in both the short and long run.

We are writing as Pākehā (non-Māori) epidemiologists and public health doctors. What interests us is the intersection of social history and medicine, the ways in which diseases are influenced by the environments that people live in, and the impacts of health services and other social interventions. We attempt to bring together biological explanations for ageing with an understanding of how changes in lifestyles and living conditions may affect population health. Coming from public health, we are particularly interested in the big picture view, in what is happening to whole populations.

This account foregrounds what can be measured and compared. Some might object: don't statistical trends provide a rather thin account of the lived experiences of growing up, ageing and dying in New Zealand? We disagree – the statistics shed light on important questions of policy and practice. The archaic nature of present arrangements for superannuation, the future spend on health care, employment laws, how to share life opportunities more fairly, environmental constraints on human development, the complex relation of wealth and health, personal decisions on balancing work and other aspects of life – a statistical history of life expectancy has something to say about all these matters, and more.

At a personal level, we all reflect from time to time on the number of years that we have left on this mortal coil. This value, the age an individual might live to, is easy to comprehend even if it is, usually, unknowable. At the level of a population, we can choose from a variety of aggregate measures. Life expectancy equates to the average age at death, or 'expected' remaining number of years to live. (See text box opposite.) In this book we refer most commonly to 'life expectancy at birth', but it is possible to estimate the average years of life remaining at any age.

There are two ways of calculating the life expectancy of a population. The first is 'cohort' life expectancy, obtained by following up a defined group and recording years of life for each individual. More commonly, we use 'period' life expectancy, which is a convenient way of summarising age-specific death rates that apply at a given point in time. (Examples of an age-specific death rate would be deaths per thousand individuals in the first year of life, or the rate at which deaths occur between age 40 and 41.) As shown in the text box, the period life expectancy for calendar year 1901 would be the average number of years lived by a group (imaginary, not real) who throughout their lives experienced the age-specific mortality rates as observed in 1901.

LIFE EXPECTANCY AND OTHER MEASURES OF LONGEVITY

We use life expectancy (LE) as a marker of 'health' in this book – a common practice given that historical records of mortality are reliable, and it is hard to quibble about the accuracy of knowing whether someone is dead or alive. We visit considerations of quality of life and morbidity during the book, and particularly in our concluding chapter.

There are two types of life expectancy: period and cohort. Period is the version more commonly encountered in the literature, but it is easier to understand cohort life expectancy first.

Cohort life expectancy is the average age of death of an *actual* population followed for many years. The figure overleaf shows the survival curve for New Zealand females born in 1901, taken from Statistics New Zealand.[2] The y-axis shows the proportion of the cohort surviving to one year of age, two years, etc. The curve drops to nearly 0.9 at one year of age, due to high infant mortality (i.e., nearly 10 per cent of babies died in the first year of life in 1901), then levels off. By the age of 90 years (or 1991 in calendar years), less than 10 per cent of this cohort was still alive. The area under the curve is a measure of the average survival or the average age of death, which is the same as cohort life expectancy: 63.8 years.

Life expectancy is just one way to describe the longevity of this cohort. Another is the median age of death, i.e., the age at which 50 per cent of the cohort has died. For this 1901 birth cohort it was 75 years, considerably higher than the life expectancy of 63.8 years. Put another way, a female born in 1901 had an average age at death of 63.8 years, but a 50 per cent chance of making it to 75 years. The reason these two measures of longevity differ is the high infant mortality (which immediately lowers the average age of death, or immediately reduces the area under the curve), and the rapid decline in survival (or increase in mortality) after the median age of death of 75 years.

The figure also shows the 'synthetic' survival curve that we use to estimate period life expectancy. The period approach refers to an imaginary world, which includes a large number, say 100,000, females who were born in 1901 and who experience over the remainder of their imaginary lives the age-specific mortality rates observed for females in 1901. That is, we take the mortality rates that were in force in a particular period and apply these to our imagined population to calculate survival curves. The beauty of this is that as soon as we have the mortality rates for, say, 2010 to 2012, Statistics New Zealand can announce the period life expectancy. The downside is that if mortality rates continue to fall in the future, the (imaginary) period life expectancy will under-estimate the (lived) cohort life expectancy. Indeed, that is what we see in the figure since the 1901 female period survival curve sits well to the left of the cohort curve. The average age of death or life expectancy is 56.8 years – much less than the equivalent cohort figure of 63.8 years.

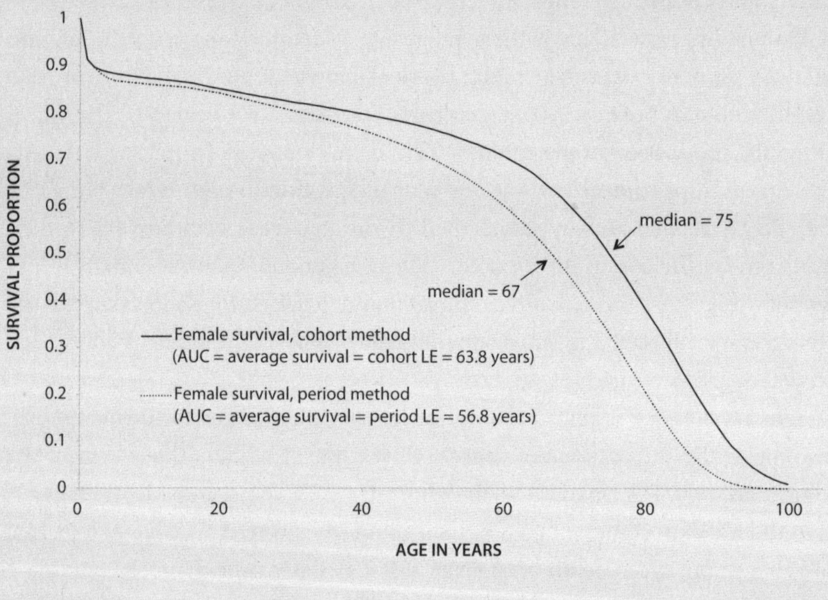

Another way to visualise a population's longevity, survival or mortality experience is to plot the frequency of death by age. (The first graph accumulated *survival* by age.) The second figure does this, using the period method for New Zealand females in 1901 and 2011. We have noted already that the 1901 period life expectancy is 56.8 and the median age of death is 66.7 years. But now we can see also the modal or most common age of death. In 1901, the distribution was bi-modal, with one peak in infancy, and another at age 77 years. The curve for 2011 is moved to the right, infant deaths are much less common and there is a sharper peak in older age (the most common age of death is now 89 years). The great majority of deaths fall within a narrower range at an older age. The median age of death in 2011 is 86.2 years, and the period life expectancy 83.0 years. (Should mortality rates keep on falling in the future, then all three figures will be under-estimates of what actually happens in the cohort.)

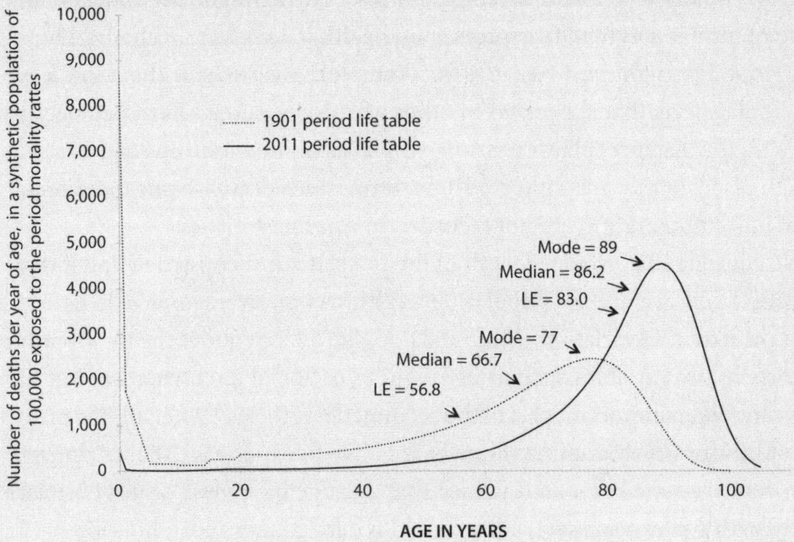

These three measures of longevity are calculated for populations, but can be applied also to individuals, in terms of their potential. For an individual female, for instance, we can talk about average years of life (life expectancy), a 50 per cent probability of living to the median age of death or the age at which she is most likely to die.

LIFE EXPECTANCY – WHAT IS IT?

Of course, quality of life is important as well as longevity, and attempts have been made to measure 'healthy life expectancy' by taking account of the expected quality of life (e.g., freedom from disability) in each year lived. But this is difficult. What constitutes good health, and how it might be measured, are simple questions without simple answers. Cultures that highlight the independent action of individuals tend to express good health in terms of mechanical functions (mobility, sight and hearing, for example). Measures of this kind leave out social aspects that are prized in other world-views: the Māori perspective of health, for instance, places a strong emphasis on relationships and connections to place, family and culture. These dimensions of well-being are difficult to put into numbers and are not recorded in routine statistics.[3]

We concede that average length of life is a statistical construct, and it does not give a full account of population health. As an average, it tells us little about the extent of variation within the population, nor about the distribution of mortality by variables such as age, gender or social circumstance. But life expectancy is an important part of the account nevertheless. After all, 'the pleasures of life are worth nothing if one is not alive to experience them'.[4] (Indeed, when countries are compared we see that average happiness scores correlate closely with life expectancy!)[5] Few would regard higher mortality (lower life expectancy) as a good thing, and death rates are measured with fairly high levels of accuracy and the information is widely reported. Therefore, comparisons of life expectancy provide a useful way of tackling questions such as: does good health result from economic progress, or is it a cause? are populations with a relatively even distribution of resources healthier than those with greater inequalities in living standards? and, what is the relative importance of factors such as medical treatments, education, public health services and 'good genes'?

Embedded in most people's conception of a good life is avoiding an early death, but what represents an 'early death'? In some villages in southern India in the 1960s, death at 40 years or more was considered evidence of a virtuous life, and the body was left above ground, on the rocks, for birds to consume the flesh.[6] A person who lived to 40 was regarded as filling their full span, and their death was accepted as natural rather than caused by malign spiritual forces (for which cremation was deemed necessary). At the beginning of the twenty-first century, there are few countries in which a death at 40 would be seen as a positive outcome. In 2010, in 41 countries, a woman who reached the age of 40 was still short of half the national (period) life expectancy.[7] (In India, life expectancy for women in 2010 was 67.5 years.)

World-wide, the long-term improvement in life expectancy at birth shows no sign of slowing down (see Figure 1, overleaf). It is not true everywhere all the time – in Russia male life expectancy has stumbled downhill since 1965; in South Africa HIV/AIDS chopped about ten years off life expectancy in two decades.[8; 9] But these are the exceptions rather than the general rule, and the rate of progress in some populations is remarkable. Some countries are gaining an extra year every four years: this is an extra six hours added to a life, every day. To put that one extra year in perspective – in the United States in the late 1980s an extra year of life expectancy is what would be achieved (in men) by eliminating all accidental deaths.[10] We are talking about a change that is one of the greatest achievements of the twentieth century.

Putting aside the intrinsic human goal of a long and healthy life, living longer contributes a great deal to economic growth (so long as the extra years of life are weighted to the 'productive' years, as has been the case in the last two centuries). Even at a relatively modest costing of the value of a year of good quality life (say £30,000, the benchmark used by the National Institute for Health and Clinical Excellence in England and Wales when making decisions about which health services should be funded first),[11] the increase in average lifespan over the twentieth century has been worth a lot of money. If we accept that there are seven billion people, the world population in the early 2000s, living on average 36 years longer than they would have if the mortality rates of a hundred years ago still applied, and the economic value of each year of life gained is £30,000, then the global extension of human longevity is worth close to £7,600 trillion. In the United States, two economists, Kevin Murphy and Robert Topel, used a willingness-to-pay approach to value increased longevity, and they also came up with large numbers. They estimated that the increase in life expectancy between 1970 and 2000 added about $3.2 trillion a year to national wealth (that's just in the United States, and amounts to about half the annual average GDP of the country).[12] Whichever approach you take, this is of course a simplistic piece of maths – apart from the knotty question of how to put a dollar value on a year of life, we are not taking account here of the costs, environmental and social, of providing for all these extra life-years. But in times when social goals are sometimes treated as valid only if they are monetised, estimates like those made by Murphy and Topel should not be set aside too quickly.

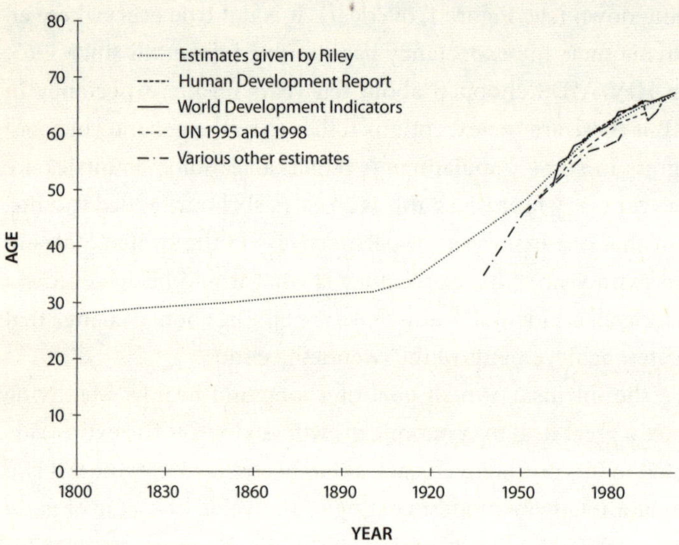

Figure 1: Global life expectancy, 1800 to 2000

Source: J. C. Riley, 'Estimates of Regional and Global Life Expectancy, 1800–2001' (*Population and Development Review* 31 [2005]: 537–43). The dip in the early 1990s in the HDR life expectancy series is due to HIV/AIDS.

The story of life expectancy in New Zealand is a fascinating one, full of contrasts and surprises, and has not been told in full before. If we want to make a reasonable stab at what the future holds for this country, it makes sense first to examine the past. We believe also that inquiry should have context: the causes of good population health and low mortality are tied closely to local circumstances.[1]

As an example of 'local circumstances', note that non-Māori New Zealanders had the highest recorded life expectancy in the world from about 1870 to 1940.[159] But there was a dark side to this achievement: Māori health statistics plunged while non-Māori prospered. It was for the indigenous population a century of 'ngā tau hekenga': decline, disease and dispossession.[13] Māori mortality rates peaked in the late 1800s, followed by a dramatic recovery. Life expectancy at birth rose by 20–25 years in the first half of the twentieth century, and the gap between Māori and non-Māori was almost halved.

We attempt to explain these trends in chapters 4 and 5. In brief, there seems to be an obvious answer for non-Māori longevity – would-be settlers must surely have been a fitter-than-average sample of the population to endure an arduous journey halfway around the world. It is true, there certainly was a 'healthy migrant effect', and some have claimed this is the sole reason for very low mortality in the early years of European settlement.[8] We disagree, and argue that the 'healthy migrant effect' is only part of the explanation. Low mortality was evident especially among infants and young children (who were mostly born in New Zealand) rather than adults (the majority of whom migrated from Europe). There are other clues. In the middle of the nineteenth century, setting aside deaths in military action, British troops in New Zealand, who were assigned by regiment not health status, were the healthiest in the Empire. Death rates were not only one-sixth those in India, but they were roughly one-third those experienced by soldiers in the home country.[14] Altogether it is plain that other factors than migration, such as crowding (or lack of it), diet, climate and housing conditions, must have played a part.

New Zealand is a country of immigrants, and since these islands were the last corner of the planet to be populated (Māori arrived first about 700–800 years ago),[15] the histories are relatively short. Adaptation is a common theme. One wave after another, settlers have struggled to reconcile the familiar with the local. The first humans brought with them dietary preferences from the Pacific islands, to a territory that was (at least, in the early phase of Māori settlement) peculiarly protein-rich and starch-poor. Europeans introduced ways of living and public health measures that were developed in industrial conurbations in the northern temperate zones, although New Zealand, with a much milder climate, had no large cities and very little manufacturing.

The timing of the migrations influences the story in important ways. New Zealand was established as a British colony after the great pandemics (such as plague, typhus and smallpox) were well and truly on the wane in the northern hemisphere. This was an advantage for the European settlers. For them, better living conditions and richer food sources were translated, uninterrupted, into lower mortality as the major causes of death at that time, such as tuberculosis and pneumonia, were nutrition-sensitive.

In some respects the timing was kind to Māori as well. Previously, smallpox had decimated indigenous populations after first contact with Europeans. In the sixteenth and seventeenth centuries, the disease extinguished entire Amerindian civilisations, and even at the end of the eighteenth century smallpox caused heavy mortality in Australian Aboriginal tribes along the east coast of New South Wales.[16] In the nineteenth century and early twentieth century, there were occasional outbreaks in New Zealand but there were relatively few fatalities. We don't know exactly why smallpox has been more damaging in some places than in others. The history of the disease is complex.[17] But European settlement in New Zealand did coincide with a global trend for the aggressive variant *Variola major* to be displaced by a milder form of the smallpox virus (*Variola minor*). The great distances that colonists had to travel to get to New Zealand may have favoured the natural selection of less virulent smallpox variants. (If the virus killed its host on board ship, the organism had fewer opportunities to be transmitted on shore.) However, it wasn't just good luck: improvements in the nineteenth century in quarantine and vaccination also contributed to low mortality from smallpox in New Zealand.

The benefit of late contact and settlement was partial only, of course. Māori were relatively new arrivals, compared with aboriginal peoples in Australia and America, but they had lived separately from the world's major population centres for long enough to be susceptible to most Old World infections. Measles, influenza and pertussis, for example, caused many deaths in New Zealand among Māori.

A small country, which for much of its history has been run by a single level of government with neither a house of review nor a formal, written constitution, New Zealand has been susceptible to rapid change. This includes social reform (ranging from universal suffrage to world-leading smoke-free laws) and changes in economic direction (including at various times the raising and lowering of trade barriers, introduction and withdrawal of comprehensive welfare provisions, and the transfers of significant assets into, and out of, state ownership). In politics as in life generally, one could say New Zealand has placed a high premium on pragmatism and demonstrated a relatively weak attachment to fixed ideological settings. If political and economic changes influence population health, then New Zealand offers a rare opportunity to observe such effects.

This country also provides raw material to test the role of health services. New Zealand has been a 'test bed' for the early adoption of some reforms (for example, child-health care in the community and accident compensation) but slow to move in other areas (such as comprehensive primary health care). New Zealand currently spends just under the OECD average on health care per person, yet has better than average life expectancy (Figure 2).

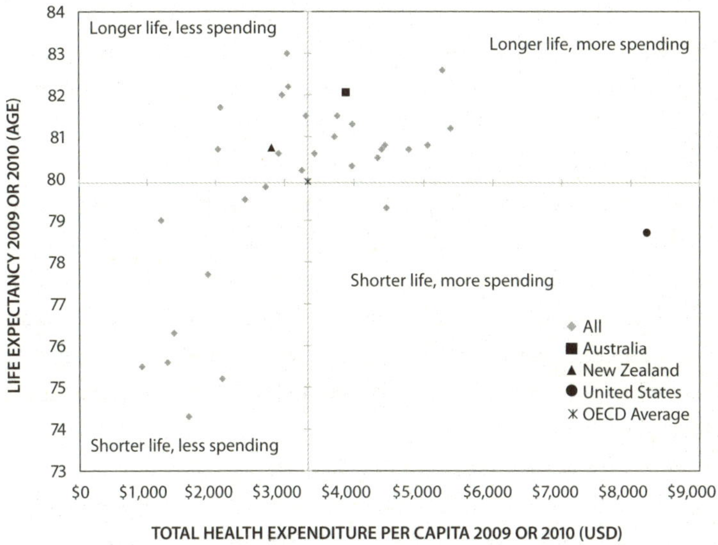

Figure 2: Life expectancy at birth and expenditure on health, OECD countries, 2009–2010
Source: Data extracted from Organisation for Economic Co-operation and Development statistics (www.oecd.org/statistics/).

In 2012 New Zealand led the way, internationally, in converting wealth into well-being, on the basis of national rankings relating the HDI (Human Development Index, a composite national measure of life expectancy, education and income) to per capita gross national income.[18] Does this demonstrate particular efficiencies that may be usefully highlighted? Or is it simply a sign that variables other than health care are most important in shaping the health of populations? We will return to these questions in chapter 6.

In this field, as we have observed already, parochial investigations have an important place. A comparison of trends in life expectancy around the world shows that there are no simple or universal explanations for mortality reduction: even factors such as income, education and social networks, which would seem intuitively to have straightforward and positive relations with health, have stronger effects in some populations than in others, and indeed, in some instances appear not to be related to mortality risk at all.[19; 1; 20]

Take migration as an example. As a general rule, people who have the inclination, the energy and the means to move from one country to another tend to be healthier than average. However, at the end of the 1800s, there was a phenomenon known as 'therapeutic migration'. This was the opposite of the 'healthy migrant effect' as long-term sufferers from tuberculosis deliberately set sail in search of a cure. (They believed, perhaps with good reason, that the New Zealand climate was kinder on the lungs than conditions in Europe.) What happens to migrants once they settle also varies from one setting to another. For example, in the 1980s and 1990s the relatively low mortality of Greek migrants to Australia showed no sign of converging on local rates with increasing duration of residence.[22] On the other hand, lower mortality rates amongst Asian people in New Zealand in the 2000s are explicable by the healthy migrant effect, with Asian mortality among long-term residents much the same as New Zealand overall.[22]

In New Zealand, mortality rates are consistently and strongly related to socio-economic position (measured by variables such as income and education). In Japan, by comparison, the relation is weak and inconsistent,[23] especially among women[24] (in some studies mortality rates increase with years of education, rather than the reverse). In the United States, regions with high densities of doctors and hospitals do not have better health outcomes than elsewhere, although health-care costs are certainly much higher than the national average. Across the Florida straits is a middle-income country (Cuba) with admirable public health statistics (infant mortality as good as or better than the US, for example), and the highest ratio in the world of doctors to population.[25]

What this means is that the findings of research elsewhere are instructive, but it is unlikely we will fully understand the local pattern of ill-health unless we examine our own histories.

FOUR WAYS OF EXPLAINING CHANGES IN LIFE EXPECTANCY

Understanding trends in mortality in New Zealand requires a framework on which we can pin explanations of the past, and which, perhaps, might serve as the basis for projections into the future. Here are four approaches to understanding human longevity, and we will make use of all of these framings in the chapters that follow.

Biological

The notion that some races or ethnic groups are biologically 'hard-wired' for long life has been discredited. Where there are well-confirmed clusters of centenarians (in Okinawa for example), the primary explanations for low mortality are found in lifestyle and environment.[26] But our understanding of how environmental shocks act on the body, and what biological changes accompany ageing, has advanced rapidly in recent decades. For instance, in 2009 the Nobel Prize for medicine went to scientists who first described telomeres, the knot on the end of the chromosomal shoe-lace. Their discovery was described as one that for the first time provided a structural explanation for ageing.

Telomeres are worn by the constant doing up and undoing of chromosomal replication, and when the knot is frayed, and the shoe-lace unwinds, then genetic damage and error is more common, and cells malfunction. This description makes sense, intuitively, to anyone who wears lace-up shoes, and may, in the future, provide valuable insights into how ageing occurs, and where there lie opportunities to intervene. But at present the application of this knowledge to increasing longevity is uncertain. One could argue that telomere shortening is a biomarker of wear and tear (and hence ageing), rather than a causal conduit itself. We will return to telomeres, and biological bases for ageing more generally, in chapter 7.

There is some truth in the saying that if you want to live to a ripe old age you should choose your parents well. Twin studies show that about a quarter of the variability in lifespan is inherited.[27] This fraction varies, depending on the age at death, and the prevailing causes of mortality. Deaths among young adults are less influenced by genetic inheritance than deaths in old age, for example.[28] But we struggle, using the biological approach, to explain trends in life expectancy. Constitutional factors such as genetic makeup determine whether individuals in a particular population are towards the top or the bottom end of the range, but they cannot explain why the average life expectancies of populations have changed so quickly in recent times.

We know that humans can adapt to significant threats in their environment. For example, most individuals in sub-Saharan Africa are immune to *P. vivax* malaria because they have a specific genetic mutation that prevents this organism entering red blood cells. But on the whole, selective pressures take a long time to change gene frequencies in human populations. (Malaria is a long-time companion of humans in Africa – the disease appeared there about 5000 years ago.) The arithmetic has been worked through for the gene for lactase retention (which provides an individual with life-long ability to digest milk). Assuming this gene (which acts in a simple dominant fashion) conferred a 5 per cent advantage in reproductive success, the lactose tolerance trait would take 350 generations (or 7000 years) to be dominant (that is, present in 90 per cent of the population).[29] This happens to approximate the time since early human agrarians first incorporated dairy products into their diets, initially from goats, sheep and cows in the Middle East.

Whilst biology, or genetics in particular, is not a likely explanation for radical mortality decline within ten generations, considerations of biology are highly relevant to the question of limits. The decline in mortality in the last two centuries has been astounding in its rapidity, but can it continue indefinitely? Will life expectancy in 2100 be over 100 years, and in 2200 more than 130 years? These are projections based on a simple linear extrapolation of the last century's progress, but the figures seem too high to be believed. If ageing has a biological basis and cannot be slowed down indefinitely, or if the lottery of cell division leads inevitably to mutations and to cancer, regardless of how clean we make the environment, then there must be a limit to how low mortality can go. We return to these questions in chapter 7.

Human ingenuity

Here we apply a technological lens as we examine longevity. Such a view highlights the successes that humans have achieved, and emphasises the recent past rather than the longer-term history. In the last hundred years, interventions, both clinical and public health, have prevented disease, improved physical functioning, provided comfort and eased suffering, increased the store of social welfare, reduced inequalities and left their stamp on human biology.[113] In developed countries, humans are 20 to 30 per cent heavier, on average, than they were a hundred years ago, due to increased caloric intakes and prevention of disease. A US college-aged male in 1900 weighed 60 kilograms on average – his counterpart in 2000 weighed 75 kilograms.[30] Compared with the members of the New Zealand rugby team in 2013, the original All Blacks, who toured Britain in 1905, were 10 centimetres shorter and 25 kilograms lighter, on average.

Fertilisers, pesticides and faster growing crop varieties have boosted the production of food. Humans now have the capacity to transport this food to every corner of the planet, so that everyone (or at least, all those who can pay the grocery bills) can be nourished by fresh fruits and vegetables all year round. The cornucopian perspective is very attractive: why shouldn't such ingenuity be applied to the challenge of ageing? Are there conceivably any limits to what might be achieved in the future?

Some argue that we already have the means to engineer 'negligible senescence', and if we were willing to make it a priority, we could fine-tune and implement powerful rejuvenation therapies that would substantially extend longevity.[31] Others contend there are fundamental biological and demographic constraints that will defy the technologists, and will prevent life expectancy at birth rising much beyond the mid-80s.[32]

Health care – whether it is aimed at prevention or treatment – has become increasingly important as a cause of low mortality. Cardiovascular disease, the most common cause of death in New Zealand for much of the twentieth century, is a good example. We do not believe that the fall in heart disease and stroke mortality was solely due to health care – far from it. But we will argue that the contribution of medical interventions has been important, and is increasingly dominating temporal trends.

Social determinants

The social determinants analysis concentrates on the allocation of resources; the role of institutions; socially determined rights, roles and responsibilities; and social systems that encourage participation and civic engagement. Economic growth is a product of society functioning in a particular way, and this covers both the causes of wealth accumulation and how wealth is distributed. Wealth (however it is measured) tends to correlate with life expectancy but the fit is far from perfect. Some high-income countries have surprisingly poor health statistics. Life expectancy in the United States, as mentioned already, is far below what might be expected, given the enormous resources this country can draw on.[33] Other populations have achieved impressive standards of health at much lower levels of economic development. Sri Lanka, the Indian state of Kerala and Costa Rica, for instance, took alternative 'roads to low mortality'.[34] The details are debated, but common to most of the 'low mortality at low cost' countries has been a deliberate emphasis on social determinants of good health, including education, poverty relief, social welfare programmes and comprehensive primary health care.[20] On the other hand, it must be pointed out, mortality rates have also improved during times of repression and hardship. Two examples of periods when mortality fell in the face of social adversity are Korea during the Japanese occupation in the first half of the twentieth century,[20] and post-World War II Portugal under the dictator Salazar.[35]

Social determinants of health are not just personal attributes such as education and income. They also include characteristics of groups, such as hierarchies of power and influence that bear down on individuals in different ways. The stress that results may 'get under the skin' through the action of fight or flight hormones like cortisol and adrenaline, but hierarchies also act by shaping exposure to classic risk factors, such as tobacco, alcohol, and high saturated-fat, salt-heavy foods. We will look closely at tobacco, alcohol and diet, and will seek to relate the timing, direction and distribution of changes in consumption to upstream social forces.

Ecological

This is the big picture view. Human societies are part of physical and biological systems that provide the resource stocks and flows for economic development, and absorb the wastes and by-products. Human well-being therefore depends on a balance between draw-downs (human use of the environment) and ecological capital, although the contribution of the natural environment to prosperity is seldom recognised in national accounts. In the short term, society may survive, even prosper, by going into ecological debt, but common sense would say that this cannot continue indefinitely. René Dubos was one of the first to write about human health and ecology, and he pointed out in the 1950s the risks to the species of living beyond its means. It was not simply a case of prudent book-keeping, in Dubos' view. It was also a matter of what was attainable. Dubos believed that the defining feature of ecological systems is flux or change, and for this reason he did not accept the utopian goals of the health technologists and social reformers. Absolute health can never be attained, according to Dubos, 'because man will never be so perfectly adapted to his environment that his life will not involve struggles, failures and sufferings'.[36]

Ingenuity permitted the spread of the species, and its success to date. But the history of civilisation confirms that there are limits to adaptation, even for clever humans, when the environmental balance gets too far out of kilter. The most famous example of a society that over-spent its environmental budgets, and could not recover, is the Polynesian settlement on Easter Island. Others who followed a similar route, hastened along by significant shifts in climate, were the Anasazi people in the south-west of the United States, the Mayan cities of central America and the Norse extension into Greenland.[37] Some argue that we face a similar threat to the sustainability of modern civilisations, on a global scale, signalled by accumulation of CO_2 in the atmosphere, rising temperatures and more extreme weather.

STRUCTURE OF THE BOOK

The book is organised chronologically. We examine first what we have called 'the long history': from the time when modern humans emerged, to the first visit to Aotearoa-New Zealand by James Cook in 1769.

The hundred years after Cook's landing was a time when Māori outnumbered European settlers, and in large tracts of the country they lived with relatively little interference from the British colonial government. The land wars that began in the 1860s signalled a new phase in New Zealand history. It was a time of very rapid immigration, of occupation territorially and culturally, and of rapid improvements in non-Māori mortality. (Records, for the first time, were based on systematic death registration systems.) Māori health of the same period followed a different trajectory, and warrants a chapter of its own.

We take the next cut-point at the end of World War II. This was the end of the period when New Zealand non-Māori had the lowest mortality rates in the world. It was a time of great social change for Māori, due to wholesale urbanisation and substantial social reform. The convergence of Māori and non-Māori life expectancy halted in the 1980s, and we devote a chapter to the so-called 'reform years', covering the period from the Lange Government to the present.

Finally, we aim to bring the threads of this story together, sum up the major influences on mortality in New Zealand, compare the New Zealand experience with trends in other countries and speculate on the future of human life expectancy. How low can mortality go? And what are the social and ecological implications of continuing mortality decline?

1

Before Cook

The Long History of Human Longevity

The old always think the world is getting worse. It is for the young, equipped with historical facts, to point out that, compared with 1509, or even 1939, life in 2009 is sweet as honey. Immersion in history doesn't make you backward looking; it makes you want to run like hell towards the future.

— HILARY MANTEL, *THE GUARDIAN*, 17 OCTOBER 2009

What is known about human lifespans prior to the arrival of Europeans in New Zealand? In this chapter, we take a long view, beginning with the work of palaeo-demographers who have attempted to piece together life tables for our hunter-gatherer ancestors. We consider the transition to agricultural societies and the consequences for population health, and then focus on conditions among Māori prior to 1769.

The best estimate for Māori life expectancy pre-Cook, based on skeletal remains and what we know about hunter-gatherer and early agrarian societies elsewhere, is about 20 to 25 years. This figure is dominated by high infant and child mortality – those who made it to the age of 20 years could expect to live, on average, another 15 to 20 years.

Finally, we turn to the much more extensive literature on mortality in Europe in the centuries preceding Cook's journeys to New Zealand. At the time of Cook's voyages, England and Wales were just starting up the steep slope of life expectancy increase and the average lifespan was around 36 years.

HUNTER-GATHERER SOCIETY

The first traces of modern humans are seen in Africa and they date to roughly 150,000 years before the modern era. For approximately 95 per cent of human existence since that time, our species operated in hunter-gatherer mode. The defining characteristic of this way of life was an exquisite dependence on local resources. How many people, how closely together they lived and how often they needed to move, all this was determined by the food, shelter and water that were nearby. Much of the time the basic population unit, the band, was no more than 20–25 people, but in times of abundance larger numbers might come together. Occasionally, the environment was so productive that lucky foragers could make a good living with what was on hand. The Portage River in modern-day Ohio supported a sedentary hunter-gatherer society about 1200 before present (BP), with ample local year-round supplies of fish, small mammals and birds. But this was unusual. Mostly, hunter-gatherers had to be mobile. However small the group, the food immediately to hand would eventually be depleted and then the band must shift. The need to be mobile conditioned technology (as there were limits on the tools that could be carried from one site to another), economics (surpluses had no value because they were not portable), and population dynamics (wide birth-spacing ensured parents on the move were relatively unencumbered).

Much of what is written about hunter-gatherer society comes from observation of survivor groups in remote areas in more recent times. As agricultural civilisations extended their range, hunting and gathering societies were overrun, absorbed, destroyed or displaced. Those that continued the traditional way of life were pushed to the margins, where food supplies were depleted and unreliable, and living conditions in general were much less favourable. As a result, we should be cautious when extrapolating from present (or recent past) examples of hunter-gathers to the far distant past. Nevertheless, this information makes a necessary and useful addition to our understanding of the long history of human longevity.

Mortality Patterns

Studies of hunter-gatherer populations in the modern era typically report high mortality in early life. Infant death rates may be as high as 300 per 1000, with perhaps half of all live-born children dying before the age of 15 years.[38] A comprehensive summary of mortality among 'ethnographic' hunter-gatherers (as distinct from Paleolithic populations) found that life expectancy at birth varied from 21 to 37 years.[39] For example, the !Kung people in southern Africa in the 1960s and 1970s had an expectation of life at birth of about 30,[40] although the figure was rather higher for those born after 1950. The commonest causes of death were infectious disease and trauma. Many of the diseases that are prevalent in modern societies, such as coronary heart disease, diabetes and cancers, appeared to be uncommon.

One might ask: how could a society sustain itself if people lived only to age 20 or 25, on average? The answer is that most of those who survived high mortality rates in childhood lived a good way beyond age 20 or 25. That is, the average age of death (i.e., life expectancy), the median and the mode are quite different in societies with high infant mortality, as shown in the text box in the Introduction. Amongst the !Kung, individuals who had survived to age 20 could expect to live on average another 30 years. Life expectancy at 45 years was around 20 years in five traditional hunter-gatherer populations studied between 1965 and 1990.[39]

Figure 3 demonstrates the impact of high mortality in early life, drawing on examples of modern hunter-gatherer groups. (Note that 'forager-horticulturalists' and 'acculturated hunter-gatherers' practise a mix of gardening and foraging.) High child mortality means that only about two-thirds of babies survive to five years of age. However, mortality reduces after this point, and roughly half of those who survive childhood live on into their 40s and 50s. Figure 3 includes information on Sweden in the middle of the eighteenth century (obtained from church records) – note the Swedish survival curve is similar to that calculated for twentieth-century hunter-gatherer populations.

Another source of information on mortality amongst pre-historic communities is studies of skeletons. Bones provide clues to the age at death, the likely cause of death, other diseases that may have been present although not necessarily the cause of death, and past injury. Information is often patchy, because there are relatively few samples. Hunter-gatherer societies, by and large, did not bury their dead in cemeteries. Over-represented are groups that lived in fertile areas (such as the Maghreb peninsula in North Africa), where population density was high and people had no cause to move around. 'Palaeo-demographers' have used other kinds of evidence too, such as archaeological pointers to the size and density of settlements, and analysis of DNA recovered from bones and teeth.[41]

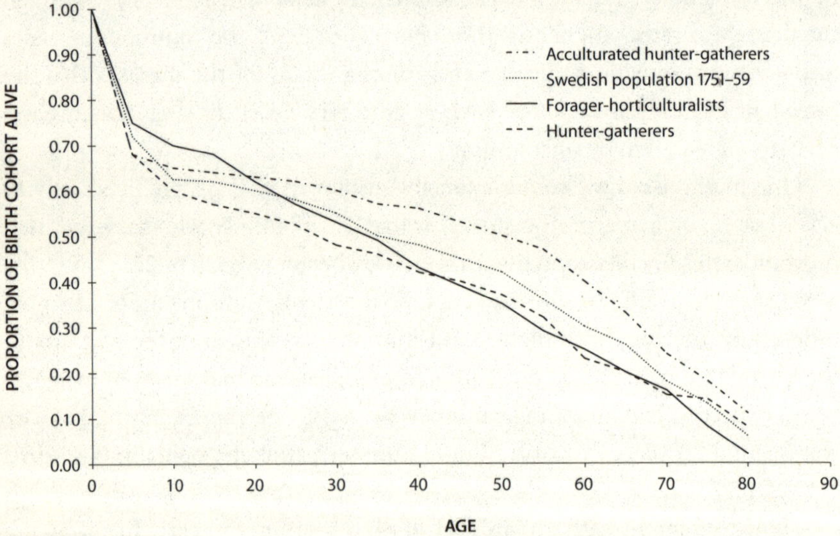

Figure 3: Average survival curves for modern (twentieth-century) hunter-gatherers, forager-horiculturalists, acculturated hunter-gatherers and the Swedish population 1751–59

Source: Based on Figure 1d in Michael Gurven and Hillard Kaplan, 'Longevity among Hunter- Gatherers: A Cross-Cultural Examination' (*Population and Development Review* 33, no. 2 [July 2007]: 321–65).

Making sense of skeletal signs depends on some big assumptions. First, the estimation of age from skeletons is accurate, to within a year or so, during adolescence, when there are obvious age-related markers of growth and development. But at older ages, dating depends on measures of wear and tear, bony re-modelling and degenerative changes that are only moderately correlated with age. We assume that the relation between changes in the bones and age has been constant over the history of *Homo sapiens*, but this may not be the case. It is possible that early hunter-gatherer populations matured more slowly than contemporary humans, as a result of low bodyweights, intermittent shortages of food and high levels of physical activity. If maturation occurred more slowly, then age at death amongst adolescents and young adults would be under-estimated using modern standards for skeletal development.

We assume also that skeletal samples give us an unbiased view of what was happening in the population at large. But there are many reasons why this may not be the case. Studies of recent burial sites, where it is possible to match results based on the skeletal remains with registers of births and deaths, find that cemetery samples are seldom representative.[41] Deaths at young ages are commonly under-counted, because children's skeletons do not endure as well as adults'. On the other hand, cultural mores relating to burial may cause some groups, those with influence and authority in particular, to be over-represented in cemetery samples.

Average age at death (the statistic available from the cemetery studies) is the same as average life expectancy at birth only when the population is in equilibrium, that is, when births and deaths balance, and there is no migration. Of course, this is hardly ever the case: when the birth rate is above replacement, average age at death will under-estimate life expectancy, and vice versa. Think about the base of the population age pyramid, and what happens if it swells (or shrinks). If the proportion of the population in younger age groups is increasing, and there is no change in death rates, there will be more deaths amongst relatively young individuals, and the average age at death will fall (although life expectancy has not changed, since age-specific death rates are the same). Imagine an extreme example, one in which three-quarters of the population was made up of pre-school-age children. Even if these children were relatively healthy, with a life expectancy of 70 years or more, the average age at death would be skewed heavily towards the under-five-years category.

As a consequence, the age distribution of deaths tells us as much about fertility as it does about mortality, especially in the range in which palaeodemographic data are most reliable.[42] The important point is that a change in the birth rate will change the average age at death if the force of mortality remains the same. Therefore life tables based on skeletal samples require not only information on age at death, but also an estimation of the population growth rate.

Bearing in mind these caveats, studies of skeletal remains from hunter-gatherer populations provide estimates of life expectancy ranging from under 20 years to the high 30s. In the Americas, life expectancies for forager populations were rather higher before 1500 BP than in the more recent period (500–1500 BP). In this latter 'classic' era, leading up to European contact, in some populations in the Americas more than half the fully grown individuals died before 20 years,[43] and life expectancies tended to lie in the range 20–25 years.[44]

Trauma was a relatively common cause of death. Up to 40 per cent of skeletons in some studies of early hunter-gatherer populations showed signs of violent death, and many ethnographic studies also report that violent deaths (including those due to infanticide, inter-clan conflict and accidental injuries) were relatively common. Samuel Bowles, an evolutionary biologist at the Santa Fe Institute and expert on the causes and consequences of ancient warfare, argues that violence has been a common cause of mortality throughout the history of forager groups. According to Bowles, trauma caused 30 per cent of deaths among the Ache, a hunter-gatherer population living in Paraguay, and 17 per cent among the Hiwi, in Venezuela and Columbia.[45] Stephen Pinker estimates mortality from violent causes in some hunter-gatherer societies approached 500 per 100,000 per year (more than three times the rate in Germany during World War II).[46] These are very high rates, although the numbers of deaths, in absolute terms, were relatively small because the populations were tiny, by modern standards. We note some anthropologists believe that Pinker exaggerated the frequency of violence in hunter-gatherer and foraging societies as a result of extrapolating too freely from present-day populations that endure in a highly modified form, to the conditions that applied in the distant past.[47]

We can speculate that patterns of infectious disease changed when humans moved from moist, tropical environments to grasslands and open spaces, and then pole-wards into temperate and sub-arctic zones.[48] Modern tropical rain forests provide warmth and moisture sufficient to sustain a rich mix of microbes, with many vectors on hand and ample opportunity for host-hopping. This ecological pressure-cooker ramps up the force and variety of infections. The epidemiology of infectious diseases among modern primates may be a guide to what the first human hunter-gatherer bands experienced: African monkeys are infected with many more species of malaria, for example, than the four that predominantly affect humans. However, being infected is not necessarily the same as being sick. After a long period of co-existence, it is likely that early humans grew to tolerate many of their microbial close neighbours, just as the microbes found ways of inhabiting humans without compromising too severely their host's mobility and longevity.

In more arid environments, much of the tropical pathogen load was shed. Population size was another important factor in determining disease profiles – forager groups were too small to sustain many pathogens that required a regular supply of susceptible individuals. Infections that persisted in dispersed, low-density populations were those that did not rapidly induce host immunity and were spread by close contact or contaminated food and water (such as intestinal parasites), and those that survived for lengthy periods buried in the host (for instance, the herpes, Epstein Barr and hepatitis viruses). There are signs of territory-limiting encounters – with the trypanosome that causes East African sleeping sickness, for example. *T. brucei rhodesiensis* lives in antelope, and is spread by the tsetse fly. In its primary host, infection causes no illness. In humans, the effects are severe, and frequently lethal. Consequently, humans steered clear of antelope country. Indeed, sleeping sickness may explain why the great ungulate herds of central Africa survived human predation.[48] (Bison in North America, and moa [the large flightless bird] in New Zealand, without microbial security guards, were less fortunate.)

Modern-day hunter-gatherers characteristically have lean body builds. This reflects the low energy-density of most foods and the amount of work that is required to obtain them. Supplies are often precarious, but food sources are typically varied and provide a wide range of nutrients.[49] For example, the diets of the San and !Kung people of southern Africa included over 150 plant and 100 animal species.[43] Energy intake of Dobe bushmen in the 1960s was estimated to be about 2100 calories per day on average, 5 to 10 per cent greater than subsistence requirements and about two-thirds of average intake in modern, high-income populations. These calories were gathered relatively economically: adults spent, on average, only two-to-three days per week gathering plant foods and pursuing game.[50] The rest of their time was available for rest and socialising:

> A good case can be made that hunters and gatherers work less than we do: and rather than a continuous travail, the food quest is intermittent, leisure abundant, and there is a greater amount of sleep in the daytime per capita per year than in any other condition of society.[50]

Other observations of hunter-gatherer groups before they were expelled from 'the better parts of the earth'[50] suggest protein intakes may have been relatively high, and vitamin and mineral deficiencies uncommon. In the 1830s Sir George Grey, later a two-term Prime Minister of New Zealand, led expeditions into parts of the West Australian interior that had not been visited before by Europeans. In his diaries he wrote:

> Generally speaking the natives live well . . . in his own district a native knows exactly what it produces, the proper time at which the several articles are in season and the readiest means of procuring them . . . I can only say that I have always found the greatest abundance in their huts.[50]

When large game was available, human populations were relatively small in number and competition for resources was light, then life expectancy at birth may have been rather better than 20–25 years. But hunter-gatherers often faced dwindling supplies, due to over-hunting or climatic changes, the advance of deserts in dry times, and crowding and competition in the most suitable habitats. In these circumstances, groups had to travel further, to rely on small game and less accessible and possibly less nutritious foods from plant sources, and they may have been more severely affected by mortality due to trauma, acute hunger and chronic under-nutrition.

AGRICULTURAL SOCIETY

Agriculture emerged at roughly the same time, about 8000 to 10,000 years ago, in the Middle East, China, New Guinea, Ethiopia and the Americas. There was a period of slow spread and patchy adoption, but settled communities relying principally on farming for their sustenance were established in many parts of the world by about 6000 years BP.

Mortality patterns

Was farming a technological breakthrough, a big step forward in human progress, or more of a lateral shift, an escape from an unsustainable roam-and-capture lifestyle, but a move with mixed effects on human welfare? The short answer is: both. Agriculture increased the quantities of food available for human consumption, and by and large reduced the energy costs of obtaining this food. With no need to roam, surpluses could be created, stored, and consumed or traded. The limits on birth-spacing and family size that acted on groups in which mobility was the imperative no longer applied. Populations grew rapidly, density of settlement increased as well, and a concentration of people and resources sparked cultural revolutions that have changed the face of the planet. However, the transition from mobile to settled societies was not straightforward. As Rousseau put it: 'With regard to agriculture, which is slower to appear, it depends upon all the arts; it ushers in property, government, laws, and by degrees misery and crime.'[51]

The change from foraging to farming was associated with an increase in the proportion of juvenile skeletons in cemetery studies. Fertility increased in settled communities, perhaps by as much as an extra two births per woman, on average, but in general the health of populations deteriorated when farming was adopted. Agricultural settlements provided opportunities for disease to move from farm animals to humans, and new parasitic diseases emerged. For example, the blood fluke *Schistosoma* has been identified in Egyptian mummies from the time when rice was first cultivated under irrigation (around 3200 BP).[52]

From about 5000 BP, towns and cities grew large enough to support micro-parasites with direct lifecycles (i.e., spreading from human to human), such as typhoid fever, rubella, dysentery and (later) influenza. Despite all the social and economic benefits of urban living, it appears that human longevity scarcely improved. Studies of skeletal remains from the early period of Greek civilisation are consistent with life expectancies of the order of 25–30 years.[38] On the basis of Roman documents setting out the calculation of life annuities, it is estimated that life expectancy at birth in the third century AD was 20–25 years.[53] Mortality may have been higher in outlying parts of the Roman Empire: skeletons of children from Roman Egypt (first to third centuries AD) show severe stunting and signs of significant nutritional deficiencies, comparable to modern populations with life expectancies of 20 years or less.[54]

Thomas Hobbes described primitive life as 'poor, nasty, brutish and short'. In fact, the average length of life in well-functioning hunter-gatherer communities may have differed little from that in 'civilised' European populations up to the modern era (Figure 3). In Europe in the seventeenth and eighteenth centuries, life expectancy at birth, which was generally in the low to mid-30s, was similar to that estimated for Iron Age communities two thousand years earlier.[38]

Explanations

With subsistence agriculture there was commonly less variety than applied in the hunter-gatherer diet, and when crops failed, sedentary communities had fewer options for recovery than their foraging ancestors.[43] Although agriculture multiplied food production, severe hunger was, paradoxically, a greater threat than in the past. Crop failures could be devastating when there were few alternatives to feeding large, settled populations. The way food was distributed also added to insecurity. As they grew in size, agricultural societies became increasingly unequal. Even when food was plentiful, powerful and favoured groups had first call on resources, and the effects of mal-distribution were particularly damaging when supplies were tight. Children were especially vulnerable, and their skeletons show signs of nutritional deficiencies and severe growth interruption more commonly after agricultural settlement than before.[55] Skeletons from the Eastern Mediterranean record a fall in average heights: early bronze age farmers were up to 12 centimetres shorter than hunter-gatherers in the same region 5000–10,000 years earlier.[55]

Chronic infections of many kinds are likely to have been more common in large settled populations than in small, mobile bands of hunter-gatherers.[56] Many organisms (hydatids and tapeworm, for instance) were acquired from domesticated animals. Egyptian mummies from the early dynasties, when settlements were less firmly established and population densities were still relatively low, had fewer parasites in their intestines than mummies from later more cosmopolitan times.[38] In the Americas, archaeologists Steckel and Rose combined a number of skeletal markers (including age at death) into a single index, based on a database of more than 12,000 skeletons. They report a decline in health status of indigenous populations prior to European contact, associated particularly with growth in populations and increased density of settlements.[57]

Epidemic infections, that on occasion caused catastrophic mortality, took hold when large, close-living populations were established. Some modern pathogens (such as the virus that causes measles) were acquired from the animals with which farming communities were in close contact (in this case it was the organism responsible for the disease of cattle called rinderpest), and then evolved to enable human-to-human spread. Diseases such as malaria and yellow fever were present amongst hunter-gatherers, but the force of infection may have been much greater in settled human populations. Clearing forests and settling close to wetland habitats, for example, would have increased contacts with mosquitoes and other disease vectors.[58] Another factor was the density of populations in farming settlements, which increased opportunities for transmission of infections.

The dynamics of infectious diseases depend not only on population density (from the pathogen's point of view, this means the distance to the next host), but also population size and the proportion of susceptible individuals, since what matters most to the pathogen is the distance to the next *non-immune* host. Measles, smallpox, rubella, typhoid and dysentery all require large, close-living populations (in the range of 100,000 to 500,000 people) to be sustained, and for this reason it is unlikely these diseases were endemic (i.e., established without the need for re-infection from outside) before about 5000 BP.[52] The first cities created opportunities for economic specialisation and innovation, but at the same time opened up new niches for nimble microbes.

In the long term, a modus operandi developed between sedentary human populations and some infectious agents. If the reproduction and spread of the organism was favoured when the host was mildly affected, there was selection for less virulent forms. But this wasn't always the case. In principle, there is no evolutionary pressure to a more benign state for cholera, for example, since the infection is spread through contaminated water supplies, enhanced by voluminous watery diarrhoea, and the cholera bacillus can be sustained outside the human body in a secure environmental phase. (On the other hand, most infections with cholera cause no symptoms or only minor disturbance, and the El Tor variant, which emerged in the 1960s, has an even higher ratio of carriers to [severely affected] cases than the so-called classic biotype.)

Once upon a time students of public health were taught that tuberculosis first infected humans 6000–7000 years ago, when a modified form of the bacillus that causes tubercular disease in cattle took hold in early farming communities. But it seems now that the disease has a much older history. Based on analysis of the genome of *Mycobacterium tuberculosis*, researchers propose that the common ancestor of the bacteria emerged in Africa about 70,000 years ago.[59] Two lines of organism may have evolved 10,000–20,000 years later, including one form of TB that passed directly from humans to humans, and another that spread to animals (leading to bovine TB) with subsequent re-infection of humans.[60; 61] It appears that many strains of *Mycobacterium tuberculosis* developed simultaneously, and this ferment of microbial evolution took place more quickly after the transition to agriculture than before.[59]

The bacteria that causes syphilis is a younger pathogen than *M. tuberculosis*, but it also took on a chronic and moderately disabling form in the course of time, less inclined to kill its host rapidly than in early manifestations.

The epidemiologist Tony McMichael suggests there were three phases in the history of infections after humans took up agriculture. These are dissemination, mixing and adaptation.[43] The first phase was local – the passage of organisms from livestock to humans, and development of unique patterns of endemic infection in settled agrarian populations. Then there was mixing between regions, as civilisations traded, crusaded and migrated. For example, smallpox is first recorded in Rome in 165 AD (when the Antonine Plague killed a quarter of the city's population). The disease probably arrived with traders from India. In the fourteenth century the bubonic plague took the Silk Road from China to Europe.

The third phase was global – when there was technology and economic muscle to extend empire across oceans to new continents, infections reached long-isolated, immunologically naïve populations, with serious consequences. Populations and states in central and south America crashed as a result of pathogens that travelled with the Spanish. Three hundred years after the Spanish conquistador Cortez, the inter-continental microbial caravan reached the south-western corner of the Pacific. The people who lived there had been isolated from the major mixing bowls of world infections for about 5000 years. Most importantly, they had decamped, from coastal East Asia most likely, before the confluence of the disease pools of Europe and Asia (the second of

McMichael's three phases). This placed Māori, like other indigenous peoples around the Pacific rim, at a great disadvantage when they eventually encountered Old World infections such as measles, diphtheria and pertussis.

MORTALITY IN AOTEAROA BEFORE 1769

As best we know, Māori came to what is now called New Zealand about 750 years ago.[62] Radiocarbon-dating of the seeds gnawed by the Pacific rat and analyses of the rat bones themselves point to a first landing in the second half of the thirteenth century of the Christian era.[15] This fits with other evidence, including dates of accelerated deforestation, species extinctions and artefacts from the oldest archaeological sites (Wairau Bar in particular).[63; 81]

The arrival of waka, the long-distance Polynesian canoes, was the finale in a series of great migrations – New Zealand was the last sizeable chunk of land in the enormous Pacific to be settled. The first push out of South East Asia occurred 30,000–40,000 years ago and populated what is now known as Melanesia (Papua New Guinea and the Solomons). Next were the Austronesian-speakers, who about 5000 BP moved into the Pacific from a homeland somewhere around Taiwan.[64] This group reached the 'portal of the Polynesia' (Samoa, Fiji and Tonga) within about a thousand years, and left their mark with the Lapita cultural complex, known by a characteristic style of pottery. After a significant pause, during which 'archaic' Polynesian culture, languages and technology took shape, central Polynesia (the Cooks, Society Islands including Tahiti, Tuamotu and the Austral Islands) was occupied.[65] Recent carbon-dating, more precise than was possible previously, tells us that settlement of the Eastern Polynesian islands occurred more rapidly and much later than most scholars had estimated. It appears as though there were two phases of colonisation: the Society islands and Tahiti were most likely populated around 1025–1120 AD, and then there was a burst of voyaging in the 1200s to the other, more remote Pacific islands, including Hawai'i, Easter Island and New Zealand. This period of intense exploration may have coincided with a temporary reversal in the El Niño weather pattern, leading to an easing in the prevailing westerly winds that made conditions more suitable for long-distance sea travel.[66; 67] It is intriguing that large-scale voyaging across the Pacific ceased soon after all the inhabitable island groups had been settled. Perhaps the change in climate was key; perhaps population pressures in the centre of Polynesia were important motivations for migration; very likely there were means of reporting back to the source islands when colonisation was successful.[68]

Tradition locates the ancestral homeland of Māori in Hawai'iki, a place to the north and east of New Zealand. Archaeology points in much the same direction.[69] Similarities in artefacts, language and burial practices indicate that the first boats to New Zealand most likely departed from the Cook or Society Island groups. The fact these boats carried men and women, domestic animals (dogs) and a variety of plants for cultivation signals that they were purposeful voyages – New Zealand was not settled by accident.

Mortality patterns

Information on mortality among Māori before European settlement comes mainly from cemetery or urupā studies. Māori oral history is rich in detail, and encompasses many generations, but does not capture lifespans in a manner that fits epidemiological calculation. Estimates have been made also from modelling of population growth, the experience of Pacific populations on other islands and the journals of the early European visitors to New Zealand.

Abel Tasman and others on his 1642 expedition kept diaries and many of these were published. More detailed accounts of Māori life can be obtained from Cook's expeditions, thanks in particular to Cook's own diaries, and Joseph Banks' observations. The French explorers who landed in New Zealand shortly after Cook (these were parties led by de Surville in 1769, and Marion du Fresne in 1772) also left detailed accounts.

In the first contact accounts, Māori men are commonly reported to be heavily built, muscular and in good health.[70] There are relatively few descriptions of Māori women, and what is recorded suggests that their health was not as robust as that of the men (see page 43). Banks reported that he saw old people in most of the places he visited, and was impressed by the vitality of the elders.

> Hardly a canoe came off to us that did not bring one or more [old people] and every town had several whom if we may judge by gray hairs and worn-out teeth

> were of a very advanced age. Of these few or none were decrepid, indeed the greatest number seemed in vivacity and chearfullness to equal the young.[71]

Marion du Fresne's party spent almost two months in the Bay of Islands, and for most of this time his men moved freely around the local villages. Le Dez, lieutenant on the *Marquis de Castries*, wrote:

> The Zealanders are commonly five feet seven to eight inches [170 to 172 centimetres] tall. We saw several who were six feet tall [183 centimetres]. They are well built and well proportioned . . . I have seen no cripples or any one with a natural defect. Very few of them are thin; they all seemed to me to enjoy good health and to have a robust constitution . . . Among the old men, who were numerous, several were extremely aged to judge by their wrinkles.[71]

It is difficult to know how much weight should be placed on these accounts. The descriptions are mostly positive, in their references to vigour, appearance, body shape and stature. But the explorers met only a fraction of the local population, and many of their encounters were with war parties, likely to contain the strongest and fittest of young men. It is impossible to tell the true age of those described as 'old'. Some of the signs referred to in the journals (such as the condition of the teeth) may have been unreliable. (Fibrous diets, particularly in communities that relied upon fern root, caused more wear and tear to teeth than Europeans would have expected.) Also, assessments of stature, robustness and vigorous good health were relative to what was expected or commonly observed, and the English and French sailors (particularly the latter) who travelled to New Zealand provided an undemanding reference point. When de Surville reached Tokerau (Doubtless Bay), there were only seven or eight healthy men out of about 150 on board – malnutrition and scurvy had disabled the remainder.[71] The average height of British (male) military recruits born in the 1740s and 1750s was about 162 centimetres (5 foot 3 inches), about 15 centimetres (6 inches) less than modern measures.[72] Most importantly,[73] these first-encounter reports were based on impressions and conjecture, and were filtered through powerful preconceptions.

Anne Salmond points out that European notions of 'primitives' in the seventeenth and eighteenth centuries had two aspects. One construction was the innocent, uncorrupted child of nature; the other was the violent, monstrous, demonic savage.[71] Both versions appear in the early accounts, and perhaps it would not be surprising if descriptions of height and strength were sometimes exaggerated. For instance, after Tasman's party had been attacked at Golden Bay in 1642, they were wary of future contacts with Māori, and in their diaries described the local inhabitants as especially fearsome. On the Three Kings Islands, one of the sailors wrote, they saw exceptionally tall men, walking with enormous strides, and brandishing 'wooden sticks about two fathoms long'.[74]

Studies of skeletal remains suggest mortality amongst Māori prior to European settlement was similar to that reported in other parts of the Pacific.[75] Fertility may have been rather lower than in other Pacific islands:[76] examination of pelvic bones has provided estimates of roughly three–four children born per woman in New Zealand.[77] Some have speculated that fertility rates and life expectancies may have been higher during the 'protein boom', the early phase of Māori settlement when seal and bird meat was readily available.[78] It is plausible but there is really no evidence to prove or disprove such a hypothesis.

Studies of individual burial sites have placed the average age at death between 21 and 38 years.[77; 79] At the largest archaeological site, Wairau Bar at the north-east tip of the South Island, 42 adult skeletons have been examined. This site was probably first occupied towards the end of the thirteenth century AD, shortly after Māori came to New Zealand. An early assessment of the age at death of these individuals reported a range from 19 to 41 years, with an average of about 28 for men and 29 for women.[80] Assuming that infant and child mortality rates were high (Sutton suggests infant mortality of between 16 and 25 per cent in the Palliser Bay settlement on the south coast of the North Island, on the other side of Cook Strait)[75] and population growth was slow, these age-at-death findings fit with a life expectancy at birth of 20–25 years.

A recent review of the skeletal remains from Wairau Bar suggests average life expectancy may have been under-estimated, although it is difficult to tell by how much.[81] The maximum age at death at Wairau Bar (41 years) is lower than expected, even in a high mortality population, and suggests that older individuals were either missing from the sample, or were systematically under-aged in the assessment of skeletons. On the other hand, the burials at Wairau Bar include only one adolescent skeleton, and no remains of children have been recovered.

In an attempt to overcome the problems of small numbers and missing data, researchers have pooled the information from archaeological sites, and estimated that life expectancy at birth in pre-European New Zealand was between 19 and 27 years (depending on assumptions regarding population growth and infant mortality).[82; 79]

We do not know whether mortality among Māori varied during their settlement of New Zealand. But we speculate that conditions were harsher in the period preceding European contact than they had been in earlier centuries, due to fewer wild game, more people and competition for the most productive gardens. Similar trends were seen in other Pacific islands. In Hawaiʻi, for instance, survivorship curves from skeletal series show higher mortality in the 200–300 years immediately before contact with Europeans than earlier. Oral history includes accounts of severe food shortages (consistent with reduced diversity of food items in midden samples) and frequent, violent conflict.[65] (Mokapu on the island of Oʻahu [Hawaiʻi] is the largest cemetery site in Polynesia from this pre-contact period. It contains the remains of about 1163 individuals, including approximately 200 infants and children. Life expectancy at birth in this group is estimated to be about 24 years.)

Estimates of life expectancy from cemetery studies must be treated with caution, for reasons that have already been discussed. Under-counting of child deaths is particularly important. Since the proportion of Māori children who lived into their teens was perhaps only a half to two-thirds, life expectancy at birth was not a good guide to the considerably higher average age of death for those lucky enough to make it through childhood.

Another perspective on early mortality is provided by attempts to model the growth of the Māori population of New Zealand. Modelling depends on assumptions that are necessary, but also influential and questionable. They include the date of first settlement, the size of the founding population, the extent of subsequent inward and outward migration during the period of trans-Pacific voyaging, and the size of the population at European contact. One such study assumed first colonisation occurred between 750 and 950 AD with an initial group of about 50 individuals, with no subsequent in-migration, and grew to a population of around 150,000 people when Cook first visited.[79] With these starting and finishing points, the arithmetic tells us that fertility must have been higher, or mortality much lower, than is deduced from the studies of skeletal remains.

However, there were probably more than 50 women in the founding population, because otherwise it is very difficult to explain the variations in mitochondrial DNA now observed among Māori.[83] Studies of the genetic makeup of kiore, the Polynesian rat, show the animal was introduced to New Zealand on more than one occasion. This implies many human voyages across the Pacific, and is not compatible with the assumption that there was no in-migration after the first landing.[84] Although it is not possible to date the first settlement precisely, it very likely took place much more recently than 750–950 AD, as mentioned already.[15] Also, although there is no direct evidence, it seems improbable that population growth was linear throughout the period of Māori settlement.

In summary, information on mortality prior to the arrival of the Europeans is not consistent. Early European explorer journals record a vigorous, strongly built population, without visible signs of significant disease or impairment. Yet cemetery studies report average ages at death of adults in the mid-to-late 20s, and on this basis, life expectancy at birth may have been as low as 20–25 years. Possibly mortality was lower in the early phase of Māori settlement than in later times, but there is little information to confirm that this was the case. From the studies of skeletal remains it appears that fertility was slightly less than in other Pacific islands.

A simple comparison of numbers of people and size of islands points to conditions being less favourable for settlement in New Zealand than elsewhere in the Pacific. At the time of European contact, New Zealand, with 16 times the land area of Hawai'i, had perhaps half as many inhabitants.[65] As we have pointed out already, it was believed that Polynesian canoes reached Hawai'i centuries before they came to New Zealand, but recent studies suggest the head-start for the northern islands may have been less than a hundred years. Tonga and Samoa, before European contact, supported 30–50 people per square kilometre: the figure for New Zealand was about 0.4.[65] Within New Zealand, the much lower population in the South Island (perhaps no more than 3000–10,000 at time of European settlement, compared with maybe 10–15 times this number in the smaller North Island)[75] shows, again, the influence of factors such as climate, crops and sources of wild foods on settlement and population growth.

What were the common causes of death in this early period? Some have speculated that kidney infections, arteriosclerosis, intestinal tumours and dental infections may have been important.[80; 85] But there is no direct evidence and these long-distance retrospective diagnoses should be treated cautiously. There are some clues, however: marks and defects in bones, the fact that we know there were risks associated with particular foods (for example, bracken includes chemicals associated with tumours in the bowel), and oral history (for instance, heavy loss of life associated with military campaigns).

On the basis of oral histories, two Māori leaders at the end of the nineteenth century, Māui Pōmare and Peter Buck (Te Rangi Hīroa), proposed that tuberculosis (TB) had preceded European contact.[86] This seemed unlikely, when the prevailing view was that tuberculosis arrived in the New World with the Spanish conquistadors.[48] But on the basis of recent developments, Pōmare and Buck may be right. Genetic studies of the *M. tuberculosis* complex, described earlier in the chapter, have uncovered diverse, ancient lineages. It is possible the bacteria moved out of Africa with the first human migrations, and then radiated eastwards in association with movements into and around the Pacific over the last 10,000 years.[61] The other important piece of evidence comes from the review of Wairau Bar skeletons, which has reported signs of chronic, destructive pathology of the ribs and vertebrae that were overlooked previously and that match the lesions of disseminated TB.[81] If TB was in New Zealand pre-1769, it would seem likely that it was a less pathogenic strain (or group of strains) than those introduced post-1769 given that florid tubercular disease did not appear to be in situ. This scenario is plausible, in light of the new phylogenetic studies.[59] It makes sense also that a strain of TB that could successfully move across the Pacific amidst small groups of voyagers would not disable its host as rapidly as strains developing in large high-density populations. However, we hasten to add, this is speculation on our part.

Leprosy or a condition that was very similar was reported by Māori to have been with them for a long time (and was known as 'ngerengere' or 'tūhawaiki').[87; 88] However, it seems from all accounts that rapidly spreading conditions with high fatality were uncommon prior to European contact.[13] For instance, early explorers commented frequently on the absence of the characteristic scars caused by smallpox, which in England in the first half of the eighteenth century infected most of the population and caused as many as one death in five.[89]

Bones examined in the urupā studies show signs of fatal injury (such as skull fracture), but these are relatively uncommon perhaps as fatal injury conferred less chance of making it to the urupā (assuming that warfare or other causes of fatal injuries occurred away from the settlements). Fractures of the long bones are seen, often with evidence of successful alignment and healing. Degenerative changes in the spine and upper limbs, as might result from digging and paddling, are seen in most of the adult skeletons.

The records of Cook's first voyage refer to the apparent absence of venereal diseases amongst Māori, although these conditions had been encountered elsewhere in the Pacific. However, sexually transmitted infections were evidently well established in New Zealand when Marion du Fresne's expedition re-traced Cook's footsteps several years later.

We conclude that most of the serious infectious diseases that were common in European populations were not present in New Zealand before 1769. Tuberculosis may have been an exception. Enteric infections such as cholera and typhoid had very likely not been experienced by Māori until Europeans visited, and illnesses such as measles and whooping cough that were sufficiently long-established in European populations to present as moderately benign disorders of childhood were also novel, and therefore were serious threats to the health of New Zealand's first settlers.

Explanations

When they stepped ashore from the first canoes, Māori had to adapt to radically different circumstances – the New Zealand islands were large, cool, steep and out of the comfort zone of most of the plants that sustained settlements in the tropics. Only six Polynesian food crops were recognised by Cook (kūmara, taro, yam, gourd, paper mulberry or aute, and a species of cabbage tree *Cordyline terminalis*), although the mulberry and the yam were no longer reported in the nineteenth century. Furthermore, the Pacific cultivars that took root in New Zealand were not as productive as they had been in the northern islands. (Kūmara [sweet potato] provided only one crop per year for instance.) Of the native plants in New Zealand, there are currently about 190 that are known to be edible, and Māori used most of them.[90] However, none gave up as much energy, as readily, as the kūmara – many of the New Zealand native plants required lengthy preparation, soaking, pulping and cooking.

If the waka set out for New Zealand with pigs and chickens (important food sources in Polynesia), then it seems none survived the voyages, or if they did land, they did not adapt successfully to the new islands. Dogs came with the first settlers and were common in most Māori settlements; on occasion they were eaten. Rats also travelled in the canoes. They flourished in New Zealand and contributed to the diet of Māori, more as a delicacy than a staple.

The first humans to New Zealand found wonderful new sources of food (and maybe this is why pigs and chickens were never imported in the early voyaging times). The South Pacific was the kingdom of birds, thanks to the lack of ground-based predators and the fact there was no mammalian competition for local ecological niches. Before human occupation, there were more than 9000 species of birds in the Pacific islands (greater than the number of surviving species world-wide).[91] Many of these birds were flightless; all were relatively easy prey as they had no experience of humans. The wealth of bird life (and the plentiful supplies of fish and other marine foods) meant 'the amount of accessible fat and protein per square kilometre on a Pacific island may have been unequalled anywhere in the world'.[68]

To get a sense of the super-abundance of bird life, consider Norfolk Island in 1790. Robert Hughes describes an island that was settled briefly by Polynesians, but had been unoccupied by humans for several hundred years before the arrival of English convicts and their military escort.[92] The ship in which they sailed from Botany Bay was wrecked, and without other sources of food, crew and convicts had to make do with the mutton bird, which roosted on the island in enormous numbers through the summer. The quartermaster of public stores counted the birds collected each day. In one three-month period 170,000 birds were captured and eaten – nearly four birds per person per day. (The convicts survived – the mutton bird colony was exterminated.)

The first Polynesian settlers in New Zealand had to change from a pattern in the source islands of established agriculture supplemented by fishing, to a lifestyle that was dominated initially by hunting, fishing and gathering. The climate in New Zealand varied greatly from one end of the country to the other. So did the fertility of the soil, and availability of fish and other game. Early settlers may have retained horticulture to a greater extent in the north where conditions were favourable to gardening, and moa birds and seal probably made up a larger part of the diet in the south.[75]

When they were available, moa, sea birds and sea mammals were rich sources of protein. At first, supplies in parts of New Zealand were probably as bountiful as those on Norfolk Island in 1790. The moa hunter campsites along the east coast of the South Island contain the remains of hundreds of thousands of birds. It is said that one of these sites, at the mouth of the Waitaki River, was 'the largest prehistoric killing site in the world'.[93] And these were not the puny mutton birds, weighing barely a kilogram each, that sustained the Norfolk Island convicts. The legs of the largest species of moa, which contained most of the meat on the bird, were the height of a man. Māori could slice off drum-sticks that 'weighed thirty to forty kilograms – each [one] the size of a full-grown pig'.[93]

However, the barbecue bonanza did not last long – perhaps only 100–150 years. Carbon-dating of moa bones in ovens and rubbish tips runs out in the late 1400s, and the nine species of moa were probably extinguished altogether in the 1600s.[68; 94] After this time moa are no longer referred to in Māori tradition (except in mythical form).[95] Moa were long-lived, slow-breeding birds, which until the arrival of humans had been threatened only by the giant eagle (*Harpagornis moorei*). Even though the numbers of Māori must have been small compared with the population of moa, the birds succumbed rapidly to ground-based predation (human mainly, perhaps with contributions from the kiore). The other factor was loss of habitat – the east coast forests on both main islands were transformed by fire in the first few centuries after Māori settlement. In the same period, seals, which had once been abundant all around the coast and an important food source for Māori, were greatly reduced in numbers, and colonies persisted only in isolated parts of the South Island.

In place of large game, Māori had to rely on relatively nutrient-sparse wild foods, such as the bracken fern, and those plants that could be cultivated. There was land suitable for cultivation in most parts of the country, and new ways were found to farm the cold-sensitive kūmara, with underground storage pits being built to hold the crop from one season to the next. There are signs that the New Zealand population increased but, even in the north, horticulture did not produce enough to meet all needs. Wild foods remained an essential part of the diet, which may help explain why early Māori populations were widely dispersed around New Zealand. The lack of a food base to support large settlements may also go some way to explaining the lack of large pan-tribal political entities such as those that emerged elsewhere in the Pacific.[68]

With the rise of agriculture from roughly 1500 onwards, settlements were concentrated in the most fertile parts of New Zealand. Tradition from about this time records tribal fights over gardens, fortified settlements appear in the archaeological record, and burial sites are for the first time concealed, presumably because of grave-robbing.[95] The climate turned also – in the seventeenth century average temperatures fell by about 1 degree C, the prevailing westerlies strengthened and storms were more common.[75] In these conditions, it must have been a struggle, at times, to support the increasing numbers of people – excavations show a diminishing variety and quantity of shellfish and other local food at some sites. At the time the European explorers arrived, disputes over access to marine resources and good land for gardening were common in densely populated areas such as the Bay of Islands and Turanga-nui (Poverty Bay), and often led to armed conflict.[71]

Studies of human teeth provide some insight into the nature of the foods consumed at different points in settlement. Before about 600 BP the findings from New Zealand skeletal remains are similar to those reported in eastern Polynesia, and fit a diet that consisted mainly of soft foods (e.g., cooked meat, fruit).[75] Periodontal disease occurred early, bony erosion followed and loss of teeth in young adult life was common.[81] Samples from later periods more commonly showed evidence of trauma including erosion of enamel, wearing away of occlusal surfaces and abscesses in the jaw bone.[80] Pathology of this kind fits a fibrous diet and frequent consumption of grit-laden foods such as shellfish.[80]

Fresh- and salt-water fish were important food sources throughout Māori settlement, but the species that were hunted, and the quantities that could be obtained with existing technology, varied over time and from one part of the country to another. For instance, the midden evidence suggests a growing dependence on salt-water snapper (in the north) and barracouta (in the south) at the time that land-based protein sources were depleted. Fresh-water eel were prized as food items but there is scant archaeological evidence of large catches prior to the 1800s, perhaps due to the limitations of pre-metal technology.[75]

William Anderson, surgeon's mate and surgeon on Cook's second and third voyages, reported on Māori in Queen Charlotte Sound:

> . . . when they dare not venture to sea, or perhaps from choice, they supply the place of fish with muscles and Sea ears [abalone, or pāua in Māori] of which the shells of great quantitys lye in heaps near their houses, and they sometimes though rarely find means to kill Rails, Penguins and Shags which help to vary their diet. They also breed considerable numbers of the dogs . . . for food, but these cannot be consider'd as a principal article of diet.[96]

Overall, considering the food sources that were available, the nutrient and energy values of these sources, and the archaeological evidence of what was consumed, diets may have been marginal for good health, for many people, and for much of the period of Māori settlement. Conditions were probably most challenging for those living in the south and in inland areas, especially in the later years of undisturbed Māori occupation.

Average heights of adults are commonly cited as a measure of population health, since they are a function of 'net' nutrition (caloric intake less the demands resulting from work intensity and disease load).[97] The records of European explorers include many references to the stature of the indigenous people. Cook wrote in his journals: 'the Natives of this Country are a Strong, rawboned, well made, Active people, rather above than under the common size'.[98] (By 'common size', Cook was likely referring to the average height of British sailors, which was at this time around 167 centimetres.)[99]

On occasion, the explorers made measurements. For example, William Monkhouse reported that Te Maro, the warrior who challenged Cook's landing at Turanga-nui and was shot, was 'a short, but very stout-bodied man – measured about 5f 3i [160 centimetres]'.[71] The chief taken the same year from Tokerau (Doubtless Bay) by de Surville was reported to be '5 feet 2 inches and squarely built'.[71] Two years later, Jean Roux, ensign on the *Mascarin*, wrote of people from the Bay of Islands who visited Marion du Fresne's ship:

> These islanders are generally tall, well-built . . . We measured some of them, who seemed to be tallest among them, and they were over 6 feet and well-proportioned. Their usual height, as far as I could see, is five foot five to five foot six inches [165–67 centimetres].[71]

On the basis of skeletal studies, it has been suggested Māori men in the

1700s averaged about 170 centimetres in height.[80] At Wairau Bar, the estimates of adult height (175 centimetres for men, 160 centimetres for women) lie towards the upper end of estimates from other Pacific island populations.[81]

We note here that the first systematic survey of the heights and weights of Māori adults was carried out by A. S. Thomson, an Edinburgh-trained Army surgeon based in Auckland with a scientific interest in climate and health.[100] In 1849 he measured 147 Māori men who attended the military hospital for smallpox vaccination, and collected the same information from 617 British soldiers under his care. The average heights of Māori and British were almost identical: 169.6 and 170.9 centimetres respectively.[101] Average weights were also much the same: 64.0 and 64.9 kilograms.

Philip Houghton has suggested that the typical Polynesian body shape (a heavy-set, muscular torso with relatively short limbs) resulted from the selection processes associated with lengthy ocean voyages and, in particular, the stress of exposures to cold on long ocean voyages.[102] But there is little evidence to support Houghton's hypothesis, and some observations count against it. For instance, body proportions differ little between skeletons from remote Oceania and those excavated from sites close to Asia, where migrations began, preceding the period of long trips across the Pacific.

Others have asked whether differences between men and women may shed some light on the strains acting on Māori populations in the late pre-European contact period (roughly 200–400 BP). Comparisons of the length of the tibia bones and the prevalence of bony changes associated with growth delay suggest that the difference in heights between men and women was greater than currently applies, and that females were more prone to interruptions in growth.[103] Comments in the journals of explorers and early settlers imply there was rather greater variation in height and build between Māori men and women than expected. For example, Julien Crozet, Marion du Fresne's second in command, commented that 'the women in general are not as well made as the men',[104] and Joseph Banks, several years before, had written, 'the men are the size of the larger Europeans, stout, clean limnd and active, fleshy but never fat . . . the women . . . are rather smaller than European women'.[75]

Regional censuses carried out soon after European settlement report greater numbers of men than women, in all age groups, and this pattern was evident still at the time of the first national Māori census (1857/58).[104]

Put together, these observations have been used to argue that females were disadvantaged in access to food, shelter and protection, at a time when there was strong competition for resources – although Ian Pool argues that this sex bias is overstated, having been interpreted and reported through the lens of Victorian prejudice.[105] As these pressures relaxed in the second half of the 1800s, sex ratios became more equal, and by early in the twentieth century the proportion of females in the child population was similar to that among newborn infants.

Even in the most populous parts of the country, in the north-eastern portions of both islands, the density of settlement was low, compared with other parts of the Pacific, and this must have reduced the risks of many infections. Within settlements, there were aspects of Māori tradition that served public health very well. For example, Māori understood it was important to dispose safely of human excrement, to avoid leaving food scraps around the village, and to avoid food supplies and waterways that may have been contaminated by corpses. These rules were framed in terms of protecting what was sacred and avoiding sorcery (makutu), and in times when people were living securely and undisturbed, traditional mores would have helped control the incidence of enteric infections. When occupation was uncertain and contested, and populations were on the move, these rules regarding hygiene must have been more difficult to implement.

Health care prior to European contact was administered by tohunga (priest or expert) and other healers. In place was a well-developed system of explanations, diagnostic processes and treatment regimes. How effective were these approaches compared with what was offered by European providers at this time? Banks was not impressed. He wrote in his diaries that: 'I am inclined to think that [Māori] knowledge of Physick is but small.'

However, most British medicine of the period relied on anecdotal and untested therapies, and there is no reason to assume the techniques were superior to those of other cultures. Rae Lange tells the story of a British soldier who fell into a boiling pool at Rotorua in the 1870s and scalded both legs. One leg was treated in the Pākehā style, Māori poultices were applied to the other, and it was the latter that healed more quickly.[86]

MORTALITY AND LIFE EXPECTANCY IN EUROPE

We now turn to Europe, the source of the second wave of migration to New Zealand.

Mortality patterns

There are few reliable, nation-wide records of mortality until the nineteenth century. The Nordic countries are exceptions – in these countries there are annual reports based on registrations of deaths as far back as the early 1700s. However, other sources of information have made it possible to estimate long-run mortality trends as far back as Tudor times (1500s). Following the Reformation, European rulers took a close interest in evidence of church affiliation: in these fractious times it was prudent for a monarch to know how many of his or her subjects supported the home team. In continental Europe, the Council of Trent (1545–63) made rules about the recording of baptisms, marriages and burials in Catholic parishes. In England, Henry VIII placed similar requirements on the new Church of England. Many of the church records have survived, and they make a valuable resource for demographers and historians.[106; 107]

In the sixteenth century, Europe was beset by crises – epidemics, famines and wars swept across the continent, and mortality fluctuated widely. At this time, in Geneva, it is estimated that smallpox killed almost a third of the city's children.[108] Between 1560 and 1660, the climate cooled abruptly, leading to crop failures, famine, population displacement, epidemics of disease and conflict.[109] The Thirty Years' War (1618–48) caused massive civilian mortality, comparable to the effects of the plague. Between the Rhine and the Elbe more than a third of the population perished due to violence, hunger and disease.[110] Mortality among men in Europe in the sixteenth and seventeenth centuries was, according to one account, much the same as it had been in Rome two millennia earlier.[111]

England was the first European country to move to a more stable mortality regime. From the 1700s onwards, fluctuations in death rates and yo-yoing in life expectancy are much damped down and the causes of catastrophic mortality are less evident. For example, plague was seldom seen in its full menacing form after around 1670 – there were outbreaks of the disease subsequently, but they were localised and less severe than the fearsome visitations of earlier centuries. Within a hundred years smallpox and typhus had also declined considerably. Malaria took longer to recede – the disease was endemic in coastal areas and in the eastern part of the country until the 1800s.

During the eighteenth century, the population of England more than doubled, though this was probably due more to increasing fertility than to a fall in the death rate. The reduction in year-on-year variability in mortality was not translated immediately into improved life expectancy, since the great epidemic infections contributed only a small proportion of all deaths. In the mid-1500s, when the parish records of mortality were first kept, the crude death rate in England was about 29 per 1000 per year. Two hundred years later, around the time that James Cook departed on his voyage of discovery, the annual death rate (not adjusted for changes in the age structure of the population) was similar at 28 per 1000.[112]

In England, life expectancy at birth was about 36 years at the time of Cook's departure for the southern hemisphere in 1768.[106] It was around this time also that strong social class differences in mortality first emerged – by the end of the eighteenth century, the life expectancy of British nobles was ten years greater than the population average.[1] Conditions for both nobles and peasants were less favourable in other parts of Europe – Fogel estimates life expectancy at birth in France to be 26 years in 1750, and 33 years at the end of the eighteenth century.[113]

Explanations

Volumes have been written on what explains trends in life expectancy in Europe.[114; 115] Here we attempt a summary, focusing on the period up to the time of Cook's voyages, and with an eye to aspects of the story that have particular salience for New Zealand.

As noted already, the first step to mortality decline in Europe was the stabilisation of death rates, as overwhelming epidemics and devastating famines became less frequent. State interventions played a significant part. For instance, national grain markets in England were established during the 1700s and these moderated prices, evened out distribution of grain, and in general led to fewer and less severe times of food shortage and hunger. High prices for grain were still associated with mortality rates above the long-run average (especially amongst poorer groups in the population), but this was less marked after the middle of the eighteenth century than in earlier times.[116] Sanitary conditions in towns and cities were still appalling, by modern standards, but during the eighteenth century local authorities took steps to improve matters. In London in the 1700s there were campaigns to pave the streets and to remove waste.[117] Drains were covered, and houses re-built in brick in place of mud, wood and thatch. In rural areas, in association with the enclosure of common lands, marshes and wetlands were drained, and these practices along with housing improvements and new methods of farming initiated the retreat of malaria from northern Europe.[118; 119]

At the beginning of the twenty-first century, living in spacious housing, receiving a high income, being a woman and working in a high-status occupation are all factors associated with low mortality and relatively long lifespans. But when Cook came to New Zealand, life expectancy of women in England was one–two years *less* than that of men, and the mortality advantage enjoyed by the English peerage was a recent phenomenon.[1] When child-birth was less risky, and the force of infectious epidemics abated, the advantages associated with being a woman or being wealthy became apparent. But for centuries, women lived shorter lives than men, and where people lived mattered more than how they lived.

In nineteenth-century France, country labourers fared better than city-living bourgeoisie, for example. In Geneva, life expectancy in the country was 45 years in the middle of the eighteenth century, and rose to 51 years for children of couples who were married between 1790 and 1819.[108] Quakers in the north of England in the second half of the seventeenth century enjoyed life expectancies of more than 50 years, almost double those of their contemporaries living in London.[1] But a century later, English cities and towns were still relatively unhealthy places for the majority of citizens. In Nottingham, it was reported that one child was buried for every two that were baptised. In Lancashire, the death rate in towns was more than double that in the villages.[120]

The risks to health of urban living that were so apparent in Europe in the eighteenth century have important implications for a New Zealand account of mortality decline, given the low population densities of settlements in the colonies. The influences of nutrition on growth, development and mortality are very relevant to our story also.

The heights and weights of English soldiers were recorded from the early 1700s. Men were small by modern standards. In the 1790s, British military recruits stood on average 165 centimetres in height, and weighed 61 kilograms.[72; 107] In 2003, a survey at New Zealand airports found the average adult male weighed 88.5 kilograms, and the average female 71.9 kilograms. This was without carry-on luggage.[121] Similar average weights have been reported in recent National Health Surveys.[122]

In Europe, there was a dip in average heights in the middle of the eighteenth century, a reduction of about 2 centimetres in the height of 20–23-year-old English soldiers.[123] The reasons for this are not clear. It may have been partly the effects of early industrialisation. With changes in the patterns of work, income inequalities widened (which may have affected food security for the most disadvantaged groups as basic items such as bread and meat became more costly relative to other commodities), and the move from rural areas to towns and cities meant that many people no longer had access to local produce.

In England and France, agricultural production increased modestly during the 1700s, and this was assisted by warmer temperatures and more consistent rainfall in the last three decades of the century.[124] Together, this meant more affordable dietary calories were available to a greater proportion of the population. Disposable incomes rose in both countries in the latter part of the century, but trends were uneven, the distribution of wealth was increasingly unequal, and the timing and size of the improvements is debated.

Better transport – the eighteenth century in Britain was the age of turnpikes and canals – boosted trade and provided the means to distribute food and fuel more widely.[120] This, together with intervention by the state in food trading, meant prices did not fluctuate as sharply as before, and quality improved also. Now that farmers could sustain their animals over the winter with feed transported by barge and cart, and livestock could be brought to market, even when the weather was foul, fresh meat was, in theory, available year round. But in practice this benefit was available only to those who could pay. For the great majority of the population in England in the 1700s meat was a luxury item.

Imports contributed to a better (calorie-rich) English diet. The quantity of sugar brought into the country increased from 10,000 tons a year in 1700 to 150,000 tons a year at the end of the century – a principal use was puddings and the preserving of fruits. Rice was imported for the first time, and the price of tea from India fell from £1 a pound in 1700 to 5 shillings in 1750.[120]

In the 1700s manufacturing on a mass scale began to get under way in England, underpinned by the flow of capital from India and the returns from the slave trade. The arrival of factories introduced industrial pollution and was socially disruptive – artisans and home workers lost their jobs. But the damage was much less than that inflicted a century later, and the upside was that the population had access to a greater range of household goods at lower prices. Some of these contributed to improvements in health. The price of soap fell, for instance, and cheap (washable) cotton clothing was more commonly available. On the other hand, countries in continental Europe that were much slower to enter the industrial era (Norway and Sweden, for instance), showed falls in mortality in the late eighteenth century that were similar to those seen in England. Economic development was clearly not the only, and perhaps not even a major, cause of improvements in population health at this time.[108]

More sophisticated quarantine arrangements may have contributed to the reduction in epidemic mortality due to plague (which had essentially disappeared from Europe by the beginning of the eighteenth century), smallpox and typhus. Interventions were sometimes crude and over-ambitious – the Hapsburgs tried to block movement of the plague out of Asia by a *cordon sanitaire* along the entire border with the Ottoman Empire. Nevertheless, from the 1700s onwards attempts to control infectious diseases were better organised, more consistently enforced and therefore tended to be more effective than they had been previously.[108]

The best evidence of an early, successful public health intervention is associated with smallpox. Inoculation, which means applying a small quantity of material from the pustules of a smallpox patient to a healthy person, in order to provoke a mild case of the disease, was widely practised during the 1700s. It was risky – sometimes patients suffered full-blown cases of smallpox, and many died as a result. But the practice prevented more deaths than it caused. Table 1 displays the history of smallpox in Boston in the eighteenth century. Out of every hundred who were inoculated, on average one or two died from smallpox. The case fatality rate for 'natural' smallpox was about ten times higher. During the century the number of people who were inoculated rose, the number of new infections dwindled and mortality from the disease fell by about two-thirds.

Table 1 Smallpox cases, deaths and numbers inoculated in smallpox epidemics in Boston, United States of America, 1702–1792

YEAR	SMALLPOX DEATHS	DEATH RATE PER 1000	NATURAL CASES	% CASE FATALITY	NUMBERS INOCULATED	% CASE FATALITY
1702	213	31.5	-	-	-	-
1721	850 (6)	77.3	5759	14.7	310	2.4
1730	500 (12)	33.3	3600	13.6	400	3.0
1752	569 (30)	36.2	5545	9.7	2124	1.4
1764	170 (46)	10.9	669	18.5	4977	0.9
1776	57 (28)	10.0	669	18.5	4977	0.9
1778	61 (19)	6.1	122	34.4	2121	0.9
1792	198 (165)	9.9	232	14.2	8114	2.0

Source: A. J. Mercer, 'Smallpox and Epidemiological Demographic Change in Europe: The Role of Vaccination' (*Population Studies* 39, no. 2 [1985]: 287–307). Smallpox deaths among the inoculated are given in parentheses and have been excluded in calculating case fatality among natural cases.

In 1796 Edward Jenner showed that similar immunising effects could be obtained, much more safely, with vaccination using material from cowpox. Once available, smallpox vaccination was widely promoted, closely followed by a reduction in smallpox epidemics and a further decline in numbers of deaths attributed to the disease.[125]

Fluctuations in mortality in Europe during this period (roughly 1560–1800) have been related to climatic conditions, and in particular the periods of northern hemisphere cooling that occurred between 1560 and 1660, and again in the first half of the 1700s. When temperatures fell across Europe, population growth slowed, and the numbers of famine events, epidemics and military conflicts increased.[109] In England, grain yields were reduced during the cold periods, and in London mortality was negatively associated with winter temperatures, independent of harvest results.[124]

Some of the causes of mortality decline in Europe were 'passive' (for instance, climate change, the reduced virulence of pathogens). Others were socially determined. Schofield and Reher comment:

> . . . the potentially negative effects of climate were eventually overcome; parents began to take care not to give rotten food or contaminated water to their children. In the long run, cultural factors were essential for the breakthrough in the fight against high mortality.[112]

CONCLUSION

At the time Cook set sail for New Zealand mortality rates in England were high, very high by modern standards, but no doubt better than a hundred years before. What caused the decline in mortality in Europe during the 1700s is not entirely clear, but important factors were improvements in the general standard of living (including more secure access to a greater variety of foods), public health interventions to control disease and the reduced virulence of some significant infections.

2

Māori Majority

The First Hundred Years After Cook

European settlement led to radical changes in Māori society, mostly to its great detriment. This chapter concentrates on the dramatic deterioration in Māori health. Impacts were severe and occurred rapidly, although relatively few Europeans set foot in New Zealand in the first 50 years after Cook. The European population grew rapidly following the signing of the Treaty of Waitangi in 1840, and reached parity, numerically, with Māori by 1860. However, the health of European settlers is touched on only briefly here – better information is available from around 1860, and forms the basis of the following chapter.

The chapter includes two periods: the time of relatively haphazard settlement following Cook's visit (1769–1840), and the first 20 years following formal annexation. In the first two decades after the Treaty of Waitangi the apparatus of colonisation was in place, but New Zealand was only nominally a British settlement. Māori out-numbered the new settlers 50 to one at the time the Treaty was signed, and remained in the majority until 1858. While sovereignty had been ceded to the Crown in 1840, in the eyes of the British at least, large areas of the country remained under Māori direction.

There is ample record, although mostly from haphazard first-person accounts, that Māori health deteriorated during this time. Deaths were not registered and there was no comprehensive population census. However, we estimate that life expectancy reached its nadir of less than 20 years, caused by the spread of novel infections, social upheaval, loss of land and the effects, direct and indirect, of inter-tribal warfare. There were glimmers of opportunity for Māori, in commerce, education and trade, but these were short-lived, swept away by the rush of new settlers from Europe.

MĀORI PRIOR TO THE TREATY

During this time there was no formal registration of deaths, nor were there any systematic censuses of the population. Official statistics in New Zealand were a product of the 1854 legislation that mandated registrations of births and deaths, but among non-Māori only. Registration of Māori deaths was not compulsory until 1913. Until then, estimates of mortality among Māori are based on local surveys, or the impressions of observers at the time, or are inferred from changes in the age structure of the population.[126]

Figure 4 (overleaf) displays estimates of life expectancy for Māori in the period 1769 to 1840 – they are very uncertain, and should be treated as a rough guide only. Shown as context also are estimates of life expectancy in England and Wales in 1769, world-leading life expectancy in the early 1800s from Norway, and the current levels of life expectancy in New Zealand (on the top right hand side of the graph).[127]

There is no way of determining precisely how many Māori were living in New Zealand at the time of European contact. Some have argued that Māori were in decline before 1769, but there is no evidence to support this view. However, there is no doubt what happened after Cook's visits. Epidemic infectious disease and an increase in lethal warfare caused a serious reduction in the population, particularly on the fringes of Māori domains where there was greatest contact with Europeans.

Missionaries raised the alarm in the early 1830s; James Busby, first British Resident, wrote (in 1837) that unless action was taken the country would be 'destitute of a single aboriginal inhabitant'.[128] Between 1840 and 1900, the period when statistics were first collected (erratically, and not on a national basis), the Māori population shrank by about two-thirds. In the 60 years prior to the Treaty, when population figures are much less certain, the reduction was probably less, proportionately, but by 1840 the number of Māori may have been only a half of those who were in New Zealand before European contact. There is no agreement over what should constitute the reference point: the population at the time Cook arrived has been estimated as 86,000,[78] 80,000–140,000,[129] 100,000 (estimate from Cook's first voyage),[130] 125,000–150,000[75] and up to 500,000.[87]

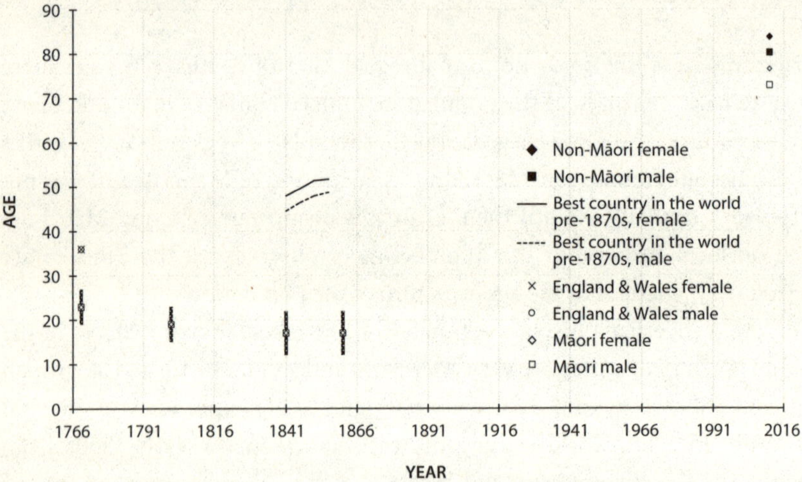

Figure 4: Life expectancy at birth of Māori and non-Māori and 'best country in the world' – 1769 to 1860

Source: 'Best in the world' data from J. Oeppen and J. Vaupel, 'Broken Limits to Life Expectancy' (*Science* 296 [2002]: 1029–31) (see also www.sciencemag.org/cgi/content/full/296/5570/1029/DC1). Prior to non-Māori becoming the top-ranked life expectancy in the world in 1876, the following countries held the top rank according to Oeppen and Vaupel: 1840–48, Sweden, Norway, and Denmark (interchangeably); 1849–60, Norway; 1861–75, Australia, Sweden, Norway and Ireland (interchangeably). Māori estimates are from multiple sources: the estimate plotted at 1769 (23, range 19 to 27) is from A. Brewis, M. A. Molloy, and D. G. Sutton, 'Modeling the Prehistoric Maori Population' (*American Journal of Physical Anthropology* 81 [1990]: 343–56), and described in chapter 1; the estimates from 1806 to 1866 are based on small surveys and case reports, at a time of epidemic infectious disease, warfare, colonisation and displacement of populations. These early Māori estimates are very uncertain.

The demographer Ian Pool estimates the population in 1860 was less than half what it had been when Cook visited.[131] Claudia Orange suggests the number of Māori men of fighting age decreased by up to a quarter between 1800 and 1840.[128] On the other hand, Belich claims the 1769 population has by and large been over-estimated, and therefore the subsequent Māori decline has been exaggerated.[78]

But even if the true reduction is only half that proposed by Pool, this represents a ruinous loss of life (comparable perhaps to the effects of civil war in the German states in the first half of the 1600s). Such a dramatic change seems out of proportion to the small numbers of European settlers in New Zealand in the early years, but it is in keeping with the effects of colonisation elsewhere. Figure 5 is based on Pool's estimates of the Māori population and shows both the early decline and subsequent recovery (which we discuss in later chapters).

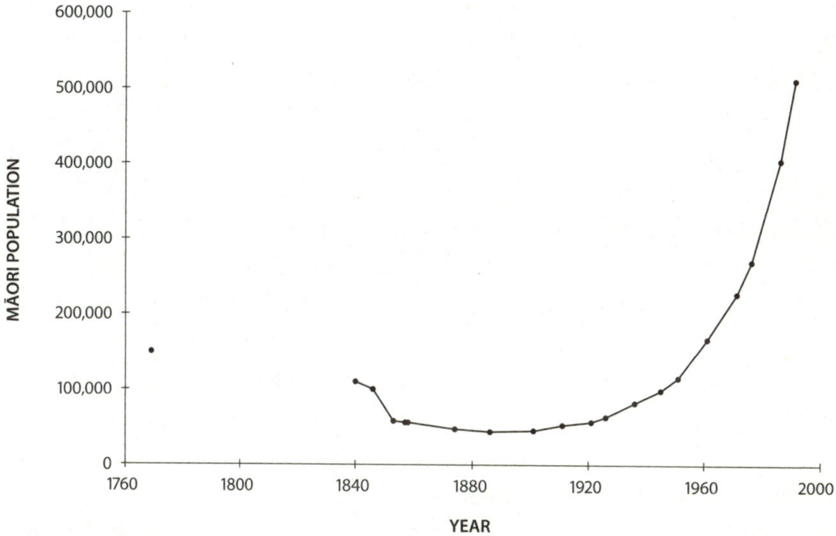

Figure 5: The fall and rise of the Māori population

Source: D. I. Pool, *Te Iwi Maori: A New Zealand Population, Past, Present and Projected* (Auckland: Auckland University Press, 1991).

In New Zealand, the two vectors of early depopulation that have received the greatest attention are microbes and firearms. We shall start with the arrival of high-lethality weaponry.

The so-called Musket Wars began when tribes from the north of the North Island (where early European settlement had been concentrated) launched armed raids on southern iwi.[78] In 1821 Hongi Hika, the Ngāpuhi leader, attacked Mokoia and Mauinaina pā, close to where the city of Auckland is now located. About half his war party carried long-barrelled firearms, many acquired by Hika earlier in the year in Sydney. Te Hinaki, the Ngāti Paoa chief, held out for two days, but the Ngāpuhi force, with their new weapons, prevailed. Some say there were 300 deaths among the defenders,[95] others claim as many as 2000 lives were lost.[132] But in any case this was killing on an unprecedented scale, and Ngāti Paoa abandoned the Tāmaki peninsula.

There followed a decade of high-fatality inter-tribal warfare, extending through both the North and South Islands, and reaching the Chatham Islands hundreds of kilometres to the east of the South Island. All the tribes scrambled to acquire firearms, and European traders were ready to oblige with supplies. By the early 1830s the market for weaponry was saturated. Indeed, it was said there were now more guns than warriors, and battles were less one-sided, raiding parties less aggressive and casualties diminished. But in the space of 20–30 years, tens of thousands of people died – perhaps one-fifth of the total Māori population, and more than the number of New Zealanders killed in World War I.[131; 133]

Rifles, even in small numbers, gave the early marauders a significant advantage, but the reach and speed of the raiding parties depended on another European import – the potato. The tuber provided more energy per kilogram than the kūmara, was less likely to spoil, and may have doubled or more the range of a war party. First planted in New Zealand by Cook, in Queen Charlotte Sound, the potato may have been introduced to Northland in 1793 by the Ngāpuhi travellers, Tuki and Huru, on their return from Norfolk Island.[134]

As well as deaths that resulted directly from fighting, there were casualties caused by the displacement of hapū and iwi. There had probably never before been such movement of large numbers of people. Some places that had previously been heavily populated (such as Tāmaki, now part of inner Auckland) were abandoned altogether. Elsewhere, communities moved to fortified pā on open ground. These settlements were more easily defended against rifle fire, but frequently the sites lacked clean water and effective drainage. Years of fighting caused serious disruptions to farming, trading and community building.[13] In the new war economy, iwi had to concentrate on activities such as cultivation of flax that would most rapidly raise funds to buy weapons. This came at a cost. Often families had to move away from their gardens and safe areas to temporary camps. Traders struck a hard bargain ('A ton [of dressed flax] fetched £120 in the Sydney market, and a ton was the price of a gun worth perhaps half that number of shillings').[135] The gathering and cultivation of food took a back seat to the arms race, and in the 1830s missionaries and government officials reported for the first time the deaths of children from malnutrition.[128]

The first major epidemics of infectious disease occurred soon after Cook's first visit. There are reports of a 'flu-like illness causing heavy mortality on the Tāmaki isthmus in 1790 and again in 1810.[95] On the Chatham Islands, Moriori were severely affected by an outbreak of measles soon after the first European ship landed in 1791.[136] Pertussis and tuberculosis were reported subsequently. By the late 1830s, regular outbreaks of respiratory illnesses affected Māori settlements, peaking in spring and autumn. Venereal diseases spread rapidly after first contact with Europeans, and very likely contributed to the sharp decline in birth rates in some Māori communities.

Māori were protected initially by the sparse settlement of New Zealand – infections could not spread as rapidly as they did on smaller, more densely populated Pacific islands. However, as European goods, services and institutions became more important to Māori, people moved to low-lying coastal areas, close to commercial centres and trading opportunities, and in these environments, crowding and poor sanitation increased the attack rates of many infections. In such settings it was also difficult for Māori to gather traditional foods, such as fish, birds, berries and kūmara, and the staple items that could be obtained by trade (bread, tea, potatoes, salted meat) did not, on their own, make a nourishing diet. The new settlements also provided better access to alcohol and tobacco, with predictably damaging effects.

Measles, influenza, dysentery, whooping cough and tuberculosis were the most significant of the lethal infections that reached New Zealand. Typhus and cholera came with the British to Australia, but as far as we know, did not cross the Tasman. Isolated cases of smallpox were reported on occasions in New Zealand in the nineteenth century, but local spread was uncommon and there were no significant outbreaks such as those recorded elsewhere in the Pacific.[126; 137] Why New Zealand escaped relatively lightly is a mystery. Without any prior contact with smallpox, Māori were as susceptible as any of the indigenous peoples, and quarantine and vaccination were introduced no earlier here than elsewhere. Timing of settlement may have helped: outbreaks in Europe had diminished in frequency and severity in the early 1800s, so there would be fewer index cases setting sail for New Zealand than headed for the older colonies. Distance may also have been protective. There is no asymptomatic carrier state, and smallpox is infectious for a relatively short time, coinciding with the vivid and characteristic rash. For this reason, when cases did occur onboard ships bound for Australasia, their trip south must have often been interrupted before reaching the final port of call. In addition, as mentioned in the introduction, New Zealand may have benefited from changes in the pathogen, with increasing prominence of less virulent strains.

Why were Māori, and other indigenous peoples around the Pacific, affected so severely by other infectious diseases that were much less troublesome amongst European populations?

There are three kinds of answers to this question: because of characteristics of the host (the patient) that may aggravate infection; features of the pathogens (bacteria and viruses) including transmission dynamics that may lead to more serious outcomes; and treatment and medical care factors.[138; 139]

Contemporary accounts focused on host characteristics, and favoured a racial explanation. The claim was that Māori, other Pacific islanders, Amerindians and Australian Aboriginals were constitutionally susceptible. Some went further, and wrote that this racial weakness was a deficiency with tragic consequences, but one that would be corrected in due course by the forces of natural selection. The fundamental shortcomings of such an approach to categorising and comparing humans have been well described elsewhere.[140] In all the work that has been done on susceptibility to disease there is no evidence in Māori and other Pacific populations of particular genes that lower the resistance of *individuals* to infections. But genetics may help explain the vulnerability of *populations* through another mechanism, as illustrated by the example of measles.

The measles virus reproduces with low fidelity, and so has the ability to change its antigenic presentation, even within a single host. This means the virus can adapt to elements of its environment, including host factors such as the histocompatibility antigens that play an important part in the immune response to infection. When successive hosts are closely related, the virus is said to be 'pre-adapted', because it is moving to a familiar immune environment. In these conditions one would expect infection to spread more rapidly and illness to be more severe. This fits with findings of epidemiological studies in Africa, which report that childhood mortality from measles is twice as great if the infection is caught from another member of the family than it is when the index case is unrelated.[141]

Francis Black proposed that the ability of the measles virus to 'pre-adapt' is the key to understanding the great measles epidemics of the New World.[142] The extent of genetic variation amongst Pacific islanders and the indigenous people of the Americas is much less than amongst Europeans, and African populations display the greatest genetic variability of all. It is thought that Māori, other Pacific islanders and the indigenous peoples of the Americas developed from relatively small 'founder' populations. (However, we note that the sequencing of mitochondrial DNA from Wairau Bar has shown up greater genetic diversity than was anticipated.)[143] There are likely to be many lines of common descent amongst those who spread out from Asia to occupy the Pacific and the American continent, and consequently the gene pool is not as deep as it would be amongst longer-established populations. For example, Black calculated that there is a 32 per cent chance that a virus passing between two South American Indians will not encounter a new histocompatibility antigen at the A or B locus, but less than a 1 per cent chance when passing between Africans.

The 'many lines of common descent' story may help to explain the speed and lethality of many of the epidemics following first contact, not just measles. But there are limits to Black's argument. For example, improvements in host resistance amongst Māori and other indigenous peoples in the Pacific occurred too rapidly to be attributed to changes in the genetic makeup of the population.

Peter Aaby, an infectious diseases epidemiologist, has suggested that the search for explanations of the severity of virgin-soil epidemics has placed too much emphasis on host and medical care factors, and not enough attention has been paid to transmission factors.[138; 139] He points out that people who receive a very large dose of virus tend to be more badly affected, and have a higher chance of dying, than those who receive a smaller dose. On this basis, Aaby proposes that high mortality on first contact from conditions such as measles was due in large part to many people getting ill at the same time. The coincidence of infection and living conditions (which were typically confined and crowded) raised the intensity of exposures for secondary cases, leading to more severe illness. People who are severely affected tend to excrete larger amounts of virus, so it is plausible that there was a cascade effect, of increasing lethality, as epidemics took hold. In support of this explanation, Aaby points to outbreaks in nineteenth-century European populations that were at least as severe as those occurring around the Pacific. Typically, these high-fatality events occurred in institutional populations and closed communities, where transmission was intense and rapid. For instance, during the Paris Commune of 1871 an outbreak of measles among the Garde Mobile killed 40 per cent of those infected.

Following the initial epidemics, it is likely there were compounding effects of disadvantage. The generally poor health status of Māori placed them at greater risk when epidemics occurred. Infections such as influenza and measles tend to be more severe when the patient is under-nourished, or is suffering from other, chronic and debilitating conditions. For instance, patients with tuberculosis and other chronic destructive lung diseases are at greater risk of dying from influenza.[144]

Poor housing conditions must have played an important part throughout, increasing the opportunities for disease transmission. In these circumstances children tend to be exposed to infections at a younger age than would occur otherwise. Both the dose of virus received, and young age at first infection, increase mortality in childhood.[145]

Contemporary reports of the health of Māori presented a gloomy picture. When Edward Gibbon Wakefield visited settlements in the Hokianga in 1839 he reported:

> I was much struck by their miserable outward appearance. They were wretchedly clothed, covered with dirt, badly supplied with food, generally speaking weak and sickly looking.[146]

James Busby wrote a few years later:

> Disease and death prevail . . . amongst the natives . . . when they contrast their own condition with that of the English families, amongst whom the marriages have been prolific in a very extraordinary degree of a most healthy progeny, they conclude that the God of the English is removing the aboriginal inhabitants to make room for them.[16]

In a letter home, published in the *New Zealand Journal* in 1848, a settler commented: 'It is singular that while Europeans enjoy such good health here, the original natives are annually decimated by disease.'[147]

How should these reports be interpreted? Some have argued that the British tended to report what they expected to see, given prevailing views on the viability of traditional societies.[78] There was certainly a strongly held preconception that dark-skinned races would give way to the expansion of European populations. Charles Darwin, passing through New Zealand on the *Beagle* in 1839 (and gestating his theory of natural selection), observed:

> The varieties of man seem to act on each other in the same way as different species of animals – the stronger always extirpating the weaker. It was melancholy in New Zealand to hear the fine energetic natives saying that they knew the land was doomed to pass from their children.[16]

It is possible also that commentators over-estimated the reduction in Māori population due to extraordinary fecundity of the early European settlers. For example, missionary marriages were indeed 'prolific in a very extraordinary degree'. The 14 couples who came to New Zealand before 1833 had 114 children between them.[78] By this standard, the Māori population may have seemed to be withering away, even if fertility and mortality had changed little from earlier times. Also, observers were prone to generalise from the areas commonly visited to the whole country, although the burden of novel infections would have been heaviest in parts of the country where the indigenous population was in close contact with traders, whalers, sailors and other visitors from overseas.

But Māori decline was not just wishful invention on the part of the colonisers. Conditions in hubs of commerce such as Hokianga and the Bay of Islands (bays on the west and east coasts of the north of the North Island, respectively) may have been a great deal worse in the early years than less accessible regions such as the Waikato or Urewera (central North Island). However, even the Waikato, which until the 1860s was mostly beyond the limits of European settlement, was affected. Francis Fenton, resident magistrate, surveyed the local population in 1844 and again in 1858, and reported a decrease of about 20 per cent, with low proportions at both surveys of children (27 per cent under the age of 14), and he found that males exceeded females by about a third.[148]

While the records of the early church missions to New Zealand may have been skewed, they do provide vivid accounts of debilitating conditions that Māori reported they had never experienced with such severity. The afflictions included suppurating infections of the skin ('scrofula', most commonly caused by tuberculosis infection of lymph nodes [usually] in the neck), acute incapacitating fevers ('influenza'), chronic respiratory infections (commonly described as 'consumption'), and severe gastroenteritis.

This description comes from the 1838 journal of John Hobbs, associated with the Wesleyan mission in the Hokianga:

> We have of late had a very uncommon degree of sickness amongst the people, and vast numbers of them have died. I have taken the principal charge of giving them medicine and great has been my distress in witnessing their miseries. Two disorders have been epidemic, one erysipelas attacking throat, face and head, of which several have died, though numbers have recovered; the other a disorder to which I cannot give a proper name. Some call it the Cholera Morbus, but it is not exactly of that description.* However, some of the people are taken and dead in a few hours.[146]

* Erysipelas is an acute infection of the skin caused by the streptococcus bacteria; and cholera morbus refers to severe, acute gastroenteritis not specific to a particular organism.

EUROPEAN SETTLERS PRIOR TO THE TREATY

In the first days, in the forgotten calendars,
came the seeds of the race, the forerunners:
offshoots, outcasts, entrepreneurs,
architects of Empire, romantic adventurers;
and the famished, the multitude of the poor
— A. R. D. FAIRBURN, FROM 'DOMINION'

European settlement was slow to get under way: on the eve of the signing of the Treaty of Waitangi, 71 years after Cook, there were '1800 to 2000 British subjects in New Zealand, of whom 158 are runaway convicts or sailors'.[130] The first settlers lived from sealing and whaling, both high-risk occupations featuring ship-wreck, injury and drowning. Then came the missionaries – the Church of England and the Catholic Church were first, and they were followed in short order by the Methodists. Later there was commercial harvesting of flax and forestry – about a third of the men in New Zealand were employed in the timber industry in 1840.[149]

The first sizeable European settlements were based around docks for the repair and re-stocking of ships, and much of the employment was in hotels and bars. Although whaling and sealing stations were established early in the far south, at Bluff and Dusky Sound, most Europeans in the early 1800s lived in the north, and particularly around the Bay of Islands. These were raw settlements, with a reputation for drunkenness, drowning and violent deaths of other kinds. Alarmed by disorder, aware of economic opportunity, and apprehensive of the growing interest shown by the French and Americans, the British government resolved to annex New Zealand as a colony. The Treaty of Waitangi was the means to this end.

AFTER THE TREATY

British occupation of New Zealand was late, compared with other edges of empire, and New Zealand benefited in some ways from advances in science and changes in social attitudes that had taken place in the 50 years since Botany Bay in Australia was occupied. The rise of the humanitarian movement made a difference. As well as the abolition of slavery throughout the British Empire (1833), there was a greater awareness of the effects of European settlements on indigenous populations. In his paper to the Statistical Section of the British Association in 1838, Sax Bannister Esq. proclaimed

> . . . the influence of this increased emigration on the millions of barbarous natives in those new lands is of the utmost importance. No human power can stop the white people: but it is conceived that they may be wisely guided, so as to become blessings to the aborigines, instead of a scourge and a curse.[130]

Reflecting the times, the British government in the 1830s was minded to expand its Empire and protect native races from undue harm simultaneously. To achieve these goals, the Treaty of Waitangi incorporated both an assertion of British sovereignty and explicit recognition of the interests of the first settlers. With hindsight, one might say the ambiguity of the Treaty documents served the colonisers well: Māori acceptance opened the doors for peaceful European settlement at a time when the military advantage (if they had chosen to exercise it) lay with the indigenous people. Then, when the demographic balance had swung decisively in favour of European settlers, the colonial government asserted a new understanding of the Treaty, one that denied special rights to Māori and highlighted the transfer of sovereignty to the Crown.[150]

But in the short term, the prospects for New Zealand appeared to be positive. Natural resources were abundant – Governor FitzRoy reported that 'the climate favours every kind of production, animal as well as vegetable, in an extraordinary manner'.[151]

Māori were well organised and keen to exploit the economic, social and military advantages that might result from engagement with Europeans. Once acquired, European products were put to effective use, whether these were farm tools, the energy-dense potato, fast sailing ships, books or rifles.

New arrivals brought with them 'elements of the European agricultural package'[152] that were of benefit to both Māori and Pākehā. They included pigs, the plough, clover seed, sheep, ducks, new cereal crops, hops and grapevines (first planted by Samuel Marsden in 1814). Māori were quick to make use of these opportunities. Early European settlements often depended on Māori agriculture, and mission stations in the north were supplied with 'potatoes, maize, onions, cabbages, peaches, sweet potatoes, pumpkins, grapes, melons, apples, and quinces, as well as flour (milled in Māori mills), fish, chickens, geese, turkeys, and goats'.[78]

In the 1830s Waikato iwi established market gardens on the Coromandel peninsula and Great Barrier Island and grew vegetables for export.[153] The trade was profitable and there appeared to be good prospects for further growth. Between 1846 and 1860 there were 49 flour mills built in the central North Island, and Māori dominated coastal shipping. In 1849 there were 43 Māori ships operating out of the Bay of Plenty.[95]

Yet Māori numbers continued to fall, and the decline accelerated in the decade or two after the Treaty was signed. The British were aware of what was happening, and made attempts to provide some kind of health care.

Missionaries such as William Williams, surgeon and evangelist to Paihia and Poverty Bay for more than 30 years, ran clinics and dispensed medicines. Samuel Marsden proposed, as early as 1826, to establish both a hospital for Māori and a medical school to train local people. This came to naught, and subsequently the matter of medical treatments for Māori, and how to pay for them, was caught up in the broader issue of how to fund public hospitals. Hospitals at this time were exclusively for the indigent, and were funded by voluntary subscriptions and philanthropy. Governor Grey proposed in 1846 that the colony establish hospitals, and facilities were opened in Auckland, New Plymouth and Wellington in the following year.[137] These were for 'the treatment of sick and destitute Europeans, and free treatment for all Māoris'.

In 1852, when provincial governments were established, a fixed amount (£7,000) was identified in the colony budget to be spent on Māori.[154] Nevertheless, government assistance was unevenly distributed and in no way proportionate to needs: in 1858, when half the population was Māori, 96 per cent of government expenditure was in the European districts.[155]

By the time Grey returned for his second term as Governor in 1861, almost £25,000 was set aside for Native Purposes, of which £3,192 was to be spent on 'Medical Attendance on Natives'. (Of this latter amount, only £50 was allocated to the South Island. This presumably was a reflection on where the numbers of Māori fell across the country.) At this time, it was resistance from

European settlers, rather than the attitude of the Governor and his staff, or the Colonial Secretary, that restricted expenditure and cut short the development of services for Māori.

A Central Board was established in 1854 to supervise vaccination of Māori populations. This arose from concerns about the vulnerability of Māori to smallpox, and the risk that infection would spread to the European population. (Also, Māori were more inclined to accept vaccination, it was noted at the time, than were European New Zealanders.)[137] Pamphlets on a number of public health topics were distributed, in the Māori language, and men who had previously acted as provincial surgeons were designated as native medical attendants. Unfortunately, these initiatives were short-lived.

Why did progress of Māori and non-Māori not proceed hand in hand? 'Nineteenth-century [British] observers were not at a loss to explain the decline of the Māori population . . . Rather, there was a surfeit of explanations, from the supernatural to the mundane.'[151] The British attributed high Māori mortality to an inadequate diet, infectious diseases, destructive and careless behaviours (alcohol, violence, mistreatment of women, inappropriate dressing), lack of health care, in-breeding and fate. ('May it not be that races of men, like individual men, have their years of growth, prosperity, decrease and decay?' asked A. S. Thomson, army surgeon, opportunistic scientist and New Zealand's first epidemiologist.)[151]

'Bad feeding, clothing and dirty mode of living' were said by missionary John Wohlers to be the cause of high death rates among children on Ruapuke Island (in the Foveaux Strait between the South and Stewart Islands) in the 1850s.[156] Thomas Chapman, in 1857, wrote: 'tobacco and filth, is in my opinion, when added to their miserable feeding, the principal cause of the death of their infants. The mother's milk and the mother's lungs . . . and the mother's food, all more or less are impregnated.'

A. S. Thomson made a list: '1st, inattention to the sick; 2ndly, infanticide; 3rdly, sterility; 4thly, new habits; 5thly, new disease; and lastly, the evil effects arising among men from intermarrying with scrofulous blood-connections.'[14]

Some of these explanations were fanciful; others, such as the 'new habits' that Thomson referred to (including consumption of alcohol and tobacco), were consequences of decline more than primary causes. The major force for change was the rapid increase in numbers of settlers. The European population of New Zealand multiplied ten-fold in a decade after the signing of the Treaty. The new arrivals amplified the risks of infectious disease, but more significant in the longer term was competition between Māori and settlers for resources and, in particular, land.

In the early days of the colony Māori could exchange land for the military, social and economic benefits of the Pākehā connection, without conceding authority. But this changed when the Pākehā multiplied. James Belich quotes John Gorst, an official of the imperial government, who wrote on the changing significance of land sales during the 1850s:

> By sale to Europeans, while Europeans were few and weak, no power or territorial dominion was parted with. The purchaser became one of the most valuable possessions of the tribe: the chief called him 'our Pakeha' . . . But as the number of Europeans increased these relations were altered; a sale involved parting with the dominion of the soil.[157]

Although Māori were attracted by the prospects of new resources, and took advantage of European mercantilism in many ways, the new economy undermined the collective core of traditional society. Some early and spectacular successes in trade were due to the skills, energy and organisational framework provided by hapū (sub-tribes). But as the English economy developed in New Zealand, the traditional social structures unravelled. Some English officials saw the weakening of hapū and iwi as a positive sign for Māori development, for example, Henry Sewell, who remarked in 1857 that 'the extinction of their tribal right and the substitution of an individual title to land is the first step, and the most important step, towards if possible, saving them'.[155]

Progress in the eyes of Sewell (member of the House of Representatives for Christchurch) and others was personal advancement (the acquisition of material goods and land ownership in particular). This was a self-serving construction of Māori aspirations – the settlers must have been aware of the political advantages that flowed to them by undercutting the Māori power base. And there were economic benefits at stake as well, if Māori were dislodged from self-sufficient rural settlements to become labourers for the colonists.

In this world-view, breaking down custom and tradition was necessary, and part of the responsibility borne by the colonising power. It appears this is what George Grey (Governor from 1845 to 1853, and 1861 to 1868) meant by assimilation: it was being cruel to be kind, breaking the shackles of barbarous and ignorant belief and practice to set free a whole race. Such aggressive evangelism was at odds with the ideals of protection that were written in the Treaty, but Grey was not alone in his construction of civilisation and Empire. There may have been others who would have been willing to explore new models of governance, new ways of grafting together English and Māori institutions, possibly even incorporating relatively benign forms of separatism. But such radical ideas held little sway compared with the forceful intentions of the Governor, and there was no benevolent force at Empire HQ that was capable (or motivated) to intervene.

Within a very short time, the political climate of the colony had turned. The rhetoric of the Treaty, early prospects for Māori development and the economic boom of the 1840s were all casualties of advancing colonisation, Likewise, the hospitals for indigenous patients, the central coordination of vaccination programmes for Māori, the use of te reo (Māori language) for education, and appointments of native medical attendants – none of these innovations survived the onset of hostilities in the 1860s.

CONCLUSION

The first 20 years post-Treaty were dominated by political events, colonisation, land grabs and the build-up to the Land Wars. This chapter says little about precise trends in health statistics because there is sparse information to draw on. The Māori population dwindled due to reduced fertility and high mortality, there seems no doubt about this, although by how much is uncertain. High mortality among Māori had colonisation and land confiscation as a root cause, upon which were heaped the effects of warfare, infectious diseases, poor nutrition, crowding, and the damaging effects of alcohol and tobacco. As to what the Māori life expectancy was, the only course of action is to (literally) fill in the dots between the pre-Cook estimates of 20–25 years and the late nineteenth-century estimates of up to 30 years. Our guess is that Māori life expectancy in the first 20 years post-Treaty was at its lowest ebb, perhaps 20 years or less.

The non-Māori population increased from about 2000 at the time of the Treaty, to approximately 50,000 by 1860. Its composition altered radically, from a motley mix of sealers, whalers and missionaries to a great variety of frontier settlers, including farmers, business and crafts folk (but not yet the itinerant gold miners). It is likely, in our view, that a combination of the healthy migrant effect and New Zealand's uncrowded and fertile landscape boosted non-Māori life expectancy above European levels, from the very beginning of British settlement. But we are speculating. Evidence of low mortality and long lifespans for non-Māori begins to accumulate around 1860, and this is the substance of the next chapter.

3

'The Healthiest on the Face of the Globe'

Non-Māori from 1860 to 1940

> *. . . the climate is most temperate and exceedingly healthy. Fruits and flowers of every description are to be found there in abundance and since house rent . . . is most reasonable . . . all the advantages of a natural sanatorium at the most reasonable rate imaginable.*[158]

In this period non-Māori life expectancy was the highest in the world, principally due to very low mortality in infancy and childhood. European settlers in New Zealand were indeed 'the healthiest on the face of the globe', but why?

Four reasons stand out. First, immigration was the dominant demographic force in this period, and new settlers were drawn commonly from rural and relatively healthy regions of Britain. Selection processes, mostly informal, tended to accentuate the better-than-average health status of those who travelled from Europe. Second, the new settlers benefited from aspects of the New Zealand environment. A plentiful and protein-rich diet, lack of crowding and scarcity of health-damaging industry stand out as likely contributors to (relatively) low mortality. Third, in the late 1800s fertility reduced earlier among New Zealand women than elsewhere, leading both to improvements in maternal health and lower child mortality (as more time and resources were available to each child). Fourth, colonisation transferred health-generating resources such as land from Māori to non-Māori: put simplistically, one group's gain was at another's expense.

Other factors played a part in pushing New Zealand non-Māori to the top of the world rankings, but we believe they were less important. Public health measures such as sanitation and protected water supplies were introduced, on average, no earlier in New Zealand than elsewhere. Child-health programmes, including the Plunket movement, and strong public health legislation were twentieth-century innovations and therefore cannot explain low mortality in the preceding century, but they may have helped New Zealand retain world-leading life expectancies up to World War II. Medical services probably made little difference to longevity until the 1940s, as coverage of the population was patchy, and anyway treatment for the diseases that were most common and most serious was seldom effective. There is no consistent short-run association between economic indicators and mortality decline. At times during this period, New Zealand had the highest GDP per head of population in the world, but the country also experienced severe economic depressions during the 1880s–90s and 1920s–30s. Perturbations in trade, employment and national wealth made no perceptible difference to the continuous improvement in life expectancy.

This was a time of radical transition in New Zealand. The population pendulum swung abruptly in favour of non-Māori, and land and other natural resources passed from indigenous ownership to the new regime. Farmers cashed in a stock of ecological credits, applying disruptive agricultural methods to virgin soils to obtain (short-lived) high yields. Then came the value-add of refrigeration, and the agricultural dividend is now the basis of a global food industry. Finally, it is notable that this period of New Zealand settlement featured a strong egalitarian ethic and a relatively equal distribution of resources (among the non-Māori population), and we argue this led to larger health gains from public investments than would have been the case otherwise.

In 2002 the journal *Science* published a paper entitled 'Broken Limits to Life Expectancy'.[159] The authors had searched death registers around the world to identify the highest recorded life expectancies for men and women, for each year from 1840 to 2000. What they found was an impressive advance, from about 45 years life expectancy at birth in 1840 to a maximum at the beginning of this century of about 85 years. Even more startling is the extraordinary linearity of the graph. The rise in record human longevity proceeded in a regular fashion for 160 years: there had been no sign of a slowing in the year-to-year improvement. The slope of the line had been flatter for men than women, although this changed recently in many countries, and as a result the gap between the sexes was reduced. Another paper, published in 2009 and adding a further seven years of data to the graph, showed that the trends continued unabated.[160]

On the graph were marked the countries that had reported the world-leading life expectancies in each period. Sweden and Japan are two countries that have commonly reported the (on average) longest-lived men and women, and recently Iceland has assumed the highest rank for men. But New Zealand had its turn as the leader of the pack. Between 1870 and 1940 New Zealand non-Māori men and women enjoyed the lowest mortality in the world.

Science was not the first to break the story. In 1882, Alfred Newman, physician and gentleman scholar, read a paper to the Wellington Philosophical Society in which he claimed this country was 'yet the healthiest on the face of the globe'.[161] Newman pointed out that the crude mortality rate was half that in England, and this was only partly explained by the younger population in New Zealand. He cites an actuary, Mr James Meikle, who had constructed a life table based on the first national census in 1874, and who observed 'an exceedingly light rate of mortality' equivalent to a discount of 8 to 10 per cent on the standard (English) life insurance premiums. Newman wasn't the only one toasting the good health of the colonisers. A local newspaper from the same period claimed conditions in New Zealand were so good that new settlers died only of drowning or drunkenness.

This chapter will investigate the nature and possible causes of low mortality among non-Māori. For the first time (in this book) there is scope for the heavy machinery of demography and epidemiology to get to work. Registration of non-Māori births and deaths began in 1848, but was not compulsory until 1858. Coverage was patchy at first, but the quality of the death records was much improved after 1876, when extra information was required at registration.

LIFE EXPECTANCY AND MORTALITY TRENDS 1860–1940

Figure 6 displays estimates of life expectancy for non-Māori men and women from 1860 to 1940, together with estimates for Māori (which are discussed in the next chapter). To give some perspective, we have included estimates for life expectancy leading up to 1860, and on the far right hand side of the graph, the 2011 life expectancies for non-Māori and Māori. Also shown are estimates for the 'best country in the world' from Oeppen and Vaupel[159] prior to non-Māori taking ascendancy in 1876. Australia held the top-ranking spot before 1876 for a few years, Ireland featured briefly, but the early low mortality countries were mainly Norway, Denmark and Sweden. We have also plotted selected estimates for England and Wales, and these reveal a ten-year gap in life expectancy from birth between the 'home country' and non-Māori in the 1860s to 1880s.

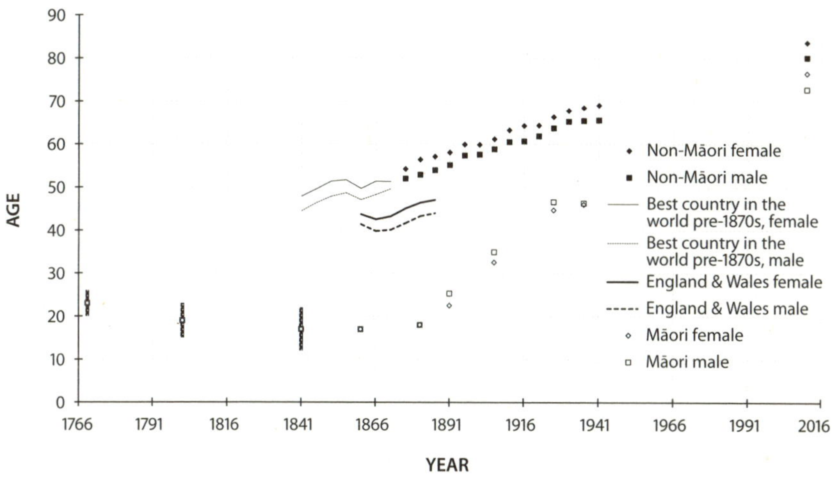

Figure 6: Life expectancy at birth of Māori and non-Māori, 'best country in the world' and England and Wales – 1769 to 1940

Source: See sources for Figure 4. Additionally, 'England and Wales' data for the period 1861–86 are from the Human Mortality Database (www.mortality.org). The England and Wales estimate for 1769 (the time of Cook's departure) is 36 (see Figure 4).[106; 107] Values for Māori from 1769 to 1866 are estimates by the authors, attempting to account for the effects of epidemic infectious disease, warfare, colonisation and displacement of populations. Māori estimates from 1891 onwards are from D. I. Pool, 'Changing Patterns of Sex Differentials in Survival: An Examination of Data for Maoris and Non-Maoris in New Zealand' in *Sex Differentials in Mortality: Trends, Determinants and Consequences*, edited by A. D. Lopez and L. T. Ruzicka (Canberra: Department of Demography, Australian National University, Miscellaneous Series No. 4, 1983: 193–219). Non-Māori estimates are from J. Cheung, *Mortality, Morbidity and Population Health Dynamics* (Hamilton: University of Waikato PhD thesis, 1999).

Non-Māori life expectancy increased by 15 years from 1876 to 1940 – nearly 2.5 years with every decade, or a year's extra life expectancy for every four calendar years. In 1881 non-Māori life expectancy was 53 years for males and 56 years for females, 35 years greater than our estimate for Māori (life expectancy at birth about 18 years). By 1946 the gap between Māori and non-Māori had closed to about 20 years.

Non-Māori enjoyed a clear advantage in life expectancy over all European countries throughout the period, although the Scandinavian countries and the Netherlands steadily closed the gap (see Figure 7). England and Wales closed from about ten years in arrears in the 1870s to about five years behind the New Zealand figure in the 1930s, and Australian life expectancy also converged on New Zealand non-Māori.

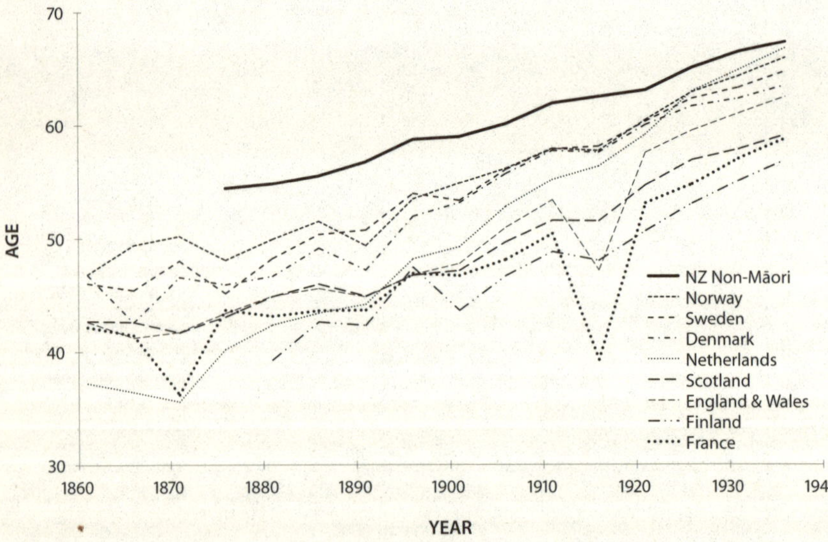

Figure 7: Life expectancy trends, sexes combined, for New Zealand non-Māori and selected European countries from 1860 to 1940

Source: Human Mortality Database. The notable dip in the 1916 estimates for England and Wales is due to inclusion of deaths from WWI; the same applies to France.

The graphs we have shown suggest a story of gradual and continuous improvement, without violent lurches and catastrophes. There are two notable exceptions: the influenza pandemic of 1918, and the First World War. The former claimed about 7000 lives in New Zealand, and the latter 17,000 lives. Deaths overseas, in this case at war, are often excluded from national statistics. Including them, however, has a significant impact on the birth cohort of men eligible to serve – in this case, the men born between 1887 and 1897 who made up more than half those who served overseas in the First World War. This cohort would have lived two-to-five years longer, on average, without the war deaths. (The Second World War claimed 12,000 lives and resulted in two-to-three years' loss of cohort life expectancy for those born in 1915–21.)[168]

Mortality rates

Mortality rates by sex and age for non-Māori from 1876 are presented in Figure 8,[162] using a logarithmic scale to ease comparisons across age. For both males and females, there were greater than two-thirds reductions in mortality from 1876 to 1936 for 0–4, 5–14, 15–24 and 25–44-year-olds. However, mortality reduced by only a third among 45–64-year-olds, and by about 10 per cent for 65+-year-olds. Infant mortality (i.e., deaths in the first year) reduced by a similar proportion as the change in combined 0–4-year-old mortality.[2] In other words, there were large improvements in infant, child and early adult mortality among non-Māori during this period, with more modest improvements in mid-life and older age groups. It was the changes in infant and child mortality that were responsible for most of the improvement in life expectancy during this time – what happened in middle-age and older-age groups made a minor contribution.

The long-run trends in infant survival (the reciprocal of infant mortality) are shown in Figure 9. Note that infant mortality was declining in New Zealand from the time that statistics were first collected, in the early 1870s, although the most rapid decline occurred later. (This is not the pattern seen in Australia and Britain, where there is no downturn evident until around 1900.) The percentage of New Zealand newborns surviving their first year of life improved from about 86 per cent to 95 per cent in the period considered in this chapter (and continued to improve subsequently – in the early 2000s infant survival reached 99.5 per cent). The greatest gains were made in the decades up to World War I, but the trend line is irregular with frequent dips in infant survival. Whether this irregular progress year by year is simply statistical imprecision, or results from true variation in the underlying rates is unclear – there were epidemics of pertussis in 1877, influenza in the early 1890s and measles in 1893.

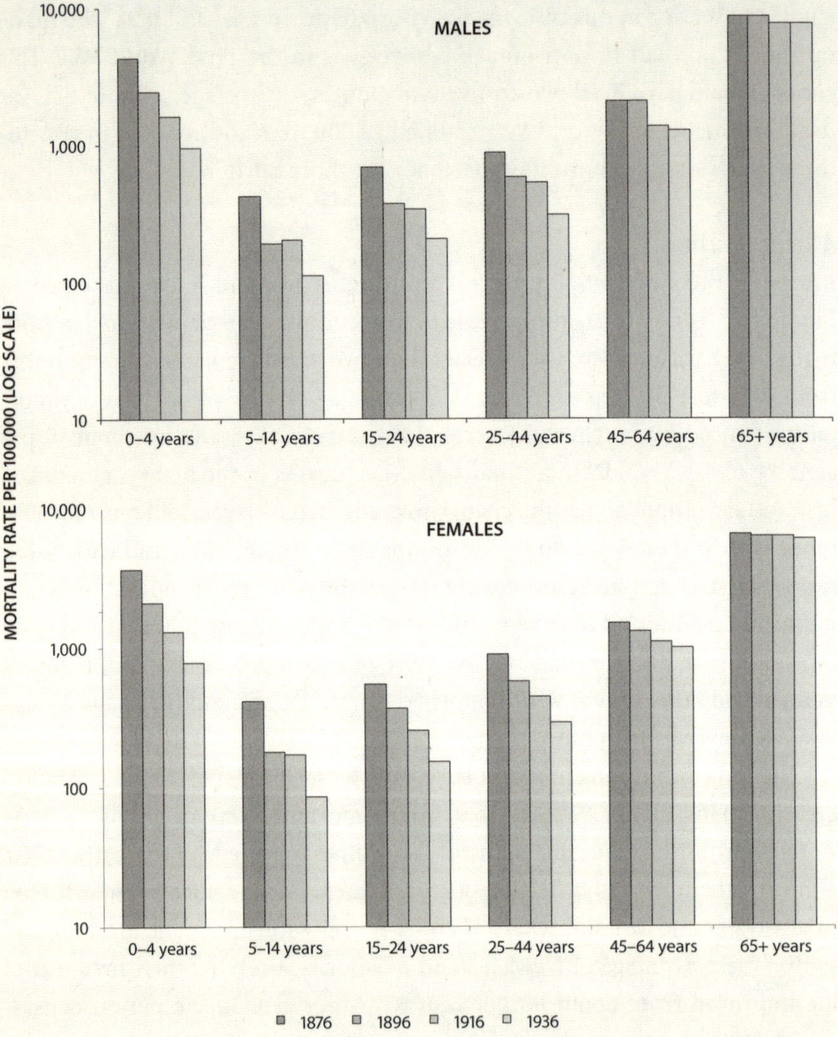

Figure 8: Mortality rates per 100,000 (log scale) by sex by age group for non-Māori, from 1876 to 1936

Source: I. Pool, 'Mortality Trends and Differentials', *Country Monograph Series No. 12: Population of New Zealand*, edited by Population Division Economic and Social Commission for Asia and the Pacific (New York: United Nations, 1985: 209–42).

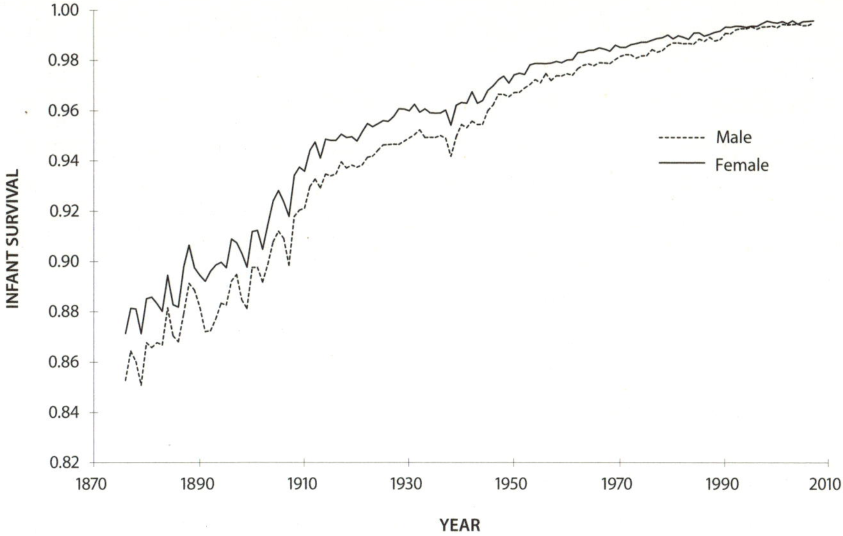

Figure 9: Infant survival, 1876–2007

Source: Statistics New Zealand, 'A History of Survival in New Zealand: Cohort Life Tables 1876–2004' (Wellington: Statistics New Zealand, 2006) (and updated data at www.stats.govt.nz). Included are Māori (who made up about 10 per cent of births between 1880 and 1930, and suffered a higher proportion of infant deaths) and non-Māori.

As we will see in later chapters, it is now difficult to extend life expectancy by forcing infant and child mortality even lower – there is not much room for improvement, and consequently what happens at older ages has greater significance. But between 1860 and 1940 most of the action took place at the start of life.

Indeed, non-Māori were at the top of the international life expectancy rankings from 1860 to 1940 solely because of their lower infant, child and young-adult mortality. Ian Pool has analysed differences between another low-mortality country of this period, Norway, and New Zealand using expected years of life remaining by age as a metric.[163; 162] Thus, life expectation at say, 40 years of age is the expected number of years of life to live if you reach the age of 40; note that mortality or death rates for ages up to 40 have no direct mathematical bearing on this statistic. Life expectation in Norway at 40 and 60 years of age exceeded that for non-Māori from 1876, due to lower mortality rates at older age in Norway. Life expectation at five and 20 years of age favoured non-Māori due to the much lower infant, child and young-adult mortality rates in New Zealand.

Considering a wider range of countries, Figure 10 (overleaf) displays mortality rates from the Human Mortality Database[164] for the 1860s to the present. Selected countries, and non-Māori and Māori, are presented for selected age groups. The logarithm of mortality rates is plotted on the y-axis, with males on the left and females on the right. Not shown in the figure, but worth noting, is that the especially low infant mortality in New Zealand was due principally to heightened survival from four weeks after birth to one year. In the first four weeks of life New Zealand mortality rates in the early 1900s were lower than those in England and Wales, but by a narrower margin.[165] This is important because it provides a clue to what was special about conditions in New Zealand. Deaths in the first month are likely to be related to events in pregnancy and around the time of birth, while 'post-neonatal' mortality (deaths after one month) is influenced mostly by external factors, such as nutrition and infection.

All countries shown in Figure 10 saw faster reductions in mortality rates among younger age groups than amongst adults. However, for non-Māori up to 1940 the rates for ages up to 40 years remained the lowest in the world. This is consistent with Pool's comparisons with Norway, but now extended to many other countries. Middle-age and older mortality rates did not decrease as much as child mortality rates – across all countries – and what is more, non-Māori rates in these older groups were low by international standards, but generally not the lowest in the world.

Causes of death

Information on causes of death is very sketchy in the early years. In the statistical returns for 1857, there are 434 deaths recorded, with a warning that registrations are known to be incomplete. Thirty per cent of deaths occurred before the age of two years.[166] Apart from a note that 60 (14 per cent) of the fatalities were due to drowning and other accidents, there is no information on specific causes of death. (In 2009 there were 29,204 deaths in New Zealand, of which 730 [2.5 per cent] were caused by drowning or other accidents.)

From 1876 onwards there is additional information on causes of death, but it is prudent to treat these as broad categories. Pool reported estimates of non-Māori cause-specific mortality from 1876 to 1976 by age group.[162] We show these in Figure 11, below. Again, we use a log scale for the mortality rate axis, in order better to see the relative rates of change for each cause of death.

Amongst those aged less than 45 years, there was more than a 90 per cent reduction in the rate of death from 1876 to 1936 in two categories: 'diarrhoea and related' and 'infectious' diseases. 'Tuberculosis' and 'respiratory' deaths both fell by about 70 per cent, and 'accidents and violence' and 'degenerative' by 61 per cent and 63 per cent, respectively. In relative terms, the reductions looked much the same when broken down by age groups and for men and women separately. Not reflected in Figure 11 is the influenza pandemic of 1918. This affected males more than females, Māori more than non-Māori, and children and young adults more than older people.

The decline in mortality from 1876 to 1936 among 45+-year-olds was less marked overall. One category, 'degenerative' mortality (i.e., cardiovascular, cancer and 'senility') increased by 61 per cent. 'Tuberculosis' reduced by about two-thirds, 'respiratory' by just over half, and 'diarrhoea and related' by 95 per cent.

EXPLANATIONS

The first question is whether low rates of mortality in New Zealand were real, or the result of errors in the records. There is no way of directly checking the quality of the data, but it is possible to look for consistency and plausibility. The New Zealand regulations governing the registration of births and deaths followed very closely the British model. Even the forms that were used to record information were almost identical to those used in Britain, and classification of the causes of death followed the same rules.[165] We think it is implausible that the non-Māori population was regularly over-estimated, hence diluting artificially and persistently the estimates of death rates. The counts from the national census, which began on the imperial model in 1881, are more likely to under-estimate the number resident in the country.

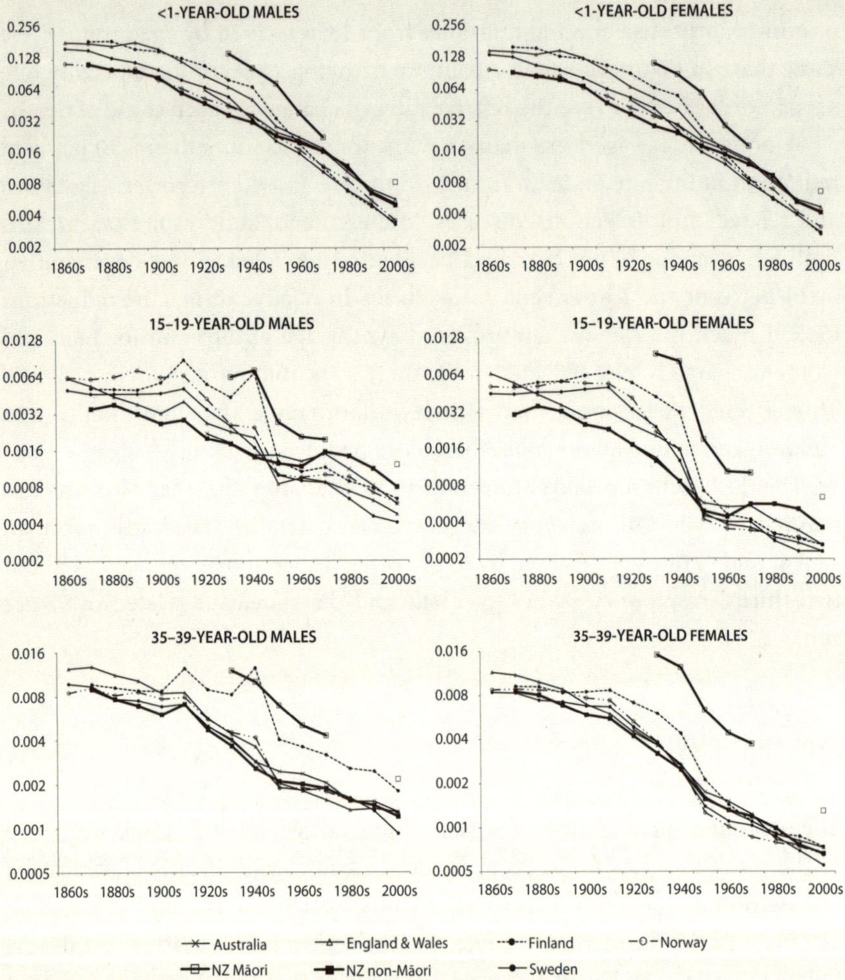

Figure 10: Selected age-specific mortality rate (log scale; y-axes) trends across multiple countries, 1860s to 2000s

Source: Human Mortality Database. Māori estimates for the 1980s and 1990s were deleted due to known under-counting of Māori deaths; such errors may exist in the 1950s to 1970s as well. Estimates for non-Māori mortality for 80–84-year-olds in the 1870s and 1880s were implausibly low, and based on sparse data; they were suppressed.

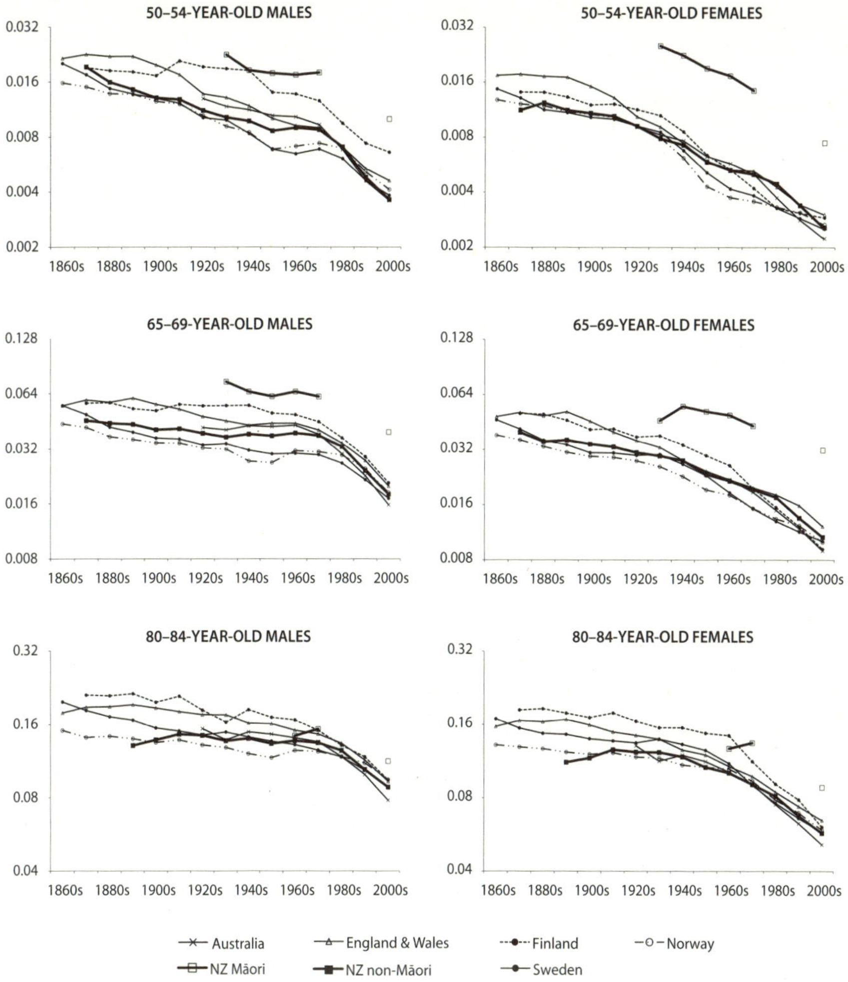
50–54-YEAR-OLD MALES
50–54-YEAR-OLD FEMALES
65–69-YEAR-OLD MALES
65–69-YEAR-OLD FEMALES
80–84-YEAR-OLD MALES
80–84-YEAR-OLD FEMALES
0.032
0.016
0.008
0.004
0.002
0.128
0.064
0.032
0.016
0.008
0.32
0.16
0.08
0.04
1860s 1880s 1900s 1920s 1940s 1960s 1980s 2000s
Australia
England & Wales
Finland
Norway
NZ Māori
NZ non-Māori
Sweden

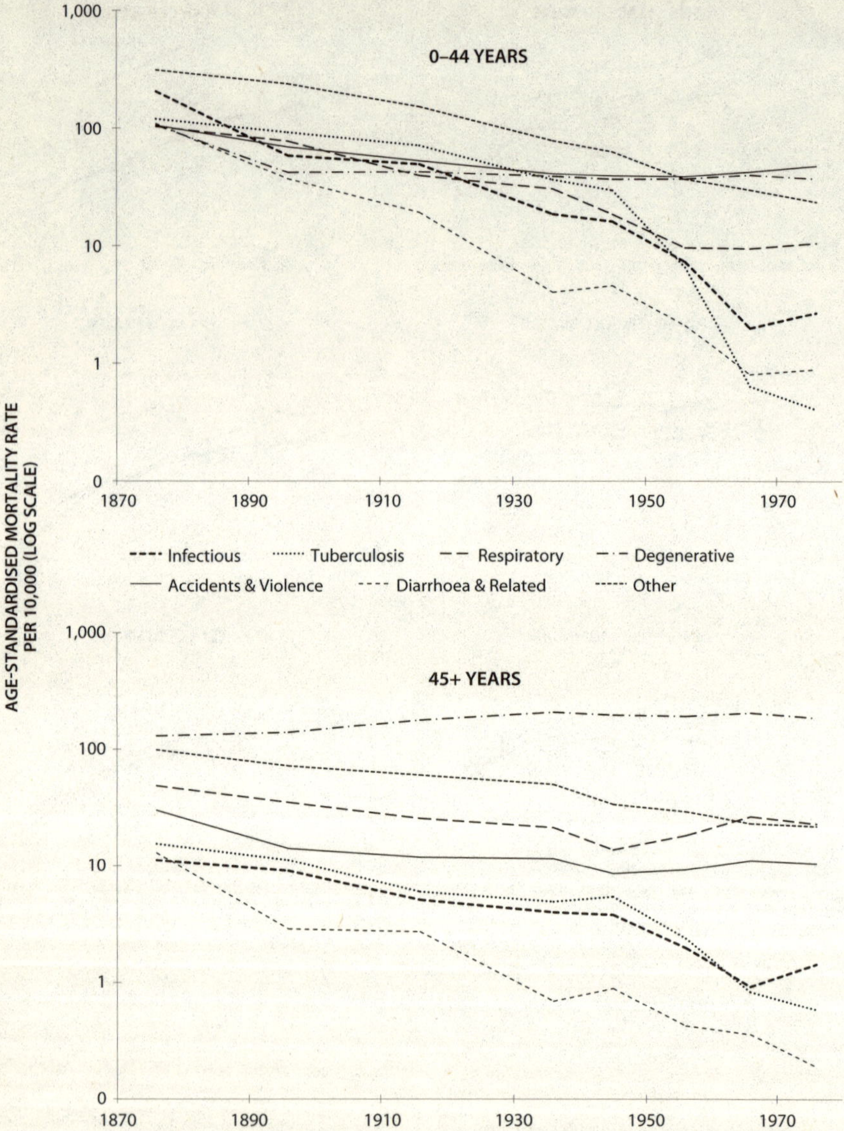

Figure 11: Non-Māori mortality rates by cause of death, for 0–44 years and 45 years and over, sexes combined, from 1876 to 1976

Source: I. Pool, 'Mortality Trends and Differentials', *Country Monograph Series No. 12: Population of New Zealand*, edited by Population Division Economic and Social Commission for Asia and the Pacific (New York: United Nations, 1985: 209–42).Three years of data used for each point. Infectious excludes tuberculosis, but includes influenza; degenerative disease includes cardiovascular, neoplasms and 'senility'. Age-standardised to WHO world population.

Deaths are most commonly missed in younger age groups, and especially in newborns. Ian Pool looked closely at the balance of reported deaths across age groups, compared with the pattern seen in this period in countries such as Sweden with well-developed statistical systems. He concluded that there probably was under-counting of infant deaths in the very earliest returns, but not to a great extent in the 1880s and 1890s.[169] Another demographer, James Gibson, also tested the internal consistency of early mortality estimates and came to a similar conclusion. He observed that recording systems improved considerably in the 1860s, and judged that the statistics for non-Māori were virtually complete by the end of the 1870s.[170]

If we accept the statistics, in broad terms if not necessarily in fine detail, then why were non-Māori New Zealanders early leaders in the mortality stakes? Here are some of the factors that have been proposed: selection of healthy migrant 'stock'; a late and relatively benign introduction to the industrial age; access to a cheap, varied and nutritious diet; low levels of crowding (in cities and within households); early introduction of an effective public health system; relatively high disposable incomes; small family sizes; and reforms in education and welfare that promoted the welfare of women and children and preceded similar interventions elsewhere.

There are two features of the nineteenth-century European population in New Zealand that are particularly relevant: the fact that the population was made up overwhelmingly of immigrants; and the rapid fluctuations that occurred late in the 1800s in marriage patterns, fertility and family size. We approach first the matter of migration.

MIGRATION

Migration accounted for more than half the annual increase in the New Zealand population until the 1880s. (In the US, by comparison, the excess of [local] births over deaths was the major demographic driver from the late seventeenth century onwards.) Because migration was so dominant, the New Zealand non-Māori population was skewed towards younger adult-age groups. Also, males outnumbered females up till the 1880s to a greater degree than occurred in Canada, the US or Australia.

Perhaps this gender imbalance influenced trends in mortality: did women have more choice, given their relative scarcity, and therefore more influence in the family, and as a consequence, provide a healthier environment for young children? James Belich thinks 'it would have been strange if women had not taken advantage of the colonial circumstances to be more selective than was possible in Britain.'[78] And Belich points out one result of the 'colonial circumstances' that favoured the health of children. Going by the census returns, the proportion of adults who were illiterate was probably much the same in New Zealand and Britain. But the female advantage in the marriage market apparently selected for literacy in the home. In 1881, 3 per cent of grooms in New Zealand signed the marriage register with a mark, rather than their written name; the county rate of 'innominacy' in England at this time varied from 8 per cent to 30 per cent.[78]

A notable feature of migration to New Zealand is the churn factor. Many new settlers stayed for only a brief period: the number of out-bound passengers each year was close to the number of arrivals for much of the nineteenth century. Transients were more likely to be migrants from Australia than from the UK, which is hardly surprising since it was relatively easy to make the return journey across the Tasman Sea to Australia. In 1857, 43 per cent of those landing in Wellington came from British colonies other than the UK itself (principally Australia); but amongst the emigrants, 95 per cent were travelling in that direction.[166] Throughout the history of New Zealand, there has been a busy traffic to and fro across the Tasman, and particularly in the 1880s and 1890s when the level of unemployment in New Zealand was high.

Over time the balance of push and pull factors, the enablers and deterrents that influence migration, won't always be the same, and this means the effects of migration on health are difficult to predict. In recent times, refugees to New Zealand, migrants from poorer communities and migrants from geographically proximate countries without stringent barriers (e.g., Pacific islands) carry mortality risks that are *higher* than those that apply in New Zealand. Such exceptions to the healthy migrant effect are now well documented.[171; 172; 173; 174; 175]

Some of the early migrants to New Zealand came because they were unwell (and in the belief that conditions in the south would benefit them). This was true famously for tuberculosis, and has been described as 'therapeutic migration.'[176] In the late 1800s many believed the climate of New Zealand (and other colonies in the south) assisted recovery from tuberculosis. Although Robert Koch identified the tubercle bacillus in 1882, pre-microbial ways of thinking persisted. Both the miasmatists (who believed ill-health was due to emanations and vapours arising from organic material) and those who held to the older, humoral perspectives (concerned with upsets in physiological and psychological balances) thought climatic influences were very important for good health. Warmth, fresh winds and regularity in the weather were commonly believed to be health enhancing.

The family of Sir Douglas Robb, Auckland surgeon and Chancellor of the University of Auckland, migrated from Port Glasgow, Scotland, in the 1890s. Robb wrote:

> Tuberculosis, which had accounted for a considerable number of uncles and aunts in their infancy and early years, overtook my father in his thirties and this led to his emigration to Australia [and then to New Zealand] . . .
>
> Such a family story of tuberculosis is a characteristic one, which could be identified many times over in the emigrants from the British Isles to Australia, South Africa and New Zealand . . . the great benefits afforded by the favourable climate and living conditions in Australasia have amply rewarded those who were either enterprising enough or fortunate enough to make their way abroad.[177]

Robb says the story of his family is 'characteristic', but there are no figures on the numbers of people who migrated in search of a cure. (However, we do know that those moving abroad on account of their disease included many doctors, and proposals in the early 1900s to restrict the entry to New Zealand of individuals with infectious diseases, including TB, were strongly opposed by the local arm of the British Medical Association.)

Selections of this kind worked against good health in the receiving colonies, and may be one reason why the New Zealand advantage in TB mortality was much thinner in middle age than in childhood or in older age groups. (In 1922 male deaths from TB were two-to-three times more common in England and Wales than in New Zealand up to age 24 and over the age of 45; between 25 and 44 years the excess was only 40 to 80 per cent.)[165] But remember that record non-Māori longevity resulted from particularly low mortality among infants and children. There are no figures on infection rates by age, but we reason that therapeutic migration was most likely to be initiated by adults with tuberculosis.

In theory, there were health checks that would have the opposite effect to 'therapeutic migration'. Migrants who came out with the New Zealand Company, or as part of later schemes of assisted passage, had to pass formal health checks before departure. These were supposed to identify and exclude people with chronic illnesses, including tuberculosis. A. K. Newman asserted, 'we must put on record the fact that thousands of people were imported at public expense, and from these many thousands all phthisics [TB of the lungs] were excluded'.[161] He was exaggerating. In practice, the health checks were often perfunctory and the screening process was demonstrably ineffective. Linda Bryder points out that amongst the 3500 individuals who died from tuberculosis in Auckland between 1880 and 1914, more than 500 had lived in the colony less than five years, and 167 died within a year of arrival.[176]

Apart from the formal health checks, there were other reasons why individuals and families inclined to migrate were, in general, likely to be more vigorous and in better health than those who stayed at home. Newspaper advertisements and posters in the UK in the 1870s called for married agricultural labourers and single female domestic servants, provided they were 'sober, industrious, of good moral character, of sound mind and in good health'.[178] Once accepted for emigration, individuals faced an arduous journey that must have been especially difficult for those who were frail. Belich claims that one in six children on some early voyages died before reaching their destination.[179]

Migrants may appear to have lower mortality rates when this is really not the case, due to the 'salmon bias'. This term refers to immigrants who return to their home country when they approach the end of their lives. When they die, the deaths are not recorded in the country in which the migrants had recently lived. This certainly happens with some groups (e.g., Hispanic Americans with family roots in Mexico), but even then is not sufficient to explain the relatively low mortality of first-generation migrants to the United States.[180] During the late nineteenth and early twentieth centuries there may have been some traffic of this kind across the Tasman, but it is unlikely that large numbers of sick colonists returned to England, simply because of the distance and cost.

When Ethel Florence Richardson, later famous under the literary eponym of Henry Handel Richardson, bought a first-class steamer ticket from

Melbourne to London in 1888, it cost her £165. For most Victorian tradesmen at the time, this was more than two years' pay.[181] Travel between New Zealand or Australia and England (and not just in the first class) was so expensive that cost discouraged many from ever returning to Europe. In the 1870s the number of people migrating from America to England was about 60 per cent of the traffic in the other direction. The proportion for Australasia was only 8 per cent.[182; 186]

> The spirit of the colonists was proved by their precipitating themselves into an untried state of existence, known to be beset with difficulties. They were almost all energetic men; the timid, the lazy and the sickly having remained in the old country.[14]

Much of what was written about and by the nineteenth-century settlers, including the passage above, has a self-congratulatory ring to it. This is scarcely surprising. People who had invested a great deal in a long and uncomfortable voyage, and had committed their future to a new and highly uncertain enterprise, naturally wanted to put the best possible spin on the story. Those who were drumming up business back in England had a more direct interest in 'boosting' the New Zealand settlements. Nevertheless, there probably is truth in Thomson's claim that migration was associated (not just amongst men, but including women too) with energy, optimism and a willingness to strive for a better life (as well as, on occasion, desperation, impetuousness and other varieties of folly).[183]

No doubt there were many factors that combined to promote 'healthy' migration.[184; 175] In important respects, migrants to New Zealand were not a random sample of the entire British population. For instance, they tended to come from the healthier-than-average parts of the country, as we shall see below.

THE NUMBERS AND CHARACTERISTICS OF MIGRANTS TO NEW ZEALAND

Nineteenth-century migration to New Zealand was a small part of a much larger international phenomenon, described by James Belich as the 'settler revolution'. Belich tackles the question of why the British Empire left deeper cultural, linguistic and demographic footprints than any of its predecessors.[179] At its root, according to his analysis, the British exodus was marked by a radical change in thinking about emigration. Previously, those who filled the ships leaving northern harbours held return tickets, metaphorically. Convicts and exiles were exceptions, obviously, but otherwise emigrants went to subdue, harvest and repatriate. Then, in the early 1800s, the focus in England shifted to long-term occupation and empire-building. The 'settler revolution' was energised by new technologies (in farming, transport, and manufacture) that enabled colonial populations not only to sustain themselves, but to thrive, as Belich says.

> Emigration ceased to be an act of desperation and became an act of hope. It sloughed off centuries of stigma, and transformed itself into settlement, the long-range reproduction of metropolitan society rather than permanent exile from it.[179]

To understand what migration meant for health status, we need to know where people came from, whether it was just adult or family migration, and who actually stayed. To these ends Figure 12 presents total numbers of immigrants arriving by year by sex for adults, and the number of children under 12 years of age (where such data exist). Figure 13 then shows what country people arrived from, and Figure 14 shows the net migration by country of source or destination.

Two points are evident from these graphs. First, immigration went through booms and busts. The early 1860s (gold rushes) and mid-1870s (Premier Vogel's nation-building migration programme) were periods of explosive population growth. The recruiting activities of the New Zealand Company and other early colonising initiatives were important in the foundation of the country, but the numbers of people involved were small in comparison with what happened after 1860. Second, the Vogel period was marked by large numbers of children amongst the new arrivals, while cross-Tasman male migrants dominated the gold-rush years.

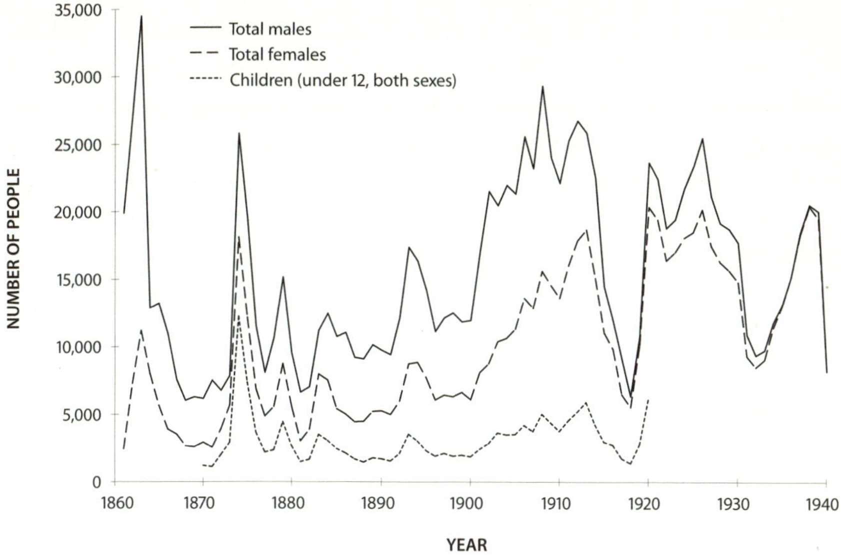

Figure 12: Immigration to New Zealand from 1860 to 1940, by sex and age

Source: Statistics New Zealand volumes. Data on children not available after 1920 or before 1870.

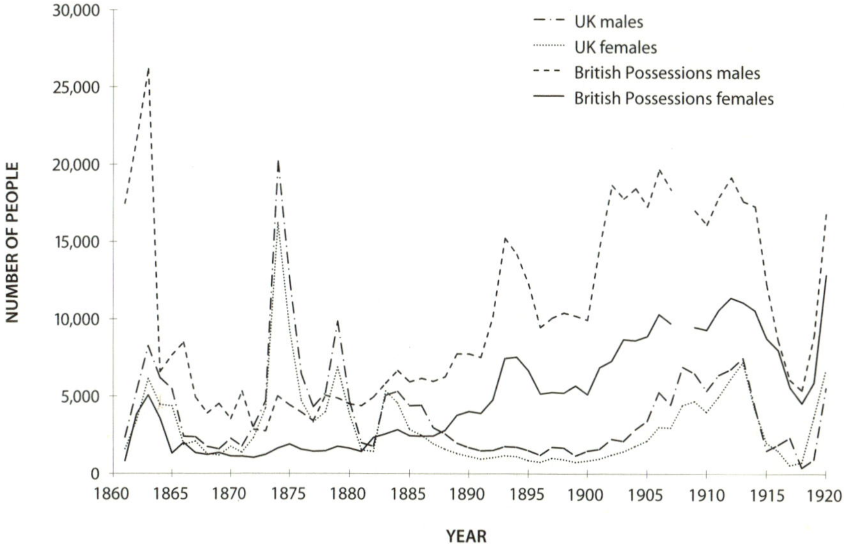

Figure 13: Immigration to New Zealand from 1860 to 1920, by source country

Source: Statistics New Zealand volumes. Data post-1920 are incomplete by country of origin, and incorrect by sex in 1908 within British Possessions, and hence are not included.

There was another surge in arrivals between 1900 and 1915, with a net population gain just over 120,000 (Figure 14). Immigration from the United Kingdom in particular boomed before the First World War, including (net) migration in 1913. The high cost of a passage to New Zealand had held people back, but numbers rose with the resumption in 1904 of government assistance.

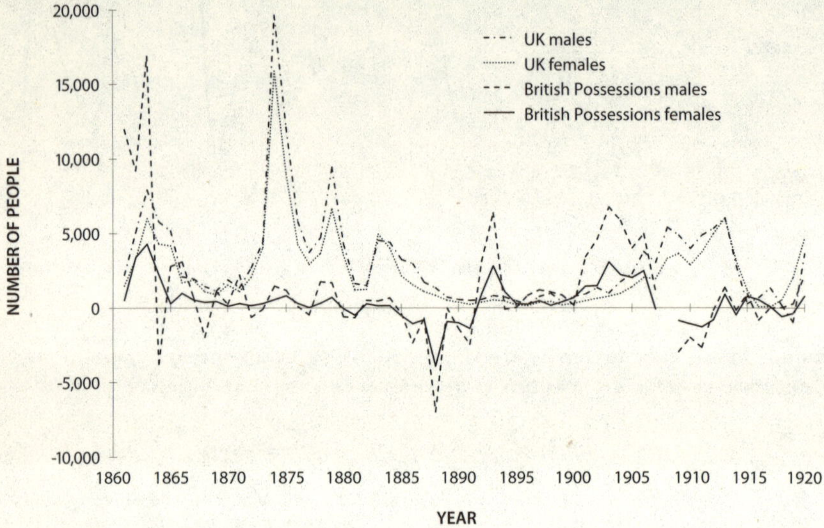

Figure 14: Net migration (immigration minus emigration) from 1860 to 1920, by source/destination country of immigration/emigration
Source: Statistics New Zealand volumes.

The overwhelming majority of long-stay migrants came from Britain. The next largest group of European migrants was from Germany – a mix of rural labourers and middle-class adventurers.[185] Other European groups were Italians (particularly following the gold rushes); Dalmatians (most prominent in the north, especially in the kauri gumfields); and Danes, Norwegians and Swedes (especially in the 1870s). Chinese immigration increased rapidly during the gold rushes. Most came as short-stay workers. The Chinese were treated very badly, and official and public xenophobia ensured that for more than a hundred years few immigrants from Asia modified the 'Britishness' of the new colony.

The backgrounds of assisted migrants differed from those (roughly twice as numerous) who were self-funded, and there were distinctive features of migration to some parts of New Zealand (the Scots being particularly numerous in the settlement of Otago, for instance). But in general, industrial workers were under-represented, some regions in Britain were favoured as sources (London, Devon and Cornwall, and the south-east, in particular), Presbyterians and those of other non-conformist faiths appeared more commonly in the migrant lists than would be expected, and Roman Catholics less so. Scots made up about 10 per cent of the UK population through the nineteenth century, but contributed almost a quarter of the migrants from the UK to New Zealand.[149] (This bias is reflected in the distribution of New Zealand government immigration agents – in 1873, there were 53 in the whole of England, compared with 78 in Scotland.)[186]

There was also a strong rural bias, particularly among the assisted migrants. Labourers, domestic servants and farm workers were especially sought after in assisted programmes. Until the 1890s, two groups, farmers and other agricultural workers and 'pre-industrial tradespeople', made up about two-thirds of the English immigrants.[149] This was partly as a result of deliberate targeting by recruiting agencies. However, the agents were pushing on an open door: economic conditions in England in the second half of the century were not kind to rural working people, and New Zealand interests were well represented by the (English) National Agricultural Labourers Union.[187] Once the first links in the migration chain were in place, family, clan and village connections played a large part in persuading would-be migrants to choose New Zealand rather than the other colonies.[182]

In the early 1850s, life expectancy in predominantly agricultural districts in England was about five years greater than the national average, and this advantage stretched to almost eight years by the end of the century.[188] Throughout the 1800s, mortality in Britain was higher in cities, and tended to be higher also in the industrial midlands and the north-west than in the south.[188]

Environmental factors such as crowding and pollution were the most powerful influences on mortality in England in the latter part of the nineteenth century. Social and economic variations such as occupation and education were more important when conditions in the cities improved, but the advantages of rural life were apparent up to the time of the First World

War. In 1910 a comparison of male adult mortality rates, by occupation, found that professional classes had lower death rates than skilled and unskilled workers, as would be expected from modern-day social-class gradients, but the lowest death rates of all, for most causes, were reported for farmers and farm labourers (Table 2).

Table 2: Age-adjusted mortality rates per 100,000 for men 15 years of age and above in England and Wales by occupational class, 1910–12

OCCUPATIONAL GROUP	PHTHISIS (PULMONARY TUBERCULOSIS)	NON-PULMONARY TUBERCULOSIS	BRONCHITIS	PNEUMONIA	DIABETES	CANCER
Professional and salaried	145	14	52	71	25	126
Skilled labour	180	14	110	81	15	131
Unskilled labour	244	19	172	149	11	159
All wage earners	172	15	122	97	12	97
Farmers	61	10	55	60	20	101
Farm labourers	85	14	67	55	7	93

Source: Table 5 in S. J. Kunitz and S. L. Engerman, 'Ranks of Death: Secular Trends in Income and Mortality' (*Health Transition Review* 2 [1992]: 29–46).

What, in particular, attracted migrants to New Zealand? For some, it was the prospect of greater religious and political freedoms (evident, for example, in William Ranstead's vision of a 'socialist Canaan' in the south).[189] Others emphasised the moral and religious governance of settlement, the emphasis in the new colony on the provision of education and better physical health for those migrated.[147]

James Barr left 'quill-driving in Glasgow' for the 'vigorous plying of the grub-hoe and axe' in the Dunedin settlement. 'We were in the pursuit of health', he wrote in his memoirs 30 years later. Barr plainly revelled in the adventure and sociability of the new settlement:

> . . . we worked, we joked, we laughed, we sang . . . and . . . reveling in such health as I had never till then enjoyed, I devoured with a wonderful gusto and relish the game that we shot, and on which we bounteously feasted.[147]

In general, living conditions in Scotland were worse than those south of the border, and circumstances in the early nineteenth century were particularly adverse in the highlands and the northern islands. However, most of the Scots who shipped to New Zealand were from the lowlands, and frequently from areas close to Edinburgh and Glasgow. (There were some exceptions – the Shetlands, for example, provided a share of the Scottish diaspora in New Zealand out of proportion to its population.)

The Irish, who made up about 20 per cent of migrants to New Zealand in the latter part of the 1800s, were less likely to be of rural origin than migrants from Scotland and England, and more often they had a military or white-collar background. Notably, they did not come from the provinces hardest hit by famine, and migration from Ireland peaked decades after the Great Hunger (1845 to 1852).

In summary, migrants to New Zealand came from all corners of the UK and to some extent further afield in Europe (especially from around the turn of the century). Not all of these sources were the healthiest areas or classes of the source country, but many of the migrants came from areas with relatively low mortality (e.g., south-west and agricultural England, lowlands Scotland).

New Zealand and Australia

If the healthy migrant effect was the only explanation for low mortality in New Zealand, we would expect to see similar mortality rates in other British colonies that were established at about the same time. This is not the case. Life expectancy in New Zealand was consistently and substantially ahead.

In 1875 life expectancy in Australia, nationally, was 47 years for men and 50 years for women.[190] (Australian health statistics excluded the indigenous population until 1967.) These figures were five years adrift of life expectancies for non-Māori New Zealanders at the same time. The Australian experience mid-century was dominated by mortality in New South Wales, the largest colony, with a history of convict settlement dating back to 1788. Consequently a better comparison may be between New Zealand and South Australia, where there was a planned approach to migration strongly influenced by Edward Gibbon Wakefield, at very much the same time as the settlement of New Zealand.

Table 3 shows mortality rates, unadjusted for any differences in the age structures of the populations, for the Australian states and New Zealand in the fourth quarter of the nineteenth century. The New Zealand statistics are better than those for any of the states, including South Australia, and it is unlikely this can be explained by New Zealand having a younger population. Age-standardisation of the death rates in the 1890s, using the Swedish population as the reference point, found that the New Zealand advantage remained.[191]

Table 3: Death rates per thousand per year, all causes, men and women, Australian states and New Zealand, 1861–1895

	1861–65	1866–70	1871–75	1876–80	1881–85	1886–90	1891–95
New South Wales	16.8	16.1	14.8	15.7	15.1	13.8	12.8
Victoria	17.4	16.5	15.6	15.3	14.1	16.1	14.1
Queensland	20.5	18.3	17.5	17.1	18.9	15.1	12.5
South Australia	15.7	15.1	15.9	14.9	14.5	12.6	12.2
Western Australia	16.4	16.3	16.0	14.3	17.1	16.1	16.1
Tasmania	15.2	14.1	15.6	16.6	15.0	15.2	13.2
New Zealand	13.7	12.1	12.1	11.8	11.0	9.9	10.2

Source: T. A. Coghlan, *A Statistical Account of the Seven Colonies of Australasia, 1895–6* (Sydney: Government Printer, 1896). Note that Māori and indigenous Australians not included.

The health of the British army in New Zealand

> . . . there are no materials among the civil population for proving their healthfulness, except the sickness and mortality among the soldiers stationed in the colony.[14]

New Zealand's first health statistics were produced by the British army. Long before there was a national census, or routine registrations of deaths, the military prepared regular reports of deaths and illnesses amongst its soldiers, throughout the British Empire.

A. S. Thomson realised how important these records were as an indication of conditions in the colony more generally. The decade that Thomson was in New Zealand (1848–58) was relatively peaceful, and there were few deaths and injuries amongst the soldiers caused by military action. The illnesses that they suffered were by and large the same as those experienced by the civilian population.

Thomson appreciated also that the soldiers in New Zealand were, by and large, a representative sample of the British army. Soldiers were assigned to New Zealand, rather than India, or Africa, or imperial garrisons in other parts of the world, according to regimental affiliation. Health screening in this instance applied at the point of recruitment to the military rather than assignment to a particular garrison. Moreover, the soldiers in different corners of the Empire were a similar mix of ages and social backgrounds, following the same military routines, and living in standard barracks.

Thomson observed that the soldiers who were sent to New Zealand were much healthier than those who served elsewhere. British troops stationed in New Zealand had mortality rates that were not only one-sixth those in Bermuda and India, but they were roughly half the mortality rates experienced by soldiers in the home country (Figure 4).[16]

When these figures were broken down by cause of death, the biggest difference between New Zealand and the other stations was for diseases of the lungs and fevers (i.e., infectious diseases). The only fatal condition that was more common in New Zealand was diseases of the brain, and these deaths, according to Thomson, were commonly a result of drinking to excess.

Thomson argued that the low rates in New Zealand could not be explained by sick men being returned to England (or what we described above as 'salmon bias'). Discharges of this kind were most uncommon. Neither were the results caused by some peculiarity in the death registrations – Thomson commented that the numbers of hospitalisations in different parts of the Empire showed a similar picture. Admissions to the military hospital in New Zealand (about 500 per 1000 per year) were roughly half those in Britain.

One thing Thomson didn't acknowledge, but a modern epidemiologist would be quick to pick up, was that the rates were based on relatively small numbers. At any one time in the 1850s, there were fewer than a thousand British soldiers in New Zealand. But even then, the maximum value of the 95 per cent confidence interval (or roughly the range in which we expect the 'true' rate to be with 95 per cent confidence) for the New Zealand mortality rate shown in Figure 15 would not include the rates for other countries. It is most unlikely that the difference between New Zealand and the other countries was due to chance.

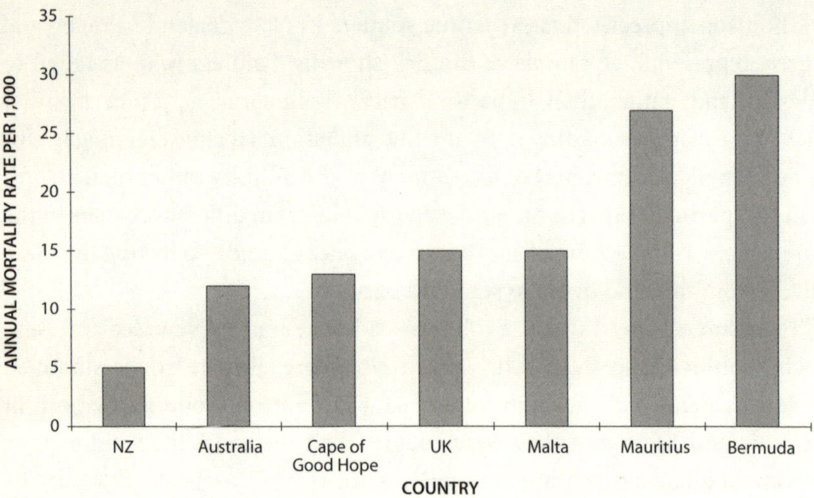

Figure 15: All-cause mortality, British infantry, around 1850

Source: A. S. Thomson, *The Story of New Zealand: Past and Present – Savage and Civilized*, vol. 2 (London: John Murray, 1859).

The New Zealand health advantage didn't apply just to young men. Thomson gathered statistics on military pensioners, former soldiers who had retired or been invalided out of the army. Two battalions of these men were sent to New Zealand in 1847, and over the following six years the annual death rate was 16 per 1000. In Britain, over a similar period, the mortality among enrolled military pensioners was 22 per thousand per year.

More information is available from the early 1860s, by which time the first actions of the Land Wars had begun, and the number of British soldiers in New Zealand had increased roughly ten-fold. Between 1859 and 1863, mortality from diseases was 7.4 per thousand in the New Zealand forces.[192] This was a period of intense campaigning, and the vicissitudes of war typically increased deaths from all causes, not just those caused by battle and accident. Yet mortality from disease in the New Zealand army was still lower than in Britain (where the military rate had improved to about 8.3 deaths per thousand soldiers per year). The local advantage was strongest for deaths from consumption, respiratory diseases and fevers (especially smallpox).[192]

Migration Summary

At the entry to the twentieth century, when the gap in health statistics between New Zealand and England was its widest, New Zealand death rates were half to two-thirds those of the equivalent age-specific English rates. Amongst the older age groups, those that contributed most of the immigrants (with the exception of the family-building Vogel years), the difference between New Zealand and England was relatively small. Infants and children, responsible for the very high life expectancy in New Zealand as we have seen, made up only a small proportion of migrants. (For example, fewer than 10 per cent of immigrants to Canterbury 1850–80 were under the age of ten years on arrival in New Zealand.)[193] This does not mean that migration was unimportant for infant and child health. There may have been inter-generational effects: if the parents of children born in New Zealand tended to be drawn from the healthiest of immigrant adults, then we would expect the offspring to benefit in many ways, including lower rates of disease and disability.[194]

In the United States in the late 1800s, infant mortality was lower than average if the mother was born abroad, and the advantage applied also in the families of second-generation migrants.[195] But interestingly, this was true only for families in rural areas. In the cities mortality was greater among the offspring of migrants than those of native-born women. If there was a transmitted healthy migrant effect, it was counter-balanced by the hazards of urban settlements.

Another test of migration as a cause of low mortality is to compare life expectancies of foreign- and local-born individuals. It is not possible to make such comparisons in the 1800s because the necessary information was not published. However, using the 1910–12, 1925–27 and 1935–37 censuses, Gibson calculated death rates for foreign and local-born residents of New Zealand and reported they were 'virtually identical'.[170] On this basis, one might conclude that local influences on health in New Zealand out-ranked the factors that acted on migration.

We conclude that the selection processes associated with migration contributed to the relative good health of non-Māori New Zealanders, but they cannot be the full explanation of low mortality. Other forces must have been at work.

FERTILITY AND THE SIZE AND STRUCTURE OF FAMILIES

In 1876, when national data were first available, the birth rate for non-Māori (46 births per 1000 population per year) was one of the highest in the industrialised world.[196] While there was a trend in many countries for fertility to decline in the last two decades of the nineteenth century, this happened particularly quickly in New Zealand, and by 1900 births to non-Māori women (27 per 1000 per year) were the lowest in Australasia.[197; 163] The total fertility rate more than halved in less than 40 years. On the basis of the 1876 fertility rates, each woman would bear 6.7 births, on average; this number fell to 3.9 in 1896, and 3.1 in 1916.[198]

Figure 16 looks at fertility trends using a 'fertility index' for Australian states and New Zealand compared to Hutterite fertility.[197] The rapid decrease for all, but especially New Zealand, is evident.

What explained this change? Changes in marriage patterns were important, given that illegitimate births were uncommon at this time. In the 1880s and 1890s fewer women entered wedlock, and the average age at marriage rose. In combination these two changes meant that one-third of women who reached child-bearing age did not have a baby.

Economic conditions may have been important. We know that when jobs are difficult to get, incomes are insecure and there is uncertainty about the future, then child-bearing tends to be delayed.[199] The long depression from the late 1870s to the early 1890s affected New Zealand especially severely, and may have encouraged couples to postpone marriage and starting a family.

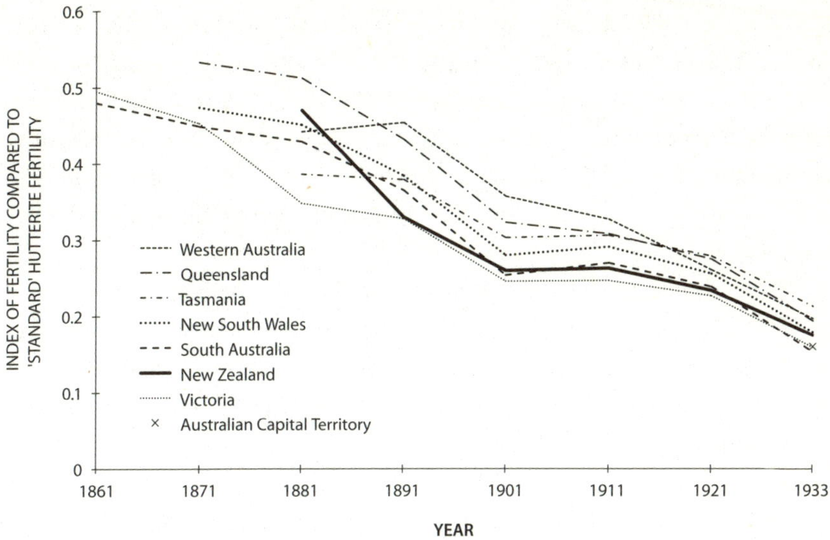

Figure 16: Fertility, Australia and New Zealand, 1861–1933

Source: E. F. Jones, 'Fertility decline in Australia and New Zealand 1861–1936' (*Population Index* 37, no. 4 [1971]: 301–38). The fertility index was created using Hutterite fertility rates, weighted by age of the female population. The Hutterites, a Protestant sect living in rural parts of the United States, are renowned for their stable and very high fertility. This group has been used as a standard in many international comparisons of fertility rates.

There was also a very important shift around this time in public views on the place and public role of women. New Zealand was the first country in modern times to grant women's suffrage; the Electoral Act 1893 declared that when it came to voting, the word 'person' in legislation included women as well as men.[200] After many years of agitation, women voted for the first time in the general election in November 1893. Raewyn Dalziel argues, 'we should not under-estimate the strength of the challenge that the women's vote posed to the status quo and the boldness of this particular "leap in the dark"'.[200] Gaining the vote was important in its own right; it was also a sign of women's growing confidence and engagement in public activities. In the same year that the Electoral Act was passed, Elizabeth Yates was elected Mayor of Onehunga: she was the first woman to gain such a position in the British Empire. This occurred against a background of high rates of literacy and female schooling – in 1877 New Zealand had been one of the first countries to introduce primary education that was free, compulsory and secular.

We suggest that these changes in expectations and public attitudes may have contributed to women delaying marriage and child-rearing. A study of fertility in Europe in the latter part of the twentieth century found that it was birth rates among the best educated women that were most sensitive to economic downturn.[199] Perhaps social reforms in New Zealand, a hundred years earlier, had in a similar way empowered women to take greater control over reproduction.

When women have their first baby at older ages, average family size is reduced. This means there is more resource and parental time available per child. Older women also tend to have longer intervals between births. Such changes in the size and structure of families make important differences to the way infections spread within households: the age at first infection of infants tends to rise, and the infective dose tends to fall. Both factors favour lower case fatality for illnesses such as measles, whooping cough and other causes of pneumonia in children.[201] Smaller and more widely spaced families have other positive effects also: in these conditions children tend to have fewer fatal accidents, and are better fed.[202]

PHYSICAL ENVIRONMENT: CLIMATE, CROWDING AND URBANITY

Geography played a part in the success of the British Empire,[203] and very likely influenced the outcome of the New Zealand settlement also. The early European colonial forays, launched by Portugal, Spain and the Netherlands, had been to tropical territories that offered quick returns in gold and silver, slaves, spices and sugar, but there was a price to pay. Tropical fevers caused many deaths, and oppressive conditions in low latitudes lowered productivity of workers. Seldom did the appearance of over-bounding natural fertility survive the first press of settlement: thin tropical soils produced for a season or two after the forest was cleared, but whatever nutrients remained were soon washed away.

By the time the British gathered an empire, the territories that were still unclaimed were in the middle and high latitudes (and mostly south of the equator). Here the settlers were fortunate to pitch their tents in climates that were less demanding (and indeed, in the case of New Zealand, provided close analogues to conditions in Britain).[16]

Some are chary of 'map determinism'.[204] Everywhere, the productivity of the soil was tested severely in the first years of colonial settlement – even in the temperate zone, it is argued, nineteenth-century farming practices could not sustain the advantage, if it had existed at all in the first place. And how much more comfortable was the climate in the so-called temperate zone? Neither Queensland in the height of summer, nor central Otago in the depth of winter, would seem, on the face of it, to be particularly health-promoting environments. For all these reasons, and others, the claims that were made for 'the healthiest place on the face of the globe' deserve close scrutiny.

The literature promoting migration to New Zealand boasted about the abundance of food, escape from excessive toil, avoidance of crowds and 'ruinous competition' at school and work, and moderate amounts of physical activity. The feature of the colony that received most attention was the climate.

The humoral theory was proposed by Hippocrates and added to by Galen and others, and was still the dominant model in early nineteenth-century medical thinking. According to this view, well-being depended on a proper balance of the four humours, each referring to a particular temperament (melancholic, sanguine, choleric and phlegmatic) and a certain disposition in the body physiology. If the balance was upset, then it was likely that disease would follow. There was a close link with climate, as each humour was thought to have its characteristic qualities of heat, cold, dry and wet. Sudden changes in weather, and extremes in weather, were some of the commonest causes of upsetting the humoral equilibrium.

Accordingly, there was great interest in the climatic conditions that would be favourable for good health. A. S. Thomson believed the lower illness rates amongst British soldiers in New Zealand than elsewhere in the Empire was due to evenness of temperature and higher degree of atmospheric moisture.[14] Others commented on the lack of excessive heat or cold, the presence of bracing winds and the 'ampleness of fresh air'. James Adam, emigration agent, included in one pamphlet in 1876 mortality tables and temperature records to show the difference between England and New Zealand (which was very much in the favour of the new colony).[147]

However, the claims that were made for the superiority of one climate or another included no evidence of the kind that modern scholars seek. There were no systematic comparisons of populations in different conditions;

no following up of individuals as they moved from one region to another. And there was no consistency. Some commentators pointed to fresh winds, others to balmy temperatures; sometimes lack of variation was a selling point, on other occasions it was the 'stimulating' contrast between seasons that was considered important. So we turn to other environmental factors that might explain the low mortality in New Zealand. Trends in industrialising Britain offer some clues.

In the second half of the nineteenth century living conditions in Britain worsened for many. From 8.9 million in 1801, the English population doubled to just under 18 million in 1851, and doubled again by 1911.[205] Most of this growth occurred in cities – Bradford, for example, grew eight-fold in 50 years. But there was not sufficient new accommodation, and crowding was severe. In the 1850s, in Liverpool, there were thought to be 40,000 people living in cellars – this was one-fifth of the city's population. In Glasgow at the end of the century, after there had been considerable improvements in housing, more than half the inhabitants still lived in 'overcrowded' conditions, defined as more than two adults per room.[205]

It is no surprise then that death rates were worse in cities than in rural areas, and this was true throughout the nineteenth century. In 1841, the national life expectancy at birth was 41 years, in rural Surrey it was 45, in London 37, Liverpool 26 and Manchester 24.[205] A study of variations in life expectancy in England in the second half of the 1800s found that two environmental factors explained the greater part of the differences between districts: crowding at the district level (population density per square kilometre) and distance to an urban centre.[188] Household crowding was important also. In Glasgow in 1911, the standardised death rate in one-room dwellings was 20.1, in two-room 16.8, in three-room 12.6 and in four or more 10.3.[205]

Throughout Europe cities were renowned for their high mortality. A tourist guide for France, written for British tourists mid-century, commented that 'all families, which from taste or necessity, pass their lives in a town residence or shop are irrevocably doomed to extinction. Those that pass the summer in the country last longer than others.'[206]

Edwin Chadwick, in his review of living conditions in Britain, reported that the average age of death of mechanics, labourers and servants in the most unhealthy parts of Manchester and Liverpool was 15 to 17 years, roughly half the figure for people in the same occupations who lived in rural areas. The sanitary conditions in these cities, Chadwick observed, were not easily forgotten:

> . . . a dunghill in one street . . . contains a hundred cubic yards of impure filth, collected from all parts of the town. It is never removed . . . it is enclosed in front by a wall; the height of the wall is about 12 feet, and the dung overtops it; the malarious moisture oozes through the wall, and runs over the pavement.[207]

The urban–rural gradient in mortality was present in New Zealand too: in the 1870s, mortality from all causes in Christchurch was twice as high as the national average for New Zealand.[208] Living conditions in some corners of Christchurch (and other New Zealand cities) in the 1870s and 1880s were perhaps no better than in the crowded settlements of the northern hemisphere. It seems difficult to believe, but some argued that in the worst instances, death rates for typhoid, scarlet fever, diarrhoeal diseases and dysentery – the 'diseases of filth' – were 25 per cent greater than in England in the 1870s.[208]

However, the scale of urban squalor in New Zealand was quite different to the circumstances in Europe. First, the settlements were much smaller. In 1881, there were only four boroughs in New Zealand with populations greater than 10,000 people.[167] These 'conurbations' were tiny compared with the cities of the northern hemisphere. The largest centre in New Zealand at that time, Dunedin (population 24,732), contained about half the number of people who were living in Liverpool cellars 20 years earlier. And the great majority of New Zealanders lived outside the metropolitan boroughs – together, Auckland, Wellington, Christchurch and Dunedin included only 26 per cent of the national population in 1882.

The disadvantages of large cities were evident elsewhere. For instance, a reconstruction of child mortality based on the 1900 US census found that the strongest predictor (after race) was living in a city of more than 25,000 people.[195] This association persisted after adjusting for parents' employment, literacy and migrant status.

Second, the density of settlement within the urban areas was much less in the New Zealand cities. This was partly a result of the balance between population pressure and land supply – the new towns tended to sprawl as land around the margins was, on the whole, readily available. But in Christchurch and Dunedin, established by companies that were strongly influenced by the views of Edward Gibbon Wakefield on desirable urban form, the low densities were deliberate. Large town blocks (up to an acre) were reserved to attract investors.[246]

In Australia, the capital cities in each state drew in a much larger proportion of the population than in New Zealand. Forty per cent of Victorians lived in Melbourne in 1901; in the same year 36 per cent of the New South Wales population lived in Sydney.[246] New Zealand was much less centralised, by comparison, and evolved as a collection of small towns servicing the regions, and slightly larger towns acting as administrative and political hubs. Given the health disadvantages associated with city living at this time, New Zealand benefited from its particular urban history.

DIET

The propaganda distributed by government agents to would-be migrants to New Zealand emphasised the abundance and low cost of food. One immigration agent working in Britain in the early 1870s, reports Jock Phillips,

> . . . described how his meetings were illustrated with large sheets of watercolour paintings which produced an 'electrical effect' on the audience. The illustrations included 'the smoking meal of joints of mutton waiting for the New Zealand workman, enough to make him dance after a hard day's work.'[186]

The prospect of large quantities of fresh meat must have been attractive. Typical working-class diets in England at this time consisted of tea, potatoes and bread as staples, with bacon, cheese and root vegetables as the main supplements. Poorer English workers consumed very small amounts of meat – 25–50 grams a day, on average, according to one estimate, and only slightly greater quantities of milk (maybe 100 grams a day).[209] Nowadays, New Zealanders and others in high-income countries eat five times that amount of meat, on average, which is more than optimal.[210] Low levels of physical activity now compound the risks of a high-energy, high-animal-fat diet, and there are other ways of obtaining the protein and micro-nutrients needed to fuel child growth and development. But at a time of high child mortality, and when there were few alternative dietary sources of energy and protein, a meat-rich diet was beneficial.

In the first years of European settlement, migrants survived on rations. But even these were an improvement for many on what was available in England. For example, the New Zealand Company promised to hand out to each of its settlers 1.6 kilograms of salt meat and 2.4 kilograms of biscuit weekly, with supplementary rice, flour, oatmeal, dried peas, dried potatoes, raisins, butter, sugar, coffee and tea, depending on supplies.[90]

As land was bought, or taken, from Māori, forest cleared and grass planted, stock numbers soared and New Zealand became a nation of unrestrained meat eaters (and milk drinkers). Until the refrigerated ships of the 1880s, there was no serious export trade in meat and farmers sold off stock in local markets relatively cheaply.[211] Consequently, 'meat in large amounts was eaten at every meal: beefsteaks or mutton chops at breakfast, cold beef at luncheon, and roast or boiled beef or mutton at dinner'.[90]

Conditions in this corner of the South Pacific for European agriculture were highly favourable. Rather like England, New Zealand is made up of long, thin islands placed at right angles to prevailing westerlies that blow over large expanses of open water. This generates a temperate, wet climate, and with the added bonus of volcanic soils in many places, New Zealand is well suited to many of the food crops from the northern hemisphere. James Cook had recognised the potential early on: 'was this Country settled by an Industrus peple they would very soon by supply'd not only with the necessarys but many of the luxuries of life'.[16]

One of the British 'necessarys', the white potato, did extraordinarily well. Brought to New Zealand by the first ships from Europe, the potato grew throughout both islands, and spectacularly out-performed the kūmara as a source of calories. In 1848 A. S. Thomson visited a pensioner who had shipped from Galway, established a garden in Panmure, just outside Auckland, and was amazed by early results: 'He told me he had got forty-seven potatoes, of excellent quality and good size, from one stalk, by simply digging the ground after the removal of the native fern.'[101]

In the early period of European settlement, pigs reproduced prodigiously. (In the Wangapeka valley near Nelson, in the 1850s, three men killed 25,000 pigs in the space of 20 months 'and still left thousands to propagate'.)[16] Once bees were introduced from Europe, clover was pollinated, grasses in cleared spaces proliferated and grazing stock thrived. Cattle were introduced first, and then sheep. Without predators, with no competition for grazing and with year-round access to pasture, the numbers of animals increased rapidly (there were about 9 million sheep in New Zealand by the 1870s). In the 1920s, a Health Department investigation reported the diet of one working-class family (parents and eight children) consisted of 'milk: 2 quarts a day, Butter: good amount, Kind of meat food: soup every day, meat nearly every day, fresh vegetables: fair amount, not many green vegetables, use of tinned foods: fair amount, fruit: very little, lollies: large amount, Eggs: plenty, has their own fowls'.[212]

The European settlers did not make full use of local food sources. (For example, fish was widely available in New Zealand, but seldom eaten, since it was regarded by many as a food associated with poverty – a dish of last resort.) But there was no need – exotic crops and livestock thrived, and calories and protein were never in short supply. 'We had come to a land without scarceness. We had no luxuries, but abundance of wholesome food', wrote Jane Bannerman, daughter of the Reverend Thomas Burns, a leading figure in the Dunedin settlement.[147]

Growth rates and attained height are two physiological parameters that provide an indirect measure of the quality of diets. They reflect net energy intake, the calories in the diet less the energy consumed in physical activity and metabolism. Height is not just a measure of quality and quantity of food – stunting may result from chronic illness and parasitic infections that consume energy that would otherwise go into growth.

Little is known about average heights of New Zealanders in the nineteenth century, apart from the survey by A. S. Thomson that we described in an earlier chapter. But information has been retrieved for a sample of the men who served overseas in the armed forces in the two world wars.[213] Average heights were slightly greater than reported for Canadian and American men of the same period, and social variations were apparent (height was positively related with education, farmers were taller than other occupational groups, rural-born soldiers were taller than urban-born). There was a dip in heights amongst soldiers born at the end of the nineteenth century, and again among those born in the 1920s. There were few Māori in the World War I study sample; amongst those who fought in World War II, average height was about half-an-inch less than non-Māori.

The social variation in soldiers' heights fits with better nutrition and health status generally, in the late 1800s, among children born in rural settings and those growing up in socially advantaged families. However, the fall in stature in cohorts born at the end of the century is difficult to explain – infant mortality was on the decline during this time, and the economy was recovering strongly from the depression of the 1880s.

Numerous studies of heights and weights have been carried out in New Zealand in the twentieth century, and they generally report the same trends that have been seen world-wide. Surveys of New Zealand school children, beginning in 1913, show accelerating growth rates, with children gaining more than 2.5 centimetres in height at each age over the space of about 20 years.[214; 215; 213] The average height of 14-year-olds was 1.50 metres in 1913 and 1.55 metres in 1934. In 2007 average height for New Zealand children of this age was 1.66 metres.[216]

PERSONAL AND PUBLIC HEALTH INTERVENTIONS

The recovery of mortality decline in Britain in the later part of the 1800s occurred when the 'urban penalty' of industrialisation was paid off. This was achieved by environmental modifications, and in particular, better drains and safer drinking water supplies were necessary to make cities safe. It is with good reason that the sanitary revolution was judged by the readers of the *British Medical Journal* in 2002 to be the most important medical achievement in 150 years.[217] (The silver medal was awarded to antibiotics, and anaesthetics won the bronze.) This section also looks at public health on board the migrant ships and we examine possible reasons for the decline in smallpox, as a case study.

Sanitation

The new cities of the industrial age were so crowded that the old arrangements for waste disposal, never terribly tidy or effective, were overwhelmed. Cholera was the tip of the iceberg, just one of a large number of diseases that flourished as a result of crowding, pollution and rampant food- and water-borne infection. The most important tasks for the city authorities were to find ways of disposing safely of human faeces and securing the public water supply.

But it is more difficult than might be expected to pin down exactly what the impact was of modern sanitation. In many cities the fall in deaths from signal conditions such as typhoid began before the construction of drains and sewers, and health statistics were not necessarily better in the cities that were early adopters of the new technology. A study of 91 American cities at the turn of the nineteenth century, for instance, found the correlation between investment in water supplies and drains and typhoid death rates was only weakly negative, and varied considerably between regions.[218] Finer grained studies, looking for effects at the level of households, have also struggled to find consistent effects. As an example, a study of childhood deaths in the Dutch city of Tilburg in the early 1900s found elevated risks for social factors, such as family size, birth-spacing and crowding, but no effect of piped water.[219]

The prime piece of sanitary technology that Britain bequeathed to the world was the water-flushed sewer. Recommended in 1842 by Edwin Chadwick (neither an engineer nor a public health doctor, but a lawyer), as part of his famous *Report on the Sanitary Condition of the Labouring Population of Great Britain,* this extension of Roman engineering practice pre-dated the germ theory of disease. The problem, as Chadwick and his colleagues saw it, was how to deal to filth: the smell of the sewer was the critical issue, in their eyes (and noses). Consequently drains were designed not only to remove waste, but also to cleanse and dilute. The expense was enormous, the use of resources might be seen as profligate, and the sustainability of the technology in the future, in a water-stressed world, is questionable. It is worth noting that other countries achieved similar outcomes by different means.

Japan reported world-beating declines in infant and childhood mortality post-World War II, but was very slow to introduce reticulated sanitation. As late as 1990, less than half the population lived in districts connected to the sewerage system.[20] Other factors in Japan that may have been important include traditional practices promoting hygiene (boiling water before drinking, for example), investment in health education, formal child-care services and improvements in housing.[220]

We touch here on a recurring theme – there were plainly many factors acting on the decline in mortality. Sewers, drains and reticulated water supplies were important, but they were not the only vehicles to achieve better hygiene. Moreover, they were not the only important influences on health in the late nineteenth century. Economic conditions, better housing standards, education, child-health services and smaller families all played a part, in both England and in New Zealand, and may have overshadowed the impact of public health engineering. For children in particular, conditions inside the home may have had a stronger influence on mortality than hygiene at city level.

In New Zealand in 1891, 28 per cent of the population lived in cities of 10,000 people or more, and there were no conurbations of 100,000 plus (not until Auckland reached this mark in 1911). In Australia at the same time, 35 per cent of the national population was found in cities of 100,000 or more, and 44 per cent in cities of more than 10,000. England and Wales showed higher levels of urban concentration (62 per cent in cities over 10,000; 32 per cent in the largest cities).

What is the ratio of benefits to harms, at different city sizes? One might suppose the lack of services in small towns was balanced, at some point, by the risks of crowding in larger settlements. In New Zealand, poor sanitation was a feature of many towns, not just the larger cities. In 1874, a typhoid epidemic in tiny Cromwell affected a third of the population. In the 1870s in windy Wellington, a metropolis by New Zealand standards, 'public sanitation was so deplorable, that on turning a street corner . . . the pedestrian was said to hold his hat on with one hand and stop his nostrils with the other'.[147]

The fastest growing city in New Zealand, Auckland, had the highest rates of enteric fever in the country, infant mortality consistently exceeded that of other New Zealand cities, and 'what information there is shows that the local authorities were allowing sanitation to look after itself'.[259] However, conditions were most adverse in Dunedin, the first urban centre and the industrial hub of the colony in the early years. Submissions to the Dunedin Sanitary Commission in 1864 reported that, in Stafford Street, 20 dwellings on two sections shared one small closet. In Maclaggan Street up to 30 cottages had no privy at all so the night soil was thrown into the street. Altogether the city produced 20,000 tons of 'excrementitious matter' a year, and most of it was lying in and around buildings. (One medical man estimated there were 8000 cubic yards of human faeces in town cesspools, with an evaporating area of 1 acre.)[147]

Christchurch suffered because the city had been established on the low-lying, water-logged Canterbury plains and in the first years of settlement there was a great deal of illness, including epidemics of typhoid and diphtheria. Between the 1870s and the early years of the twentieth century there was a dramatic improvement – mortality from all causes fell by two-thirds, and there was an even greater reduction in the 'filth' diseases.[208] The greatest part of this improvement occurred in the years immediately before the city-wide system of drains and sewers was operating. The historian G. W. Rice suggests one reason was a vigorous campaign to stop people using cesspits.[208] The 1875 Public Health Act had named cesspools and cesspits as public nuisances, but local ordnances were required before the Board of Health could act. The Christchurch City Council took this action in 1878, and within two years all households were using pan-closets with arrangements for night soil removal.

Secure water supplies, with a high-pressure mains supply, were not provided until 1909 in Christchurch (which again, post-dated much of the reduction in infectious disease mortality). There remained periodic spikes in mortality for under-fives, particularly in summer, and these were most likely related to contamination of food and milk and poor household hygiene. A study of infant mortality on the other side of the Tasman, in Adelaide, Australia, found that locations with particularly high rates at the turn of the nineteenth century were distinguished not by neighbourhood factors (such as crowding, drainage and cleanliness of the streets), but by conditions inside the house. Food preparation, infant feeding practices and the numbers of people per room were the strongest predictors.[221]

Ship-board disease

In the early years of European settlement of Australia there were often heavy losses on the voyages south, especially amongst children, reflecting the crowded, unsanitary and dangerous conditions that applied.[222] Typhus, diarrhoeal diseases, measles and scarlet fever were common causes of death. However, conditions were improving by the time that migration extended to New Zealand. We know that mortality rates on convict ships to the Australian colonies fell sharply after 1815, and there were evident improvements in the records of ships containing assisted migrants, from about 1830 onwards.[223]

The reduction in deaths was not due to generic improvements in population health. In Britain, the improvements in health on ships occurred at a time when public health was making little headway, and indeed conditions were deteriorating in some of the early-industrial cities. Maritime mortality decline resulted from deliberate interventions that in many respects anticipated the land-based 'sanitary revolution'.

At the instigation of the Colonial Office, every ship on the Australia run after 1831 had to employ a surgeon superintendent who was responsible for vaccinations, pre-embarkation screening, and enforcement of public and private hygiene on board. Surgeons were backed up by volunteers whose job it was to ensure that the rules on crowding were followed, that kitchens and dining rooms were cleaned, clothing washed twice weekly as regulated, latrines were in good order and waste was disposed of. Reports were compiled on each voyage, and surgeons were paid a bonus if there were few deaths, but penalised when mortality was 'excessive' and when crew and passengers identified deficient service. At this time surgeons had little to offer by way of effective medical treatments; rather they played a policing role, ensuring not only that the ship was scrubbed and cleaned, but also that there was order, discipline and purpose on board.[223]

Simon Szreter has argued that effective public health interventions in the nineteenth century had the following characteristics: central direction; energetic local agency; and accountability, both to the central authority and to the public.[224] These were all features of the steps taken on board British migrant ships, and were well timed, as far as New Zealand was concerned. The maritime reforms coincided with European settlement of the last colony off the block in the nineteenth-century race of empires.

Smallpox – example of an epidemic disease that did not plague New Zealand

Putting aside basic sanitation, vaccination against smallpox was perhaps the first effective public health intervention. The disease was easy to recognise, and often fatal, so it offers an opportunity to test the contribution of health services to mortality trends. As mentioned already, New Zealand was little affected by smallpox, although the disease was a common cause of mortality in Europe and other parts of the world at the time of Cook's voyages. From the first national registration of deaths in 1876 until 1900 there were only eight fatal cases of smallpox registered in New Zealand (excluding fatalities among individuals in quarantine).[259] Was this success accidental, the result of medical action or were there other reasons? It is difficult to claim that medical action ashore was effective. Vaccination of infants was made compulsory in 1863, but the law was never popular and those children who were vaccinated were probably always in the minority.[259] In 1911 there were 26,354 births registered in New Zealand, but only 1078 vaccinations registered.[137] (Resistance was not unique to New Zealand. In many countries people objected that compulsory vaccination was a violation of civil liberties. In the United States opponents called it 'De-Jenneration'.)[225]

More importantly, New Zealand benefited from effective quarantine, and a waning in the pathogenicity of smallpox globally at the time of settlement in New Zealand. (Again, good timing favoured New Zealand settlement.) A less virulent variant of the smallpox virus, *Variola minor*, predominated world-wide at the end of the nineteenth century. Additionally and not fully understood, other sub-type evolution or 'drift' was probably occurring, shifting smallpox to a less deadly disease.[17]

CHILD HEALTH

New Zealand was one of the first nations to introduce a comprehensive home-visiting and education programme, focused on mothers and children. This was run by the New Zealand Society for the Health of Women and Children, also known as the Plunket Society, founded in 1907 by Sir Truby King.

Plunket was a voluntary organisation, although the costs were heavily subsidised by the government. Its services were free at point of use, and were intended for all women, although in practice few Māori were included. Plunket was strongest in urban areas where non-Māori greatly outnumbered Māori, and Māori mothers were served by a parallel system of child nurses employed by the Health Department.[226] The society aimed to promote breast-feeding and the care of babies based on best scientific principles. The backbone of the organisation was a network of local committees. These committees raised funds and employed the Plunket nurses who were based in neighbourhood clinics. The nurses ran well-baby clinics, provided antenatal care, and visited the homes of mothers with newborns. Training was provided by Truby King at the Karitane Hospitals, first in Dunedin and then in other cities, and the educational material that nurses distributed was prepared specifically by Plunket. By the middle of the twentieth century, around 85 per cent of non-Māori mothers were seen by Plunket nurses.

The strengths of Plunket were its presence in all the major population centres, the community involvement that shaped this as a service 'for women by women', high-level political support and professional networks. There were disagreements with the medical profession, and particularly at issue was the autonomy of nurse practitioners, but Plunket had the backing of senior paediatricians (some employed by the society). Another feature of Plunket was that the nurses took on a variety of welfare roles. Plunket's Director of Nursing Services in the 1980s explained, 'Roll a social worker, housing officer, arbitrator, chauffeur, home economist, nurse and friend into just one person and you'll get an idea of the work the nurses do'.[227]

An inquiry into the welfare of mothers and children in New Zealand, commissioned in 1918 by the New South Wales government, reported that the Plunket Society 'had taken the rather unusual course of appealing primarily to the better-to-do and more intelligent women of the community' (rather than concentrating on the poorest and most needy women, which was typically the approach taken by charities and other private initiatives).[228] This may well have been one of the society's strengths, politically, given the resources it could draw on from its membership, and the relationships Plunket enjoyed with politicians and the medical establishment. However, there was from time to time criticism that the service did not suit everyone. Māori were seldom included, as mentioned already, and some said that Plunket was more attuned to middle-class urban women than mothers from less advantaged backgrounds.

What was the impact of Plunket? Linda Bryder refers to an address from the Governor-General, Lord Bledisloe, at the 1934 Dominion Conference of Plunket. He said:

> . . . the present infant mortality from all causes in New Zealand is approximately one-half of that in England and Wales and the US, one-third of that in Germany, one-fourth that in Italy and Spain, one-fifth that in Egypt, one-sixth of that in British India, and one-seventh that in Chile. For this highly favoured position New Zealand and her people of all classes have to thank the Plunket movement and the man of vision who founded it.[226]

The strong support Plunket nurses gave to breast-feeding must have been helpful at a time when diarrhoeal disease was the major cause of deaths in the first year of life. In addition to discouraging bottle-feeding, Plunket gave instructions on hygiene in the home and offered material support to poor mothers, as part of its welfare remit. Infant deaths from diarrhoea and enteritis in New Zealand fell by about 70 per cent between 1922 and 1938; in England and Wales over the same time the improvement was much less (about 20 per cent).[165]

However, the good health of non-Māori children was apparent long before Plunket was established, and the decline in mortality was well under way when 'the man of vision' shifted his gaze from animal husbandry to baby management.[229] Indeed, improvement in child survival (to age ten) was twice as great in the 20 years before 1896 as in the 20 years subsequently.[169] There is a similar pattern in Australia – the decline in infant mortality began a little later than in New Zealand, but almost 20 years before the maternal welfare movement was well established.[230]

In England, on the other hand, infant mortality was essentially unchanged until around 1900, suggesting there were different causes at work. The abrupt downturn in infant mortality (which occurred at about the same time in all districts) fits with a sudden and wide-ranging alteration in infant care with a rapid effect. A possible candidate is the introduction of pasteurisation and other improvements in the quality of cow's milk used for infant feeding (although it must be noted that these measures were certainly not applied consistently throughout the country until World War II).[231]

A rather special example of the effectiveness of public health interventions comes from a study in Melbourne. Records were extracted for a sample of 16,000 women who gave birth at the major charity hospital in the city between 1857 and 1900, and details were linked with registrations of deaths.[232] This was not a typical group of Melbourne women. Many were unmarried and itinerant, and all were poor by the standards of the income means test applied by the hospital. But there was a notable reduction in death rates in the 1890s, coinciding with improvements in hospital hygiene and much reduced infection rates on the wards. A system was introduced for registering and monitoring those, other than mothers, who provided infant care outside hospital. This was a response to the cottage industry of 'baby farming' and was enforced through police inspections. Also, information on infant feeding was circulated, and there were for the first time mandatory coronial inquiries in the case of infant deaths. Many of these reforms were introduced in New Zealand at about the same time. For example, the Infant Life Protection Act, passed in 1893, required foster homes to be registered, and empowered police to enter and inspect these premises (but enforcement of these rules was weak).

TUBERCULOSIS

TB was a common cause of death in the second half of the nineteenth century amongst European New Zealanders (Figure 11). Māori must have been affected similarly, but there was no systematic study of causes of deaths among Māori until the 1930s when H. B. Turbott carried out a community survey on the East Cape, and reported TB mortality that was roughly ten times the figure for Pākehā at the time.[203]

Although the infectious nature of tuberculosis had been shown in Germany in 1882, there was no organised response to TB in New Zealand until almost 20 years later. Passage of the Public Health Act 1900 initiated a flurry of activity including compulsory notification of TB (applied in 1901, more than a decade in advance of Britain), and the launch of the sanatorium movement – an initiative powered by good nutrition, rest and fresh air.

How effective were these measures? Doctors were not pleased with the notification requirements – few could see the public health value, many feared (rightly) the stigmatising effects of the new law and many cases of disease went un-reported. Sanatoria tended to admit the relatively well, those with mild and slowly progressing cases of disease, who in any event had a good prognosis. These institutions were of little value in limiting infection. Patients with advanced disease, who were likely to be most infectious to others, were specifically excluded from admission.

Other public health measures included education campaigns, focusing on the constitutional factors that defended against the illness. For instance, a prominent New Zealand medical man claimed in 1911 that 'the strong healthy person living a healthy life has nothing to fear from consumption'.[203] The School Medical Service was established in New Zealand in 1912 and health camps for children began in the 1920s. The camps applied the principles of sanatoria, introducing children considered to be at particular risk of disease to open-air plain living with nutritious meals. (These services were not available to Māori for another 20 years. Even in the 1930s health authorities emphasised education and self-help, rather than medical treatment and investments in better living conditions. Housing for Māori communities, for instance, was not a government priority until after the Second World War.)

New Zealand did not lead but followed the rest of the world in the introduction of new forms of treatment. Thoracic surgery was applied to TB in the 1940s, screening by mass miniature radiography was introduced after World War II and effective chemotherapy was not widely available until the early 1950s.

Nevertheless, New Zealand was consistently ahead, internationally, in the TB statistics. In the early 1900s death rates from tuberculosis among non-Māori were a half to a third of those in England and Wales.[165] Around 1940 deaths from TB in New Zealand were 20 per cent less than in Australia, half those in Ireland, a third of mortality in France and a quarter of Italy.[110] What explained these differences?

In New Zealand, less crowding and freedom from lung-irritating air pollution may have slowed the transmission of infection. But most people who are infected do not suffer the disease (the ratio presently, world-wide, is about ten infected to one person manifesting disease). What matters most is whether being exposed to the TB organism is translated into illness. This depends on factors that may undermine the resistance of the host, such as chronic debilitating diseases, acute viral illnesses (especially measles in childhood), smoking and heavy alcohol use, and protein-calorie malnutrition.[233] The role of nutrition should be noted: the milk- and meat-rich diet that most New Zealanders had access to in the nineteenth century may help explain why TB death rates were lower, at all ages, than elsewhere.

There are two other possibilities, both speculative. Perhaps the belief that New Zealand's climate was particularly suitable for those affected by TB included a grain of truth. Not the bracing winds, nor the gentle temperatures, but strong sunlight may have been an important factor. Vitamin D, which is formed in the body as a result of exposure to ultra-violet B radiation, plays an important part in activating the immune reaction to *M. tuberculosis*, and individuals with low levels of Vitamin D have an increased risk of active clinical TB.[234; 235] Indeed, the combination of cod liver oil (which contains plenty of

Vitamin D) and sunlight was popular as a treatment of TB before specific chemotherapy was available.[236]

This is relevant because the amount of biologically active ultraviolet radiation reaching the Earth's surface in New Zealand not only exceeds that received in the UK (which is further from the equator), but is much greater than at comparable latitudes in the northern hemisphere. Reasons include the recent erosion of ozone in the stratosphere, but also the tilt and orbit of the Earth (which mean the southern hemisphere receives more solar radiation in summer than does the northern hemisphere) and differences in cloud cover.[237] We don't know whether there were therapeutic effects, but it is conceivable that the southern hemisphere sunlight contributed to reduced susceptibility to TB. (This would not have explained the advantage over Australia of course, since UV exposures there are even higher than in New Zealand.)

It has been suspected that exposure to bovine TB, a related but generally less severe infection, may provide humans with some protection against disease caused by *M. tuberculosis*. For example, in Sweden in the 1930s there was a gradient for tuberculosis, with the highest rates of human infection in counties with low prevalence of TB amongst cattle, and least human disease in the parts of the country with the highest rates of TB in cattle.[238] Bovine tuberculosis has been present in New Zealand since the late 1800s, if not earlier, and it has been more difficult to control than in many other countries because of frequent re-infection from wild deer and possum.[239] Early New Zealand was essentially one large farm, with millions of stock, relatively few people and plenty of opportunity for close contact with cattle. Perhaps there were some health-enhancing aspects to this agricultural intimacy.

SOCIO-ECONOMIC FACTORS

Some argue that in the big picture of things it is the economy that matters most.[240] The case is made on the basis of the links between economic growth on the one hand, and employment, disposable incomes, government investment in welfare and the consumption of life-enhancing goods and services on the other.

The period covered by this chapter includes golden times for New Zealand, economically. The first leg of New Zealand lamb to be eaten in England was thawed, cooked and served at Jesus College, Cambridge, in 1882.[74] New technologies to process butter, cheese and meat fundamentally altered farming practices in New Zealand. They also provided foreign earnings that lifted New Zealand towards the top of the international wealth ladder. Just as meat and dairy farming boomed, the breakup of large estates in the 1890s encouraged closer settlement and boosted productivity, and from 1890 to 1940 New Zealand GDP per capita grew by an average of 1.3 per cent per year.[241] When the Second World War broke out, New Zealand was one of the wealthiest countries in the world in Gross Domestic Product per head (adjusted for purchasing power) (Figure 17).

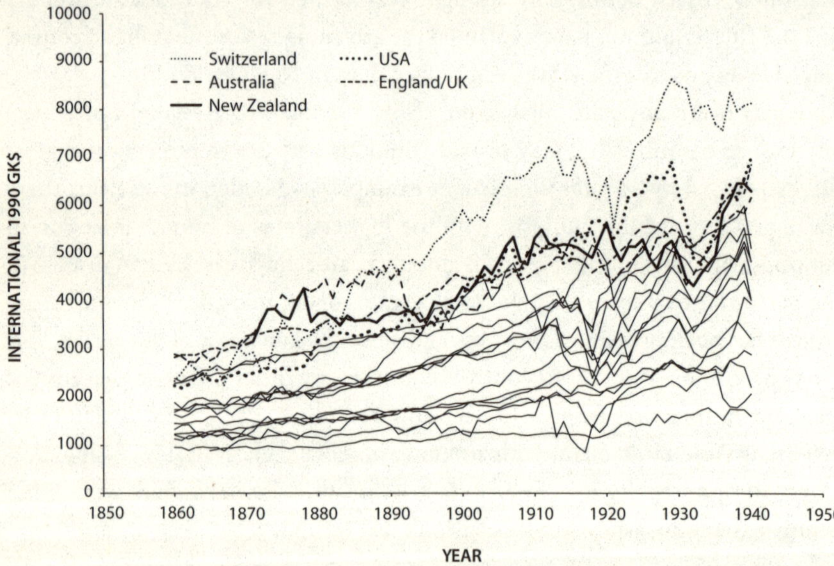

Figure 17: International GDP per capita for multiple countries (selected countries labelled), 1860–1940

Source: J. Bolt and J. L. van Zanden, 'The First Update of the Maddison Project; Re-Estimating Growth Before 1820', *Maddison Project Working Paper* 4 (2013). GDP is purchasing power parity adjusted, and in 1990 'Geary–Khamis' dollars.

But it wasn't always golden times. Economic conditions were volatile, and New Zealand was affected by several long depressions (e.g., in the 1880s and 1920s). In simple terms, the trends in economics and life expectancy are not well matched. New Zealand's position at the top of the health ladder was taken up 20 years before New Zealand became a powerhouse of agricultural exports, and the irregularities in economic fortunes since 1860 are not matched by fluctuations in mortality (e.g., New Zealand's improvement in life expectancy did not falter during the 1880s/90s and 1920s/30s despite grim recessions).

In Australia, there was a similar pattern of regular improvement in health statistics, over a period when economic conditions varied considerably. Between 1880 and 1940 all-cause mortality (age adjusted) fell by two-thirds. The decline was steady and continuous, with only minor perturbations, most significantly that due to influenza in 1919.[190] However, over the same years the Australian economy boomed, stalled, recovered and crashed. Per capita GDP fell by a quarter in the 1890s, and while there was improvement subsequently, GDP and real consumption expenditure were barely 15 per cent greater in 1940 than in 1880.[242]

We pointed out earlier in this chapter that height is related to nutrition and health status in early life, and since child nutrition is a product of how much food families can afford, height has also been treated as a biological marker of economic well-being.[107] The average height of men recruited into the Australian Army was just over 173 centimetres for those born in 1868, and almost exactly the same for the 1918 birth cohort, but men born in the 1880s and early 1890s were almost 2 centimetres shorter on average[242] – another indicator that while life expectancy improved, for an appreciable period living conditions stagnated in Australia. However, the Antipodean growth advantage persisted: school-children born overseas were shorter than those born in Australia to migrants, and the tallest children of all were those who were local-born, and whose parents were also Australian-born.[242]

Social equality within the non-Māori population, and the absence of a large urban poor population, have been claimed as reasons for low mortality in New Zealand.[170; 162] Is this plausible? It is a British epidemiologist, Richard Wilkinson, who has most forcefully advanced the argument that the *distribution* of wealth is in general at least as important as the *average level*. He argues that countries in which wealth is shared relatively equally do better, in many respects, than those with greater inequalities in wealth.[243] Others have questioned whether this is always the case, pointing out that the strength of the association between income inequality and population health is strongly influenced by the selection of data points.[244]

Two mechanisms could be at play. The first is mathematically derived.

The effect on health of gaining a dollar of income depends on the starting point. A dollar more for someone in poverty has a greater impact than an extra dollar for someone of average income. Thus, lifting people out of poverty through transfers of income from the well-off to the poor will almost certainly lower a society's average mortality rate. The second mechanism is structural: it is proposed that an unequal society simply operates differently, and the social dynamics tend to be less favourable than in conditions where wealth is more evenly shared. Examples include invidious social comparisons working through psychosocial and behavioural pathways, less egalitarianism and therefore less efficient use of resources, and an undermining of welfare provisions when the rich segregate themselves from the rest of the population.

Was New Zealand in the nineteenth century a more equal country than other 'new Europes' and the metropolitan states of Europe itself? There is plenty of anecdotal evidence that social gradients were flatter in this colony than elsewhere. An Englishwoman writing home in the 1850s reported:

> The look and bearing of the immigrants appears to alter soon after they reach the colony. Some people object to the independence of their manner, but I do not; on the contrary I like to see the upright gait, the well-fed look, the decent clothes (even if no-one touches his hat to you), instead of the half-starved, depressed appearance, and too often cringing servility of the mass of our English population.[245]

New Zealand cities were described by William Pember Reeves as 'communities of busy people, seldom very rich, as seldom miserably poor'.[246] Sidney and Beatrice Webb, British socialists, visited New Zealand in the 1890s and noted approvingly, 'a pleasant impression of general comfort among the working population who seem to enjoy themselves as much as the well-to-do and have agreeable independent manners: assuming equality of treatment by all of all'.[247]

Historian Erik Olssen has spent a professional lifetime studying Caversham, one of the oldest suburbs of Dunedin. He found the divides between social classes in the nineteenth century were much less evident than in England. About a third of upper-middle-class men and women, for instance, married partners from unskilled occupational groups, a much greater degree of mixing than was seen at this time in England. Olssen and colleagues propose that conditions in a migrant society tended to flatten perceptions of social status:

> In a colony where ditching was more important than most intellectual or artistic activities, men with physical strength and dexterity were admired. This helped to dissolve any stigma attached to unskilled labour in England. Navvies and wharfies were respected. So were the tough men of the rural frontier and the runs, the drovers who shepherded the flocks along the Main South Road and the shearers who wintered over.[248]

There was a corresponding egalitarianism in incomes.[170] The distribution in New Zealand in the nineteenth century was truncated at both ends – there were few individuals with great wealth, and the country lacked also a large, impoverished lower class. The great majority of the population were salary and wage earners of moderate means, with a bias towards employment in primary industries. In the first half of the twentieth century, agriculture accounted for 50 to 60 per cent of New Zealand's economic production: twice the proportion in the United States. (As late as the 1960s, agriculture's contribution to the economy was twice that in Australia, and seven times the figure for the UK.)[170]

BRITISH CULTURE AND INSTITUTIONS

Other explanations have been offered for the success of the English settlements in the 'new' world. They include the transplantability of Victorian institutions (banking, police, education, public health); the good luck of being first into the industrial revolution; and the superiority of British traditions, skills and character. The last argument can be disposed of quickly for its inconsistencies (why didn't these innate attributes sustain expansion before the 1800s, for instance?). But does the success of New Zealand, in its health statistics at least, bear some relation to the particularly British form of Empire? Would there have been similar outcomes if the country had been settled, say, by the French, as could have easily happened?

At the time James Cook and Jean de Surville were, simultaneously, circumnavigating New Zealand, England and France were more or less on the same footing as European Great Powers. But in the next hundred years England surged, given the impetus of American independence and industrial expansion, while France was set back on its heels by revolution and Napoleon's wars.

This gave the English colonies significant advantages: they were members of a global club that was borne along on the Anglophone wave, and were boosted by a patron that was the dominant economic force internationally. England was hungry for raw materials, and had a navy to ensure that both materials and people could be freely transported around the world.

CONCLUSION

We all like a simple explanation – or a contest made simple between two explanations. For instance, we could pit Thomas McKeown's argument that mortality decline in the nineteenth and early twentieth centuries was largely due to increasing standards of living and diet,[249] against Samuel Preston's argument that technological advances and diffusion of knowledge caused increases in life expectancy.[250] But reality – especially the reality of societies as they evolve – is more complex than that. McKeown and Preston were not really on opposing sides: sharper technologies on the farm, for instance, played a big part in boosting food production in England in the nineteenth century.

We can *describe* what has happened. Millennia of meandering oscillations in life expectancy within a reasonably narrow range among our hunter-gatherer forebears were followed by larger lurches in mortality rates in the time of agricultural and pre-industrial societies. Higher population densities and trade-freighted transport of microbes between communities generated pandemics and plagues on top of a considerable burden of endemic disease. Then infant mortality fell as societies better organised themselves, fertility was restrained and disease profiles featured non-communicable diseases in place of infectious conditions. This is the conventional rendering of the American epidemiologist Abdel Omran's 'epidemiological transition'.[251] The transition continues today, across the globe, although in a less regular fashion than Omran proposed, leading to the co-existence of 'old' and 'new' health problems (AIDS and heart disease, under-nutrition and obesity).

Different countries have achieved mortality decline through different means: some countries invested heavily in sanitation, some in education and social policy. And in all cases, no one single 'thing' provides an explanation. Rather, it is a package of 'things'. The right combination of new innovations and policies to achieve mortality decline will differ depending on what resources and natural endowments a society already has, and what causes of death are prevalent.

So, for non-Māori, what was the winning package? We believe that natural advantage, good luck and tactics all contributed. Three causes of rapid health improvements stand out, in our assessment: health selection, physical environment (most notably low crowding, high-protein calorie-rich diets and lack of polluting industry), and early and rapid fertility decline.

Good for non-Māori. Not good for Māori. The expropriation of land and other natural resources (such as water) from Māori provided the means for non-Māori mortality decline, but led to population collapse for Māori. The loss of land brought poverty, hunger and broken communities, and the remoteness of New Zealand was to the detriment of Māori. Centuries of isolation meant susceptibility to introduced pathogens was high. This is the essence of 'fungibility': health stocks were transferred from one to the other. We will explore this more in the next chapter: suffice to say here that as soon as one invokes the physical environment reason on the one hand, you need to put out the other hand and say 'at the expense of Māori'.

The settlement of New Zealand coincided with, and was to some extent shaped by, a streak of egalitarianism and desire for societies without large inequalities and extreme poverty. Without the severities of poverty, crowding and squalor that existed in European cities, New Zealand mortality rates (amongst children especially) declined early. The timing of settlement also coincided with a better understanding of the control of infectious disease, shown by more effective arrangements for quarantine, extended vaccination programmes and the dramatic improvement in ship-board survival.

Other features of New Zealand probably assisted, but were not critical to non-Māori having the highest life expectancy in the world. They include comprehensive child-health programmes (for example, Plunket) and a relatively robust economy. During this period, economic success was not correlated closely with mortality in the short term, but over the long run New Zealand's high GDP made it possible to invest in hospitals, schools and other social services, and these investments yielded significant returns for population health in the second half of the twentieth century.

4

Decline and Recovery

Māori from 1860 to 1940

There are two parts to this story: an extension of the decline in Māori health that was first apparent soon after the arrival in New Zealand of Europeans; and the recovery that took place in the first half of the twentieth century. This was a pivotal time in New Zealand history. Infectious diseases were the commonest cause of death, fanned by social disruption, poverty, loss of land and displacement. But what many had assumed to be the finale for Māori was in fact followed by an astonishing resurgence. It is difficult to tease out the reasons for the turnaround in Māori mortality because the numbers and causes of deaths were still not recorded consistently and comprehensively.

Increasing fertility was important for population growth, but insufficient by itself as an explanation. The burden of infectious diseases started to lift in the late 1800s, probably due to a mix of biology (increasing host resistance) and environmental improvements. However, the recovery of life expectancy proceeded ahead of economic development, in the face of continuing loss of Māori land, and without a serious attempt by government to provide appropriate services to the rural areas where most Māori lived. Māori asserted leadership in local communities and in national governments: Buck, Āpirana Ngata, James Carroll and Pōmare were prominent in health. Important also were growing understanding and acceptance of public health principles, better access to more effective health care, and improved housing and better living conditions generally.

DECLINE

In the nineteenth century much was written about 'the demise' of the Māori.[252; 156; 131] European observers referred to large numbers of deaths among children, evidence of poor nutrition among the young, the heavy burden of respiratory diseases (and particularly 'phthisis') and frequent outbreaks of febrile illnesses with high fatality. But reliable statistics are in short supply. One reason was that parts of the country were essentially closed to Europeans until the end of the century, and as James Belich says, 'a feature of persistent Māori independence was that you did not let the government count you'.[78] As a result, estimates of Māori life expectancy in this period (1860–1940) are based largely on occasional surveys, inference and comparisons with the experience of other indigenous peoples.

The first official, national census of Māori took place in 1857/58 (there were informal, local counts of Māori populations undertaken previously).[104] Vital registration for Māori, including births and deaths, began in 1913, but the coverage was very patchy for some time. From 1926 the same information was obtained on Māori in the national census as for the rest of the population. The proportion of deaths that were registered increased as Māori made greater use of the mainstream health system, but some age groups were not well covered until very late. (In particular, neonatal and infant deaths were much under-reported until the 1950s.)

Derek Dow[154] estimates that even in the 1930s, only 60 per cent of deaths among Māori were registered. Judith Binney has written an account of the settlement of Maungapohatu, established in 1907–8 in the heart of the Urewera ranges by the prophet Rua Kenana Hepetipa.[253] Between 1924 and 1936, Presbyterian missionaries and teachers at the local school kept records of births and deaths. Not one of the 57 deaths that occurred was officially registered, according to Binney, and only three of those who died were visited by doctors.

National censuses during this time may have missed Māori, especially in rural areas, but probably not to the same extent as the deficiency in death registrations. Ian Pool argues the under-counting was so great that published mortality rates in the pre-1940 era need to be adjusted upwards by at least 20 to 30 per cent.[126] Even when deaths were registered, it is debatable whether ethnicity was recorded accurately. There is good evidence from later periods that this information was often missing or inaccurate, and Māori deceased were more often labelled as non-Māori than the other way round (see chapter 6). All in all, the deficiencies in the official records from 1860 to 1940 mean that our figures for Māori life expectancy probably over-estimate the true values (that is, conditions may well have been even worse than shown here).

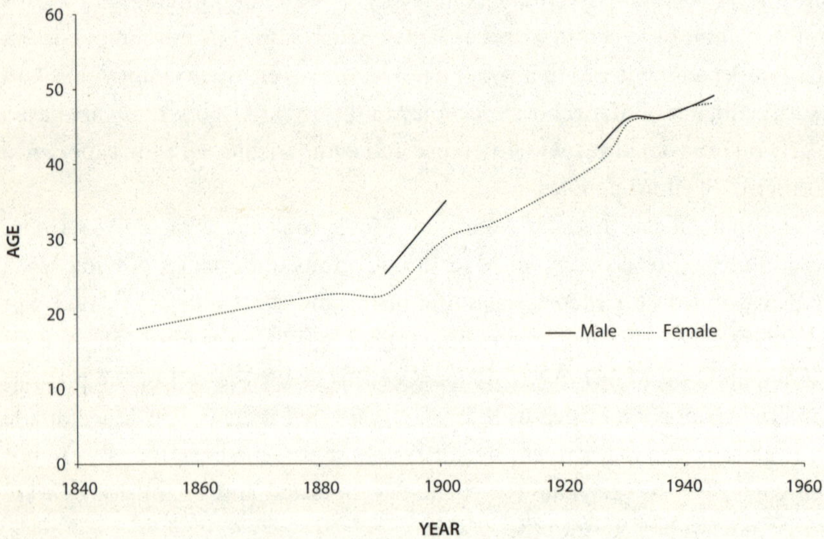

Figure 18: Lange and Pool's estimates of life expectancy at birth, for Māori, circa 1850–1945

Source: R. Lange, *May the People Live: A History of Maori Health Development 1900–1920* (Auckland: Auckland University Press, 1999).

Figure 18 shows Lange and Pool's estimates of Māori life expectancy, based on local surveys of births and deaths and estimates of survival based on the age structure of the population.[86] This series differs from what we show elsewhere in the book. There are more data points for females than for males, the reason being that life expectancy was inferred from the ratio of children to adult women at times when data from death registrations were not reliable.

Mortality among Māori at the turn of the twentieth century was probably similar to that experienced in the most distressed parts of Europe. In Russia, the infant mortality rate in 1910 was about 250 per 1000, suggesting life expectancy at birth around 30 years.[127] In New Zealand, infant mortality for Māori in the 1890s may have approached 400 per 1000.[162] This means that fewer than half of Māori live-born children would have lived to age 15 (by 1936 this fraction was more than three-quarters).[198]

We can say little about the causes of death, because coding was unreliable, and the labels that were applied were not meaningful. It appears that tuberculosis, which was perhaps reported more accurately than other causes of death on account of the long time course of the disease and its characteristic presentation, caused up to a quarter of all deaths in some years.[162] Other infectious diseases appeared frequently in epidemic form. Whooping cough was estimated to cause 60–80 deaths per 1000 persons infected in 1877–80.[126] Reports from teachers in the Native Schools in the 1880s and 1890s refer to what were probably, with hindsight, sizeable outbreaks of measles, typhoid fever and influenza.[254] Indeed, so many deaths were caused by influenza in the 1890s, Ian Pool argues, that the apparent turnaround in Māori mortality rates at the turn of the century was, at least in the first instance, merely a return to usual conditions.[198]

There was an inverse relation between the numbers of new New Zealanders and Māori: the greatest depopulation of Māori occurred at the time that inflows from Europe were at their peak (see Figure 5.2 in Ian Pool's *Maori Population of New Zealand*[131]). Surges of newcomers off the boats refreshed the local pool of disease carriers. (While the selection, formal and otherwise, of migrants may have discouraged some with chronic health problems, conditions prior to shipping, on board and immediately after arrival were all conducive to the spread of infections. Perhaps for these reasons, TB was less common among New Zealand-born Pākehā than those born overseas.)[255] But the most important consequence of 'swamping immigration' was the rocketing demand for land. Whatever the angle of approach, the transfer of land from indigenous ownership to British control stands at the centre of New Zealand history.

Earlier chapters have described the tide of European settlers that flowed into New Zealand after 1840. The high water mark was set in the 1870s, following the Immigration and Public Works Act (1870). The government of the time, led by Julius Vogel, argued that population growth was a powerful vehicle for national development and, in a sense, Vogel and his colleagues were right. The influx of settlers provided muscle and money for nation-building, and the improvements paid for themselves as the engine of the economy turned over more rapidly. Moreover, well-developed railways, schools and roads attracted fresh waves of migrants.[78] But what was needed to keep this virtuous cycle turning was land.

The New Zealand Settlement Act and the Suppression of Rebellion Act, passed in 1863, opened the way to new stretches of Māori land, aided and abetted by further legislation, including the Native Lands Act (1865, 1873) that essentially abolished customary title. From the government's point of view, collective ownership made it too difficult to connect willing vendors with eager purchasers, and the new laws accelerated land sales. Prior to the 1870s, most of the territory the Crown had confiscated, or purchased, was on the margins of the Māori heartland. But military campaigns opened up the centre of the North Island, including large tracts of potentially rich farmland. Entry to these territories was essential in Vogel's vision, and to make it happen many of the European settlements south of Auckland and in the Waikato were deliberately located to consolidate the military successes of the previous decade.

These strategies, legal and otherwise, achieved their purpose, and Europeans gained most of the land in New Zealand that was fit for economic development. (Figure 19 shows the proportions of the North Island held by Māori, around 1860 and 1960.) By 1920, when most of the large sales had been completed, Māori holdings in the North Island were about 4.8 million acres, roughly one-sixth of the total land area, and most of that was rough hill country.[256]

Where land alienation occurred early, and where the losses cut most deeply, one would expect the health of Māori to be affected particularly severely.[257] Mason Durie[13] argues there was no serious diminution in numbers in the Waikato tribes, for instance, before inroads were made into the King Country, land was confiscated and settlements were dispersed, after which population declined markedly. Tūhoe were perhaps the last iwi to engage with the Native Land Court and to lose large areas of land by sale and confiscation, and Durie suggests their numbers were not affected until the 1890s.[13]

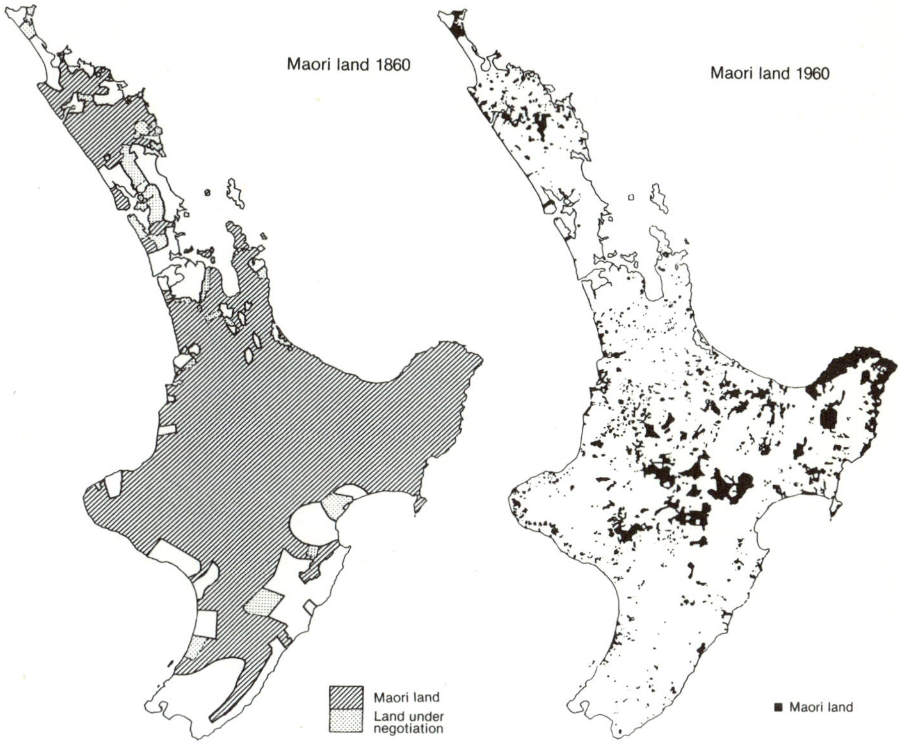

Figure 19: Māori holdings in the North Island 1860 and 1960
Source: from R. Walker, *Ka Whawhai Tonu Matou: Struggle without End* (Auckland: Penguin, 2004).

Is there evidence of differentials in mortality related to dispossession? Pool has proposed that a surrogate measure for mortality in Māori communities in the 1800s (when deaths were particularly common early in life) might be the ratio of children per 100 women 15 years and over.[126] The reasoning here is that when child mortality is low, the number of children is high in comparison with the number of women of reproductive age. It is assumed here that fertility (the other influence on child numbers) did not vary as strongly between iwi as did mortality.

Child:woman ratios certainly did differ between iwi and over time (Figure 20), and there does appear to be a link of some kind with the timing and extent of land losses, although it is not entirely consistent. The lowest ratios (and by implication, the worst child health) in the last quarter of the nineteenth century were seen in Taranaki, where alienation of land was late but severe. The highest ratio of children to women was observed amongst Ngāpuhi, from the far north, and the South Island iwi. These tribes were not subject to confiscation in the same way as Taranaki, but only because their lands had been lost very early in European settlement.

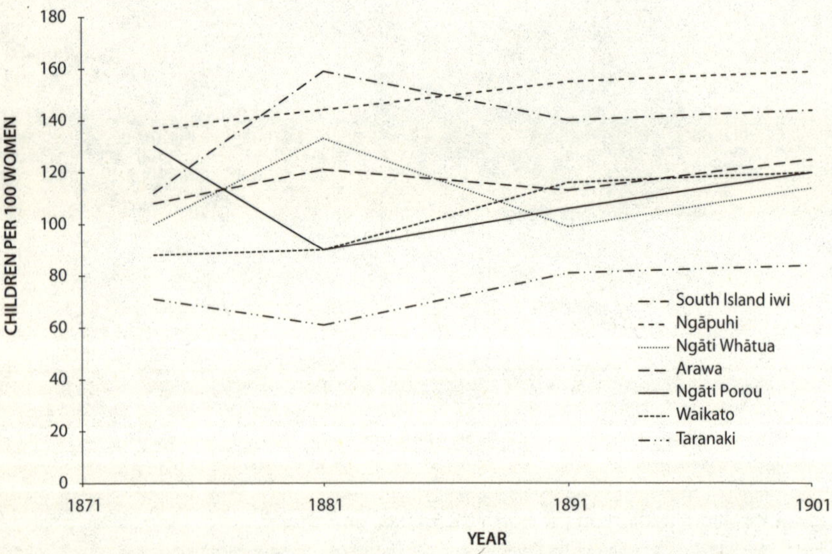

Figure 20: Children per 100 women 15 years and over, by iwi, 1874–1901

Source: D. I. Pool, *Te Iwi Maori: A New Zealand Population, Past, Present and Projected* (Auckland: Auckland University Press, 1991).

There is no obvious 'ripple effect' seen in modern-day Māori mortality – in 2010 the highest death rates were recorded in the East Cape (Ngāti Porou territory, where iwi have retained much of their land), and the lowest rates applied in the South Island (where Ngāi Tahu's losses began soon after European settlement). However, regional comparisons of this kind need to be treated with caution, as the large-scale migration of Māori to urban areas after World War II affected different parts of the country in different ways.

In general, iwi that fought with the Crown in the Land Wars, including most of Te Arawa, Ngāti Porou and Ngāti Kahungunu, held onto their land for longer than those who took up arms on the other side. However, it is not evident in Figure 20 that mortality trends for these tribes stand out in any way. We note also that land transfers continued in the early 1900s, although at a slower rate than before, and this was a time when mortality fell and life expectancy among Māori increased substantially.

The wider history of what happened across the Pacific lends some support to Mason Durie's argument. Stephen Kunitz has examined the impact of colonisation on indigenous populations in the region, and points out that the effects were uneven. Some countries fared much better than others.[258] For instance, in Samoa and Tonga the decline in populations following European occupation was slight; Hawai'i was affected even more severely than New Zealand. The differences cannot be attributed to infectious disease – all the Pacific islands were exposed to new pathogens, and at roughly the same time. But the intensity of contact and manner of occupation did vary. Samoa and Tonga did not provide the opportunities for plantation settlement that were obvious in Hawai'i, nor were these territories suitable for the agricultural industries that thrived further south in New Zealand. Samoa and Tonga were colonial outposts and trading hubs, strategic holdings rather than centres of production. As a result, interaction with Europeans was limited, and traditional owners kept their land, by and large. In Hawai'i, where the geography and indigenous governance structures enabled rapid transfers of large blocks of land, dispossession occurred more rapidly than almost anywhere else in the Pacific.

The loss of land may not have been the whole explanation for the reduction in Māori numbers, but it must have played an important part. As the best land passed into the hands of European farmers, kāinga made do with less desirable locations that were liable to flooding. There are many reports of crowded and poorly ventilated housing (Āpirana Ngata spoke on this topic at the first Te Aute meeting in 1897).[86] Water was taken from shallow wells, or from streams, that were often contaminated by sewage or other wastes. In some settlements, there were no latrines at all, and in others, the sanitary facilities were inadequate. (Raeburn Lange quotes a report by a Native Sanitary Inspector of a settlement in 1908 with 2995 people in 107 kāinga and a total of 26 'closets'.)[86] These conditions certainly favoured the rapid spread of infectious diseases such as typhoid fever, but poor hygiene was not confined to Māori settlements. Some typhoid outbreaks were caused by discharge of raw sewage from European settlements into open waterways, which then polluted traditional gathering sites for shellfish and other kai moana.[259] All these problems were worse when large numbers of people moved to temporary housing, pursuing opportunities for employment (in the gum fields, for instance), or attending the Native Land Court.

At the time, the poor state of Māori housing was sometimes attributed to loss of traditional knowledge. Riapo Puhipi, a sanitary inspector, wrote in 1908 that 'the Māori no longer knows how to build these houses properly, like their ancestors did'.[86] There may have been some truth in this, but lack of money was also an important factor. Pākehā institutions, law and custom placed Māori on the margins of the national economy, and without cash it was difficult to build safe settlements in the western manner. There were no state subsidies, and the banks would not provide credit – indeed, Māori were excluded from all provision for housing finance until the 1930s.[153]

In Māori diets, wheat, corn and potatoes were added to the traditional staples. Old ways of processing and preserving food were applied to the new items (e.g., kānga pirau or fermented corn followed the same approach taken to treating karaka berries). When food was plentiful, it is unlikely that this transitional diet had a great influence on the health of the population. But often food was not plentiful, and then children and infants were particularly at risk of under-nutrition. For instance, early weaning using bulky and indigestible milk-substitutes may have contributed to high mortality in the first year of life.

Alcohol contributed also. Drink cost money that would otherwise be spent on food, it caused violence and disrupted family life, and in many ways compounded the poor living conditions that Māori experienced at the time. Archdeacon Walsh, in his 1907 paper on 'The Passing of the Māori',[135] laid much of the blame on those who supplied the grog:

> The evil would not have been as great as it was had the liquor been of even average quality; but a special brand was supplied for the 'Native trade', which was maddening in its immediate effect and poisonous in its ultimate results.

More important was tobacco, which was widely used by Māori and was often included by European observers in their descriptions of harmful habits. This was a case of double standards, since tobacco use in other contexts was accepted. A. K. Newman, for example, who probably would not have batted an eyelid when a colleague at the Northern Club lit up his pipe, claimed –

> . . . the incessant smoking of the most fiery brands, by men, women and children, is certainly productive of a lowered vitality, which shows itself in an enfeebled progeny, and renders all classes more accessible to evil influences.[252]

Certain Māori cultural practices were regarded by non-Māori as health-damaging. Tangi (funerals) were singled out in particular, since they attracted large numbers of people, who (through European eyes) congregated in poor living conditions, imposed a significant economic burden on their hosts and presented excellent opportunities for outbreaks of infection. Clothing habits were also blamed for poor health. This was a time when Māori were shifting from traditional garments to European clothing, but did not always follow European norms. 'Overclad one day, half-naked the next, is there a wonder Tamati dies?' wrote Māui Pōmare.[86]

The focus in European reports on archaic and harmful traditions, inappropriate clothing, unhealthy diets, and the use of alcohol and tobacco neglected the underlying causes of decline, which were political, cultural and economic. But they did point to important signs of Māori in transition. Māori were moving from old ways of organising their settlements and making sense of the world to new ways of living; in between, they were at risk. We suggest this shift was at the heart of both the nineteenth-century decline in Māori health and the subsequent recovery.

RECOVERY

When did decline in the Māori population end and recovery begin? The life expectancy figures graphed in Figure 18 suggest there may have been modest improvements in life expectancy in the 1870s and 1880s, followed by the influenza-driven dip of the 1890s, and consistent gains thereafter. The child:woman ratios (Figure 20) also are evidence that conditions were improving before the turn of the twentieth century.

Belich argues that birth rates were improving from the mid-1800s but were not reflected in population growth until the 1900s because mortality was so high.[256] It seems to be the case, from observations made at the time, that fertility recovered before there was a substantial improvement in mortality rates, but again, good information is lacking. One explanation for the rebound in births might be an increasing reproductive span for women, secondary to steady improvements in diet through the 1800s (albeit with frequent disruptions due to displacement, epidemics and economic depressions). The potential range, variety and quantity of food that was available to Māori communities benefited from the introduction of European cultivars and domesticated animals (the pig especially), and technologies that allowed more efficient harvesting of traditional foods (e.g., metal hooks and spears, and stronger and lighter nets).[162; 85]

Infectious diseases were the dominant cause of mortality amongst Māori throughout this period (and were still responsible for more than half the deaths among Māori in 1936).[126] Therefore the improvement in life expectancy from the late 1800s must signal a decline in the incidence or severity of infections. To some extent this may have been due to specific improvements in nutrition, housing and the standard of living. But the reduced virulence of what had been novel and devastating infections might also be part of the general process of adaptation as human populations respond to new pathogens.

The historian William McNeill has studied the impact of infectious diseases on immunologically vulnerable groups in other parts of the world, the Americas especially. He observed that typically it took 100–150 years for populations such as the Inca to reach a new demographic equilibrium.[48] Whatever the important biological and cultural components of adaptation might be, it took roughly four to six generations, McNeill reports, before population decline was halted and recovery began. The timing certainly fits with our best estimates of the fall and rise of Māori (see chapter 2), although the extent of de-population was much less in New Zealand. At the lowest point, the number of Māori was perhaps a sixth of that pre-contact; McNeill estimates that Amerindian numbers were reduced to a 20th to 25th of the pre-Columbian era.

Infections continued to be a serious cause of ill-health: in 1938 a measles epidemic is thought to have caused one in ten of the deaths among Māori in that year. The largest outbreak of smallpox in New Zealand occurred in 1913. This was concentrated in the Auckland province and affected Māori disproportionately (there were about 2000 cases and 55 deaths, compared with five deaths among non-Māori).[259]

But the influenza epidemic of 1918 was the most serious setback to Māori recovery. While Māori deaths were not fully counted, it is estimated that the death rate nation-wide was five to ten times greater than for non-Māori.[260] Young adults were particularly badly affected: Pool estimates as many as 10 per cent of Māori men aged 30–34 died in the three-month period October to December 1918.[162] There was great variation by region. Fatalities per year varied from eight per 1000 in Hawke's Bay to over 80 in Thames and South Taranaki.[261] Nursing and symptomatic care helped blunt the force of the disease, but did not equalise mortality rates. In the 1919 'flu epidemic, Māori and non-Māori soldiers were treated side by side in the same military hospitals. The difference in outcomes by ethnicity was less than that seen in the general population, but Māori soldiers were still twice as likely to die from influenza (Figure 21, overleaf).[262] Māori remained at a disadvantage in the 1957 and 2009 outbreaks, although the absolute level of mortality was two to three orders of magnitude less than in 1919.

The single biggest contributor to the fall in mortality amongst non-Māori in the first half of the twentieth century was the reduction in deaths due to tuberculosis. Was this the case for Māori also? It is difficult to tell, because although notification of pulmonary tuberculosis was made compulsory in 1901 and the first sanatorium for treatment of the disease opened in 1903, all efforts in the early years focused on non-Māori.[263] There were some changes after a Parliamentary Committee of Inquiry (1928) recognised that Māori were affected particularly severely, but they were still not included in the regular statistics nor were they given access to treatments. As a consequence, the first systematic survey of TB amongst Māori was not undertaken until 1933, in Waiapu on the East Coast. H. B. Turbott, who led the study, reported that disease was common (more than 1 in 20 of those in the survey were suffering from tuberculosis) and the death rate was ten times the non-Māori rate nationally. Nevertheless, few cases of TB were reported to local doctors, and few deaths from TB were recorded correctly in the official statistics.[264] (There was reluctance also among non-Māori to identify as 'consumptives', given the social stigma and practical disruptions that followed official notification, with little evidence at this time that diagnosis greatly benefited the individual patient.)

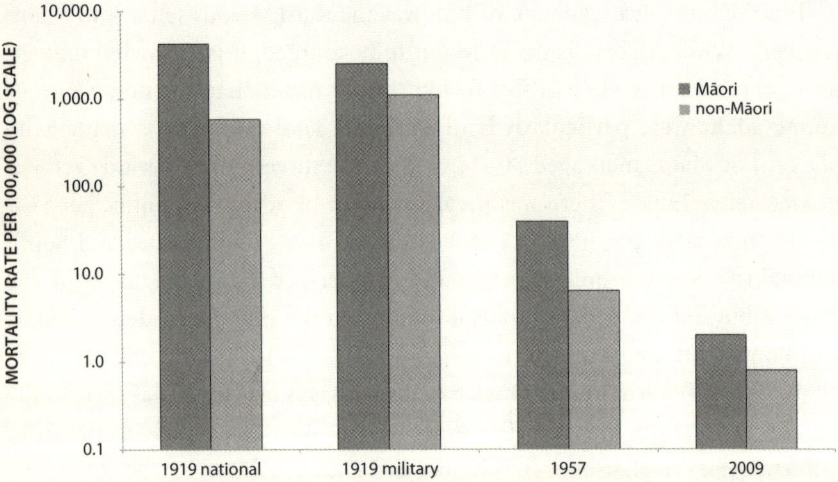

Figure 21: Mortality from influenza per 100,000 population, New Zealand, in three epidemics (1919, 1957, 2009)

Source: N. Wilson, L. T. Barnard, et al., 'Differential Mortality Rates by Ethnicity in 3 Influenza Pandemics Over a Century, New Zealand' (*Emerging Infectious Diseases* 18, no. 1 [2012]: 71–77).

Steps taken following the Committee of Inquiry included an increase in the number of district nurses working with Māori communities, and education that urged Māori to improve their housing, avoid crowded conditions, take a healthy diet and seek treatment early if symptoms of disease occurred. Some attention was paid to 'upstream' factors that affected the living conditions of Māori (the Native Housing Act of 1935, for example, and removal of the barriers to bank credit for housing), but these interventions were implemented only slowly. In the five years after the Housing Act was passed, Linda Bryder writes, only 478 houses had been built nation-wide, although there were about 45,000 Māori thought to be living in inadequate accommodation.[263]A survey in the South Auckland Health District in 1938 found that 80 per cent of Māori houses had an unsatisfactory water supply and 62 per cent lacked sanitary facilities.[259] The factors that deterred Māori from using treatment facilities (including location – few services were placed in the areas in which the bulk of Māori lived) received little attention prior to World War II.

In the 1940s mortality in south India was similar to that experienced by Māori at the end of the 1800s. One close observer of the rapid improvement that was made in India post-independence (roughly five years of life expectancy added each decade), Jack Caldwell, has argued that the root cause was a paradigm shift in views of the natural world.[6] He called it modernisation, but this meant more than physical changes, such as buildings and services, electric power and better transport systems (although all these improvements certainly did contribute to health gains). Caldwell argued that modernisation was essentially a change in thinking, driven to a large extent by the extension of formal education, to conceive of illness as amenable to human intervention:

> Declining mortality has been part of a profound social revolution, and even a theological one in terms of moving ever more areas of behaviour into the secular domain.

and

> The progress of modern medicine is even more a question of demand rather than supply. For many diseases the growth of that demand has been made possible only by a reinterpretation of the essentially religious concept of illness and its cure.

The immediate causes of death in south India differed from those that applied in New Zealand among Māori. Old World infections such as measles and whooping cough did not have the same devastating effects in India, where malaria and other 'tropical' illnesses were prominent. However, the social changes that cause populations to be more resilient, wherever they are placed and whatever the local pathogens may be, bear some similarities.

In south India, Caldwell nominated social changes and interventions that he believed made an important contribution to mortality decline. He emphasised the more effective use of health care, resulting largely from the education and empowerment of women, who were not only provided with specific knowledge but also gained a more confident world-view. Associated with the extension of education and social change more broadly, was the secularisation of illness – people resorted less frequently to magical explanations. Caldwell reported that the allocation of food in times of shortage was more equal, and this benefited especially women, who traditionally received less than other members of the family. Smaller families meant that more attention could be paid to each child, whose health benefited as a result. Public health improvements, especially in water and sanitation, were important, but Caldwell noted that before these technologies could be effective, there had to be a shift in thinking, and in particular putting aside caste notions of pollution.

In New Zealand, 50 years earlier, one can point to greater acceptance of western technologies, treatments and explanations for illness; more effective involvement of Māori communities in public health interventions; expansion of primary education and a drive to open up opportunities for women (e.g., through nurse training); and improvements in housing, sanitation, infant nutrition and other aspects of primary health care. These changes did not take place in a regulatory vacuum. Enabling legislation included the 1900 Public Health Act and the Maori Councils Act of the same year.

The Caldwell thesis is anticipated in the writings of Sir Peter Buck (Te Rangi Hīroa), who argued that the turnaround in mortality in New Zealand resulted largely from a change in popular attitudes to disease.[87] The commonest explanation of illness, in Māori tradition, was that there had been a violation of sacredness, and this had resulted in an intervention of the spirits. Buck contrasted the rapid and generally uncomplicated recovery from injury that Māori were familiar with, and which required no supernatural explanation, with the impact of diseases that need not be fatal, but were seen as beyond human intervention. The beliefs that underlay traditional health care provided coherent explanations, a rationale for treatment and reassurance. But when Europeans occupied New Zealand the old explanations could not account for the nature and magnitude of the problems that Māori faced, and in some respects, the persistence of traditional attitudes may have blocked opportunities for recovery.

This argument should not be pressed too far. There is ample evidence that Māori recognised, early on, the value of western technology, including medicines,[265] and it is apparent from letters to early missionaries that Māori actively sought interventions such as vaccinations, drugs and surgical treatments.[266] However, Buck's point was that as Māori engaged more and more with new value systems and knowledge, the fear of tapu and sorcery declined, and people were more willing to accept other explanations for illness. As Caldwell observed in India, such a change in mind-set would be empowering in many ways. It opened the door to using facilities and services where these were available, and the new world-view prompted individuals and communities to agitate for services when they were not provided.

The Young Maori movement is one of the best-known examples of late nineteenth-century agitation for change. It began with the Te Aute College Old Boys' Association, formed to improve Māori welfare, and Āpirana Ngata was the secretary. (At the first meeting, held at Taumataomihi in Ngāti Porou territory, one of the suggestions was to insert windows in the back wall of meeting houses to improve ventilation. There was strong resistance from traditionalists, but the reformers won the argument.) The Old Boys' Association developed into the Young Maori Party, and students from the three Māori boys' secondary schools, Te Aute, St Stephen's and Three Kings, were active in the work of the Party. Amongst other issues, the Party agitated for government grants to support education – Buck and Tūtere Wī Repa were awarded the first of these, and both enrolled in the medical school in Dunedin.

Changes in health administration assisted the modernising agenda. When the Department of Public Health was established in 1900, Māui Pōmare returned from the United States to take the position of Medical Officer of Health to the Maori. Maori Health Councils were established to draft health and sanitary by-laws that were adapted to the local conditions. Rules were drawn up specifically for funerals, and instructions were given on how to protect marae water supplies and to dispose of waste safely. Village committees had the job of putting the by-laws into practice, guided by health inspectors (sometimes chiefs were appointed to add their mana to the endeavour) and district nurses. Temporary field hospitals were established when there were epidemics, so that patients could be cared for without leaving their villages. Extended use of new technologies (such as the typhoid vaccine, first prepared in Europe in 1896) was carried out on a village-by-village basis by Māori health workers.[86]

The success of the sanitary and health reforms depended on gaining the trust and acceptance of Māori. Ngata, Pōmare, Buck and Wī Repa were well-placed since they had a scientific education and knowledge of te reo and Māori culture. (Buck describes an argument in which he was involved over the building of latrines. An elder objected that these were Pākehā inventions. Buck responded with references to legend and to local history, which included specific mention of the importance of latrines in traditional settlements.)[87] Nevertheless, the reformers struggled to overcome barriers that stood between Māori and the health system. Hospitals were much distrusted, often with good reason, given the attitudes of staff to Māori patients (and the frequency of cross-infection). There was also some resistance to compulsory registration of deaths, since with registration came post-mortem examinations, and these were seen as mutilating procedures that handicapped the deceased in the afterlife.

Buck, Pōmare, Ngata, their mentor James Carroll and others in the reform movement were only partially successful. They wanted the benefits of western thinking and technology while advancing simultaneously Māori identity and Māori culture, and they made greater progress towards the first aim than the second. The official position of the Young Maori Party was that identity and culture was the platform on which the Māori recovery should proceed. However, members of the Party did not have a common view on how far traditions needed to bend to fit the new age. Ngata, according to Ranginui Walker, 'was the one most steeped in Māori culture', while Pōmare perhaps was the figure who identified most closely with European values.[95]

The truth was that New Zealand society in the early 1900s had little sympathy for Māoritanga in any form. Use of the Māori language was actively discouraged; Māori religions were side-lined; and Māori practices of diagnosis and healing were not merely discouraged, but outlawed (the Tohunga Suppression Act was passed in 1907). There was a strong antipathy to notions of self-determination and community control, particularly when they were practised by Māori. The Health Councils and village committees that were established as mechanisms for administering public health had very little power in any other respect and survived in their original form for only a decade. Education on health and health care aimed to reshape Māori attitudes and behaviours – there were no efforts to challenge the cultural presumptions of non-Māori until many decades later. Compulsion was freely applied by public health authorities to over-ride Māori reluctance. The Taranaki Hospital Board, for example, in 1911 called on police to ensure that people suffering from typhoid were admitted to hospital.[86]

However, there were also important changes for the better. In the first third of the twentieth century the District Nursing Service expanded its work among Māori, water supplies were secured in many settlements (often through the initiative of local communities) and housing was greatly improved in many places. H. B. Turbott, Medical Officer of Health, reported from the East Cape in 1929:

> . . . the tendency is to get away from the pas. Better houses are being built, tanks are coming into favour for water supplies, the adoption of privies, general in some areas, is extending rapidly in the remainder. Huis and tangis are conducted in a satisfactory manner, suggestions for the betterment of sanitary arrangements being always attended to promptly.[259]

In some accounts, the Young Maori reform movement is synonymous with modernisation in the early 1900s. This overlooks other significant players, such as the Maori Parliament (Kotahitanga, 1892 to 1902) that preceded the Te Aute group by a decade, and was instrumental in setting the agenda of the Health Councils and helped slow down the attrition of Māori lands. There were other Māori leaders who played important parts in the recovery. Typically they placed greater emphasis on sovereignty and Māori autonomy than did Pomare and Buck, and felt the path of 'engagement and adaptation' gave away too much.[267] Those who took a rather more robustly independent approach to the state included Te Puea Hērangi, one of the foremost leaders of the Kīngitanga (King Movement) in the early twentieth century; Tahupōtiki Wiremu Rātana, founder of the Rātana church in 1918; and Hōne Heke Ngāpua, leader in the Kotahitanga movement.

CONCLUSION

We know that Māori mortality was high in the second half of the nineteenth century. It is difficult to discern trends, but the rapid and severe decline in the population must mean that life expectancy for Māori deteriorated during this time. The reduction in numbers of Māori occurred too quickly to be explained by low fertility alone. From around 1890 onwards, we believe life expectancy rebounded, and the improvement continued through the first half of the twentieth century, despite influenza epidemics, economic recessions and the assimilationist policies that prevailed in health and social welfare. The deterioration in Māori health had occurred alongside dispossession, impoverishment and displacement. The recovery in life expectancy proceeded ahead of economic development, in the face of continuing loss of Māori land, and without a serious attempt by government to provide culturally appropriate services. The most persuasive explanations for the turnaround include adaptation to serious infections (through biological and behavioural mechanisms that are not well understood), a growing understanding and acceptance by Māori of public health principles, better access to more effective health care and general improvements in living conditions. Māori communities were engaged at a number of levels, from councils to parliaments, aided by Māori leaders who worked successfully in both their traditional culture and the post-colonial world.

5

Post-World War II

Convergence

New Zealand non-Māori fell off the top of world rankings in life expectancy about 1940, the entry point to this chapter. In order to understand the trajectory of mortality after World War II, we focus on cause-specific death rates, since for the first time there is sufficient information for such fine-grain analysis. We include some data from before 1940 (non-Māori only) and also go forward in time, in some instances, beyond 1980, to prevent unnecessary duplication of material across chapters. We undertake only a cursory analysis of the impact of health systems on mortality trends, given that this matter receives close attention in the post-1980s chapter.

Social influences continue to shape upstream causes of health and disease. The period starts with implementation of the 1938 Social Security Act. New Zealand was the first country in the British Commonwealth to establish the principle of public responsibility for health services, and to provide free care for all based on an income-related social security levy. The chapter finishes with the economic crisis of the 1980s, which was caused by rupture of the export umbilical cord to 'mother England'. In this setting we investigate ways in which economic and social change influenced mortality. For instance, New Zealand's role as a major exporter of meat and dairy products may have affected the country's capacity to adopt new paradigms of healthy behaviour when the predominant causes of mortality changed from infectious diseases to chronic conditions such as heart disease and stroke.

Māori life expectancy over this period increased markedly, compared to modest improvements for non-Māori males and females. Thus, there was tremendous convergence. Many factors may have contributed to the reduction in ethnic inequalities, including non-Māori encountering the full force of the cardiovascular disease epidemic, making the previous astounding declines in mortality rates unachievable; rapidly decreasing infectious disease and infant mortality rates among Māori; and underlying social trends such as urbanisation and improved socio-economic conditions for Māori.

LIFE EXPECTANCY AND ALL-CAUSE MORTALITY TRENDS

Māori life expectancy continued to rise, increasing by 18 years for males (from 46 in 1936 [there are no 1941 estimates for Māori] to 65 years in 1981) and by 23 years for females (from 46 to 69 years) (Figure 22). Put another way, there were four years of life expectancy gained for every decade among Māori males, and an extra five years per decade among females. That is, with each passing calendar year, female Māori life expectancy increased by half a year.

We note another important milestone: around 1940 female Māori life expectancy overtook Māori males, most likely due to a dramatic improvement in maternal mortality (more on this later in the chapter).[268]

The rise in life expectancy among non-Māori slowed, and for men, there was barely any improvement at all between 1956 and 1976. In the 40 years after 1941, non-Māori male life expectancy increased by 5.2 years, from 65.6 to 70.8 years. Female non-Māori life expectancy increased by 7.8 years, from 69.1 to 76.9 years. Overall, this was about a third of the improvement of Māori.

A third of the gain in Māori life expectancy between 1950–52 and 1960–62 was due to falling infant mortality, about 20 per cent can be linked to reductions in child deaths, and just about all the rest was due to improvements in the 15–44 year-old-age group (Figure 39, in next chapter).[2] This pattern changed during the 1970s, when roughly half the increase in Māori life expectancy was due to improvements among those aged 45+, and infant and child (1–14-year-old) mortality only contributed about 10 per cent each. These estimates by

Statistics New Zealand are prone to error in the coding of ethnicity, but they are probably about right – and certainly are consistent with what we would expect to see during an epidemiological transition that shifted the force of mortality to older age groups.

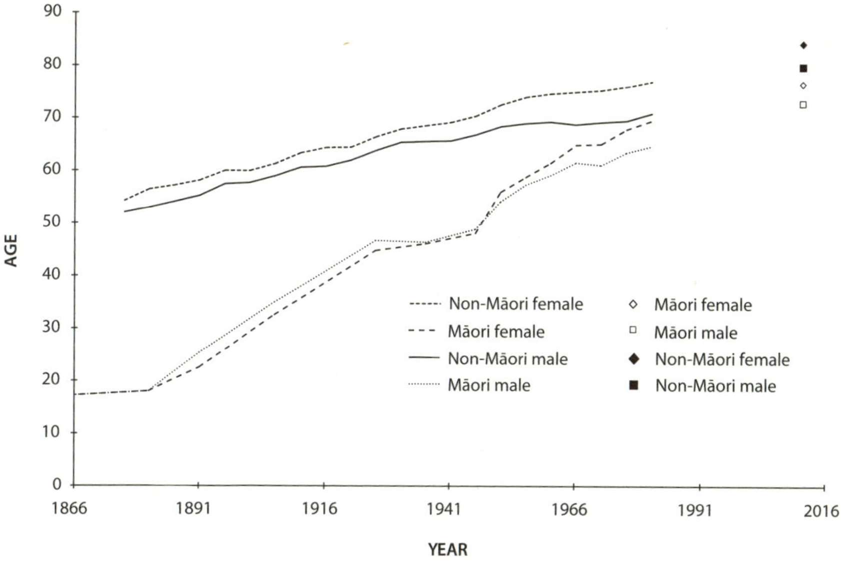

Figure 22: Life expectancy of Māori and non-Māori, 1860 to 1980, and 2011

Source: Data drawn from I. Pool, 'Mortality Trends and Differentials', *Country Monograph Series No. 12: Population of New Zealand*, edited by Population Division Economic and Social Commission for Asia and the Pacific (New York: United Nations, 1985: 209–42).

Figure 23 displays mortality rates by age group, sex and ethnicity, abstracted from data by Ian Pool.[162] We employ a log scale, so parallel lines should be interpreted as similar percentage or relative reductions over time. The starting point for Māori is 1945 because there are no reliable age-specific mortality data available before that date. Note that the steepest rates of decline are for 0–4 and 5–14-year-olds among Māori, consistent with these age groups driving most of the increase in life expectancy. Some of the apparent lack of decline in mortality rates among 65+-year-olds will be due to this group's average age increasing over time (rates are not age-standardised within age bands). All the same, it is clear that most of the action in this period was occurring in younger age groups (children and young adults especially).

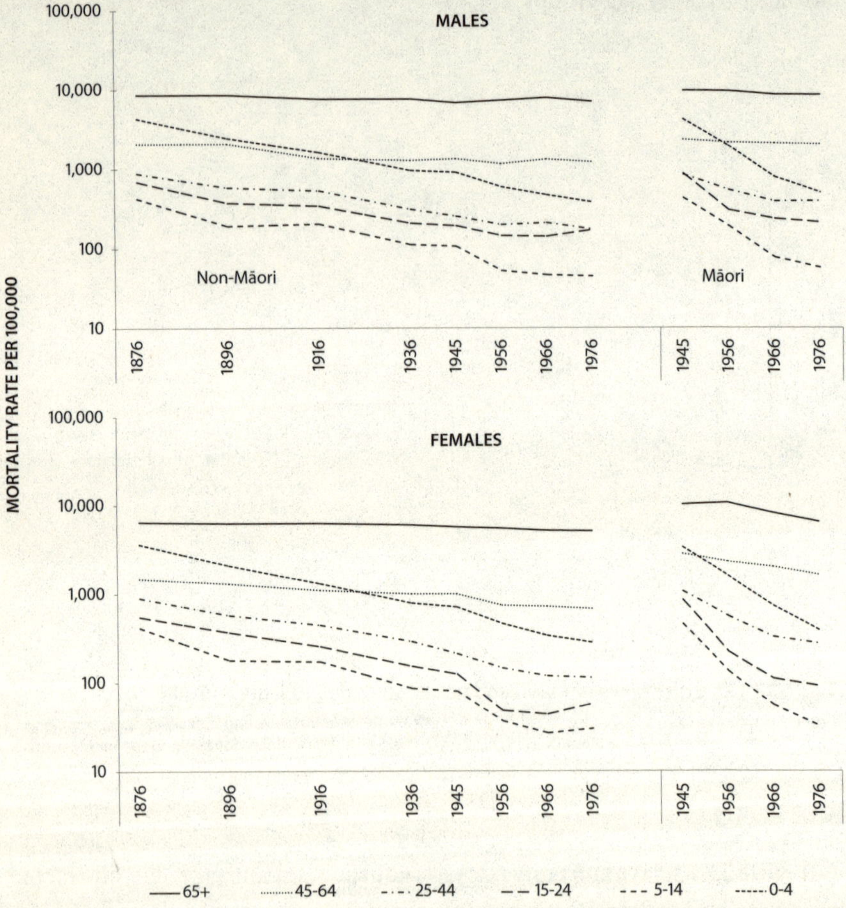

Figure 23: Māori and non-Māori all-cause mortality (log scale) by age

Source: I. Pool, 'Mortality Trends and Differentials', *Country Monograph Series No. 12: Population of New Zealand*, edited by Population Division Economic and Social Commission for Asia and the Pacific (New York: United Nations, 1985: 209–42).

There were similar changes among non-Māori. For example, infant mortality decreased by about 60 per cent from the 1940s to 1980s. However, there was little change in 45+-year-olds' mortality rates, and modest gains (and sometimes reversals) among 15–24-year-olds, which combined to put the brake on what had been a long-term improvement in life expectancy. We pin the blame on the ischaemic heart disease epidemic, which peaked among middle and older age New Zealanders, and the effects of road traffic crashes and suicides among young adults.

Other rich countries had the same experience – steep declines from 1940 to 1980. However, there are some important differences. From the 1940s to 1980s non-Māori infant mortality slipped from being the best ranked in the world, and now trailed countries such as Australia, Canada, Denmark, England and Wales, Finland, Norway, Scotland and Sweden (Figure 10). For example, female infant mortality among non-Māori reduced from 24 per 1000 in the 1940s to 9.5 per 1000 in the 1980s, but other countries' rates fell even further (5.6 to 8.7 per 1000).[164] Among 15–19-year-olds, mortality rates actually increased over this period in New Zealand (due to road traffic crash deaths in particular) compared to some decrease or no change in other countries. In older age groups, the ranking of New Zealand non-Māori remained much the same over time. Of note, Māori had consistently higher age-specific mortality than all other countries.

There was a striking convergence of life expectancies during this period. Amongst so-called MDCs (more developed countries), what was a 40-year spread in life expectancy in the 1940s between the highest- and lowest-ranked countries shrank to a 5–10-year range in 1980.[8] One possible explanation for this coming together is that while critical improvements in social circumstances and living conditions occurred sooner in some places than others, the health benefits diffused rapidly. This meant rapid gains initially for pioneer countries, followed by even faster gains by late-adopters (and hence convergence). Before the Second World War this life expectancy 'catch-up' followed the emergence, and subsequent dispersion, of knowledge and technologies to control infectious diseases. After the war the main barrier to further mortality decline was the chronic diseases, and the next surge in life expectancy was led by countries that first worked out how to control problems such as ischaemic heart disease and stroke.

Japan's recovery after 1945 began with the eradication of malnutrition, thanks in large part to the American-sponsored whaling industry that in 1947 provided more than half the meat consumed in Japan.[269] The subsequent, sustained decline in mortality (22 years of extra life expectancy in four decades) resulted from concerted public health interventions, aimed first at infectious diseases and then at the prevention of stroke. Stroke was overcome by cutting the amount of salt in the diet, and increasing the use of anti-hypertensive drugs population-wide, via a comprehensive health insurance system.[270]

New Zealand was not a complete laggard when it came to tackling chronic disease mortality, but it was not at the front of the pack either. We speculate that what acted in New Zealand's favour in one period (pre-World War II) may, in some respects, have held the country back subsequently when it was faced with a different range of diseases. A diet rich in meat, dairy products and protein may be a positive factor when food is limited and infectious diseases are the major cause of mortality, but by virtue of the associated high levels of saturated fat such a diet is a liability when food is plentiful and heart disease is the number-one cause of death.

Māori were a step behind in this transition. In the first 30 years after World War II, Māori achieved strong increases in life expectancy because of continuing improvements in infectious disease and child mortality, and these resulted in gains in life expectancy despite the lack of progress with chronic diseases.

Period or cohort effects?

An increase in life expectancy might be explained by mortality rates falling at the same (or a similar) rate across all age groups, or by a particularly healthy birth cohort reaching an age when their better-than-usual mortality figures influence average life expectancy for the whole population. An example of the first scenario (a 'period effect') would be population-wide falls in the amount of saturated fat in the diet, causing a decline in cardiovascular disease (CVD) rates in all age groups in parallel. An example of the other (the 'cohort effect') might be seen when individuals born at an adverse time in history (e.g., when food was scarce, or tuberculosis rates particularly high) carry the effects of this early adversity (e.g., higher rates of heart disease in adult life, or re-activated TB when immune function weakens) into older ages. Period and cohort effects do get blurred. For example, a change in tobacco consumption can have rapid effects with short time lags (e.g., an increase in heart attacks; a period effect), and delayed effects for a cohort who have a longer and more intense exposure to tobacco over their lifetime resulting in particularly high cancer rates in old age (a cohort effect).

Disentangling period and cohort effects can be challenging mathematically. However, sometimes the effects are so marked that they stand out in a simple display of age-specific rates by calendar year. Figure 24, overleaf, shows such a graph for New Zealand for Māori and non-Māori combined, using data from Statistics New Zealand.[2] Each connected line of points is for mortality rates for a five-year age group (at death), by calendar year from left to right. For example, 60–64-year-old male mortality rates are much the same from 1946 to 1971, then decrease steadily to 2006. Note that the 60–64-year-old series only commences around 1946, the time at which the first birth cohort included in this data (those born 1876–81) had aged into the 60–64-year age group. This explains why each advancing age-group line starts a further five years to the right, and indeed one can track a birth cohort step-wise by going up one line, and five calendar years to the right.

To reduce clutter, we have excluded infants and 1–4-year-olds, and mortality rates (on the y-axis) are plotted on a log scale. Note also that the graph includes war deaths; these show up as large spikes in young adult male mortality in 1914–19 and 1939–45. Steep reductions in child mortality (5–9 and 10–14-year-olds) are present throughout. However, there is an obvious levelling-out in young adult mortality (15–19 to 30–34-year-olds) between roughly 1961 and 1991 – we see here the impacts of road traffic crash fatalities and suicide deaths (presented in more detail below).

The feature of special relevance is the simultaneous downturn in mortality in all the middle-to-older age groups – especially among males. For 40–44 to 75–79-year-olds up to 1970, there was little improvement. After 1970, the mortality graphs for all the older age groups turn and decline at similar rates. This is a classic period effect. (A cohort effect would manifest as staggered inflection points, such as 1971 for 40–44-year-olds, 1976 for 45–49-year-olds, 1981 for 50–54-year-olds, and so on as a 'healthy cohort' traversed its way diagonally up the graph, jumping from line to line.) This pattern matches the fall in mortality rates for cardiovascular disease that was also observed in all age groups.[271] It tells us that the causes of reduced mortality (e.g., declines in smoking and consumption of saturated fat) changed right across society, not just within some birth cohorts. There may be subtle cohort effects as well. For example, people born about 1950 reached teenage years just as the full knowledge of tobacco's harm was becoming apparent, and therefore this cohort may have been less likely than those who were teenagers before them to ever try smoking. But if effects such as this are present, they are too subtle to show up in Figure 24.

The pattern is less obvious among females. There may be an inflection point c.1970 for 55–59 to 70–74-year-olds, but it is really only visible given prior knowledge from looking at the male figure first. But this is not too surprising, as we know that the CVD epidemic was slower to get under way, and was less pronounced, among females.

Cause-specific mortality and risk-factor trends

We suggest that the history of life expectancy provokes a natural sequence of questions:

1. What are the overall trends?
2. What are the predominant changes by age group?
3. What causes of death act most strongly on trends in life expectancy?
4. What changes in risk factors and lifestyles explain the cause of death trends?
5. Has the health system had any role, either through prevention or treatment?
6. What upstream social forces (e.g., economic conditions, migration) influence risk factors and health services?

We have reviewed the first two questions (overall trends and mortality by age group), and now turn to questions 3 and 4 (which are more pleasing to tackle together). Cause of death data are definitely of better quality than in the nineteenth century – but information on Māori is inferior still to that for non-Māori, at all points in time. Figure 25 presents mortality trends by cause of death (again, note the logarithmic scale). This information comes from the work of demographer Ian Pool.[162] The trends – for non-Māori– agree closely

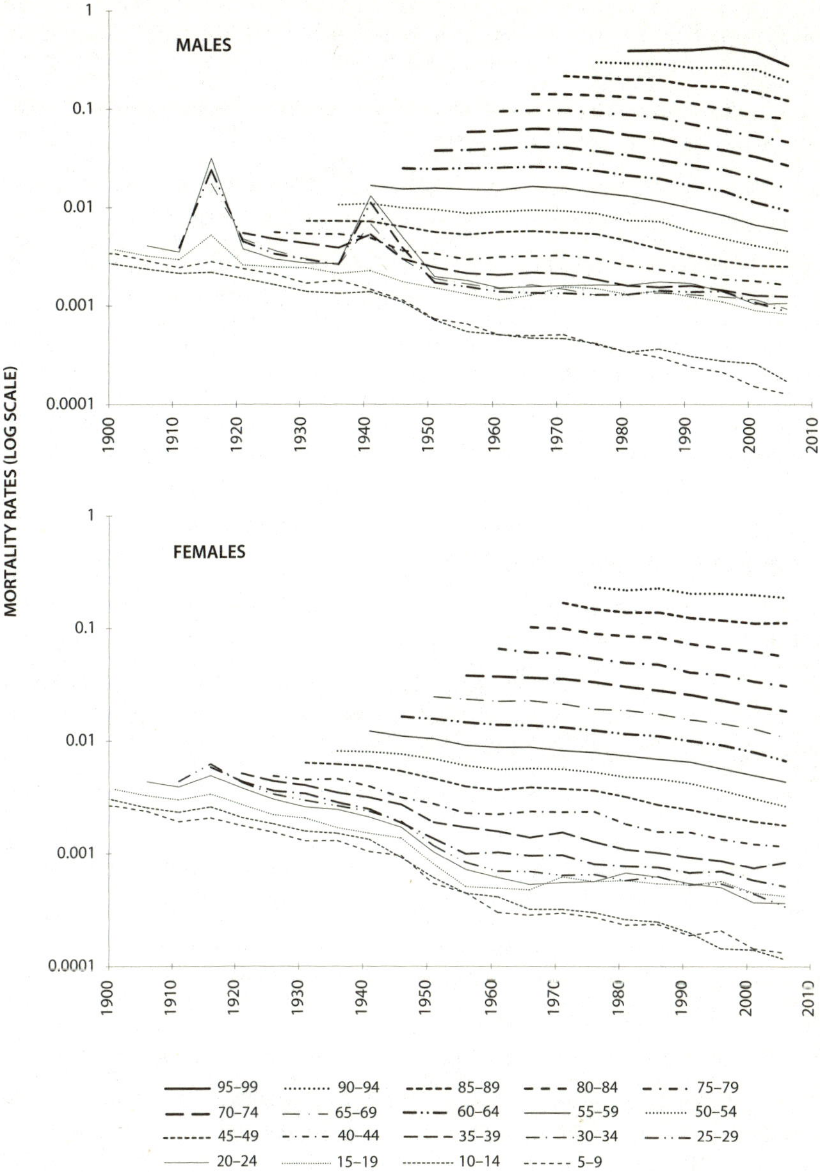

Figure 24: Mortality rates (log scale) by five-year age group by quinquennium from 1900 to 2010, by sex

Source: Statistics New Zealand, 'A History of Survival in New Zealand: Cohort Life Tables 1876–2004' (Wellington: Statistics New Zealand, 2007).

with reports by other researchers (e.g., the detailed and thorough analyses of Lancaster and Donovan).[272; 273; 274] What distinguishes Pool's work is that he went to particular effort to construct cause-specific mortality time series for both Māori and non-Māori.

There are three points to bear in mind. First, it is not possible to create reliable Māori time series pre-1945. Second, the rates for Māori are probably all prone to under-counting, and the degree of under-counting may also vary over time – we simply do not know. For this reason it is prudent not to place too much emphasis on the precise value of each rate estimate, but rather to look for broad-brush patterns. (The use of a logarithmic scale, whilst principally to accommodate diseases with large absolute variations in mortality rates, also encourages us to look at general patterns rather than precise rates.) Third, the coding of causes of death was constantly improving over time, meaning that there are very likely errors in attribution of cause of death that were more pronounced in earlier years.

Pool uses an aggregate category of 'degenerative' diseases, encompassing cardiovascular disease, and cancer and other chronic diseases. For our purposes, we want to tease this apart into cardiovascular disease (and again into ischaemic heart disease and stroke), and cancer (and again into major types of cancer). We attempt this unbundling later in the chapter.

Figure 25 illustrates remarkable reductions in mortality from many causes from 1945 to 1976 – and usually the decline was stronger among Māori. Tuberculosis mortality for 0–44-year-olds fell by a staggering 99 per cent for both Māori and non-Māori, with 80 per cent of this reduction happening in the decade 1945–55. The nosedive in TB death rates coincides with the arrival of antibiotics such as streptomycin, and other improvements in health care (such as better screening by chest X-ray).

Infectious disease and diarrhoea and related disease mortality fell by 97 per cent among 0–44-year-old Māori, and by 80 per cent for non-Māori. Rates of deaths due to accident and violence and degenerative conditions did not change. Among 45+-year-olds, reductions were not as large in percentage terms, but were impressive nevertheless. For example, tuberculosis mortality fell by 95 per cent for Māori and 90 per cent for non-Māori, and infectious disease mortality by 80 per cent and 60 per cent, respectively. However, reductions in so-called degenerative disease mortality were modest only for Māori and trivial for non-Māori, and respiratory mortality actually increased by two-thirds among non-Māori and perhaps 25 per cent among Māori (presumably a function of the tobacco epidemic). Accident and violence mortality also modestly increased for both ethnic groups.

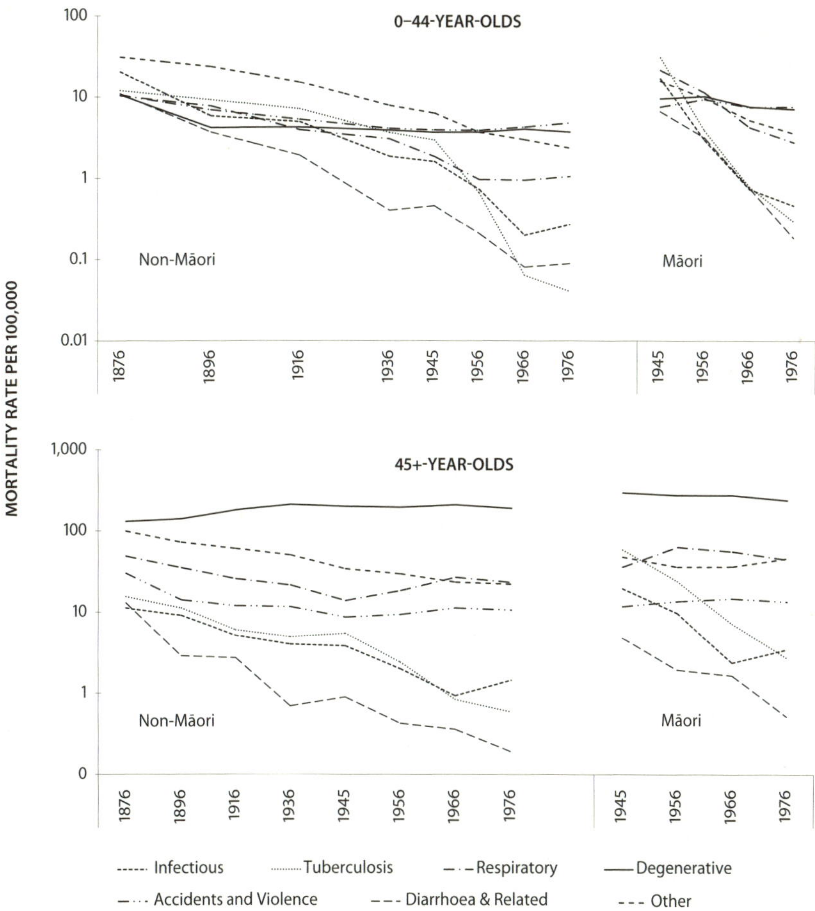

Figure 25: Māori and non-Māori cause-specific mortality (age-standardised; log scale) by age and ethnicity, sexes combined

Source: I. Pool, 'Mortality Trends and Differentials', *Country Monograph Series No. 12: Population of New Zealand*, edited by Population Division Economic and Social Commission for Asia and the Pacific (New York: United Nations, 1985: 209–42). Data have been age-standardised to the WHO World Population.

Figure 25 shows that the changes among non-Māori continued on the path that had been apparent since national statistics were first reported in 1876. Exceptions were tuberculosis, which hastened its rate of decline post-World War II, and deaths due to accidents and violence and respiratory diseases (45+-years only), which had been declining before World War II but levelled off subsequently.

In all categories Māori have higher cause-specific mortality rates. This is most evident for infectious disease, tuberculosis, respiratory and diarrhoea-related mortality among 0–44-year-old Māori, which were all at least ten times greater than among non-Māori in 1945. Positively, though, and consistent with generally faster relative declines among Māori, the ratio of Māori to non-Māori mortality was only two-fold (approximately) in 1976. An exception was deaths from tuberculosis, which remained about ten times more common amongst Māori throughout the period.

Richard Taylor and colleagues were able to construct a longer-term mortality series in Australia by reviewing and recoding death registrations back to 1907.[190] They found steep declines in infectious and 'other' mortality, offset by the massive cardiovascular disease epidemic that peaked about 1970 (as it did in New Zealand).[275] Rates of cancer rose among males, and to a lesser extent among females. In both Australia and New Zealand, 'external' deaths lingered at a high rate, especially for males, post-World War II, largely due to high road traffic crash mortality.

Cardiovascular disease mortality and risk-factor trends

The post-Second World War trends in life expectancy – across countries and sub-populations – depend heavily on what happened to cardiovascular disease mortality. The two major categories are stroke and coronary heart disease. We know enough about what causes CVD to understand the part played by personal behaviours and health services, and the underlying social determinants.

Figure 26 shows trends in coronary heart disease and stroke mortality for 'middle-age' (35–69-years-old) New Zealanders, from about 1950. (This figure – and some subsequent figures – was created by Gary Whitlock, a New Zealand-trained epidemiologist who worked at Oxford University. He created a website – www.mortality-trends.org – that generates figures for mortality trends for dozens of countries, for numerous combinations of sex and age.) The coronary heart disease epidemic peaked in New Zealand about 1970. We do not have an accurate idea of these rates before the Second World War, so we cannot confidently describe when the epidemic started and how rapidly mortality rates rose. But we can describe its fall – a startling 80 per cent reduction in middle-age mortality rates from c.1970 to the mid-2000s.

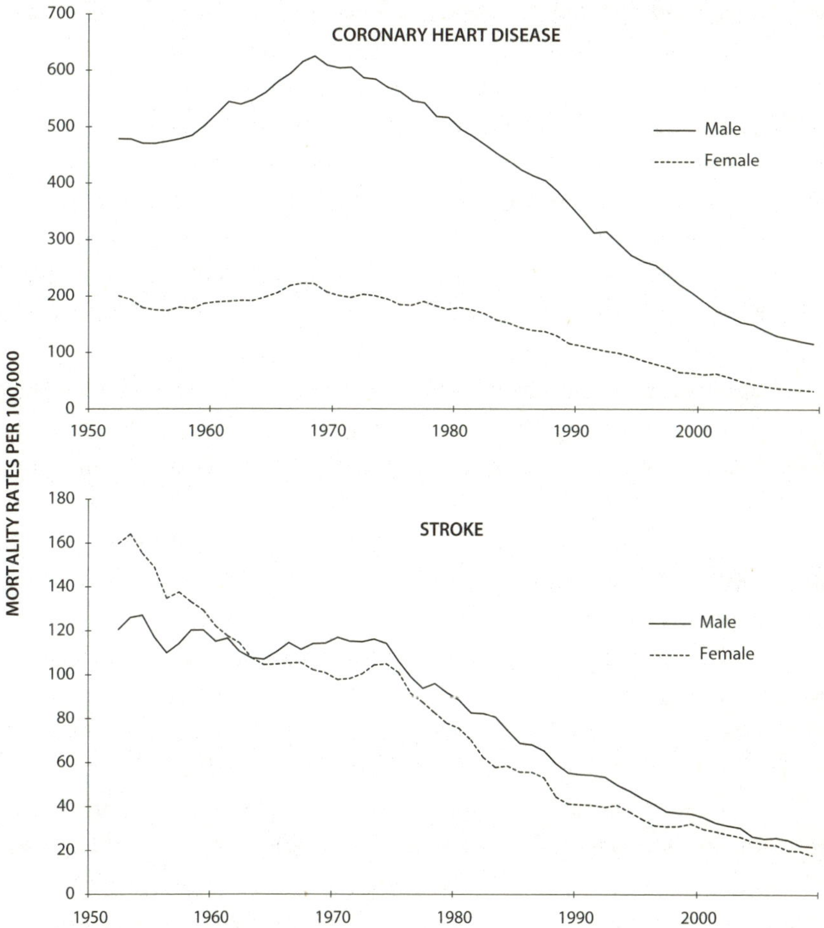

Figure 26: Coronary heart disease and stroke mortality rates for 35–69-year-olds, New Zealand, from c.1950

Source: G. Whitlock, Mortality Trends website (www.mortality-trends.org).

Male Māori mortality rates from coronary heart disease between the 1950s and early 1970s matched non-Māori males – and continued to rise when the rate for non-Māori levelled off.[276] Māori female rates appeared to be at least twice those of non-Māori females up to the age of 65 years, and up to 50 per cent greater among 65+-year-olds.

Why did coronary heart disease rates rise and fall so quickly? The 'classic' risk factors such as tobacco smoking, saturated fat and cholesterol all played a part. Rod Jackson and Robert Beaglehole – two Auckland-based epidemiologists – have examined the coronary heart disease epidemic closely. In an early analysis of rates from 1968 to 1980, they examined national food balance data and tobacco sales. (Food balance sheets give an estimate of the average consumption of various food items after taking account of exports, losses in food preparation, etc.) Using these data, and equations that link nutrient intake with cholesterol levels in the blood, Jackson and Beaglehole estimated that saturated fat consumption per capita peaked in the early 1960s and cholesterol in the 1960s to mid-1970s.[277] Population serum-cholesterol levels may have fallen by only 3–4 per cent from 1968 to 1980.

We note that a dip in beef exports from New Zealand between 1972 and 1974 boosted (temporarily) the quantities of cheap red meat in the domestic New Zealand market, and may be related to the rise that occurred at the same time in average blood cholesterol levels.[277] Without this twist of export fate, it may have been that cholesterol levels – and hence coronary heart disease rates – would have declined earlier and faster.

On the basis of a 3–4 per cent reduction in mean serum cholesterol and a 15 per cent reduction in per capita tobacco consumption, Jackson and Beaglehole estimated that '[b]etween 38% and 51% of the observed decline in CHD mortality in men aged 35–64 years in New Zealand between 1968 and 1980 could be accounted for by changes in serum cholesterol and tobacco consumption'.[277]

In the absence of reliable nutritional survey data, one can use statistics on the quantities of food thought to be available per head of population, allowing for imports and exports, and use for animal feed and seeds (Table 4). It is not possible to measure per capita consumption precisely, but some patterns are evident. Consistent with earlier reports, sporadic data from around New Zealand, and anecdote,[275] indicate that butter and animal fat consumption in New Zealand declined from about 1961 (but was always greater than in

Australia), and vegetable oils were used more frequently (but always less than in Australia). Total red meat consumption was much the same in the two countries, and modestly increasing over time. Poultry consumption increased dramatically.

Table 4: Food supply quantity (kilogram per capita per year) in New Zealand and Australia, for selected years

	NEW ZEALAND			AUSTRALIA		
Food item	**1961**	**1980**	**2007**	**1961**	**1980**	**2007**
Vegetable oils (total)	0.6	3.6	10.6	3.3	12.2	19.7
Olive oil	0.1	0.1	1.2	0.5	0.3	2.1
Meat (total)	107.6	110.5	116.8	103.7	108.7	122.7
Bovine meat	47.1	57.4	32.1	41.2	52.6	44.0
Mutton & goat meat	42.2	31.3	23.3	46.0	20.1	14.5
Pig meat	15.3	11.5	22.9	10.3	14.6	23.3
Poultry meat	2.7	9.6	34.7	4.8	20.8	39.8
Animal fats (total)	22.1	23.5	13.9	15.5	8.2	8.6
Butter, ghee	17.2	14.2	9.3	11.2	4.5	3.9
Fish, seafood (total)	20.6	15.6	26.4	12.8	14.0	24.2

Source: Food and Agricultural Organization of the United Nations website (http://faostat.fao.org/).

Subsequent work post-1980, in New Zealand and elsewhere, has confirmed the role of risk-factor changes in the decline of the coronary heart disease epidemic.[278] In broad terms, it appears that at least half the reduction was due to changes in diet and smoking, and up to half due to treatment.[279] (We will pursue the influence of health services on CVD and other diseases in the next chapter.)

High blood pressure is the main risk factor for stroke, and is in turn influenced by factors such as salt in the diet, alcohol and physical activity. We lack reliable trend data on hypertension, which makes it difficult to pinpoint specific explanations of the huge falls in stroke mortality up to 1980.[280] Hypotensive drugs may have contributed – and perhaps more so among women who were more likely than men to receive these medicines – and in-hospital acute treatment may have assisted too.[280] However, the most important factor was population-wide reduction in blood pressure (that is, a fall in blood pressures for everyone, not just those diagnosed as suffering from 'hypertension').[281]

Thanks to studies in the 1960s by Ian Prior and colleagues on the East Coast and in the Wairarapa, there is some information on early Māori/non-Māori differences in cardiovascular disease and risk factors. Prior found that CVD was more prevalent among Māori – especially hypertensive disease and disease among Māori women. In the Wairarapa at least, cholesterol levels were higher among non-Māori, but most other adverse risk factors were higher among Māori. For example, diabetes prevalence was 7–8 per cent among Māori, compared to 1.5–3 per cent among Europeans. Dietary fat intake was 25 per cent higher among Māori, due to greater consumption of butter and fat meats (and making the converse cholesterol findings curious). Hypertension and hyperuricaemia (reflecting a predisposition to gout) were more common among Māori.

Prior concluded that '[i]ncreased mortality from infectious disease [among Māori] is now replaced by an extraordinary predisposition to the chronic endemic diseases that beset western civilisations'. (Note the Anglophonic interpretation of 'western civilisation': CVD epidemics did not occur in Greece, Italy, Spain or Portugal.)

Considering Polynesian people more widely, Prior also undertook studies in remote islands (Pukapuka and Tokelau) and more developed parts of the Pacific (Cook Islands).[282; 283] Hyperuricaemia was elevated even in the remote islands, strengthening the suspicion of a genetic predisposition. Blood pressure levels were not elevated in remote islands, but they were in more westernised settings and, in particular, hypertension was associated with migrating to New Zealand.[283; 284; 285; 286; 287] These studies demonstrated that environmental factors influence risk of cardiovascular disease, and that Polynesian people may be particularly susceptible.

Prior's work is a reminder of the different ways in which migration can influence population health statistics. When health and wealth are not selection filters, and immigrants are particularly sensitive to the risks of the new environment, the 'healthy migrant effect' does not operate. In these circumstances, migrants may have *worse* disease rates than the population of the destination country.

Between 1968 and 1984, mortality in New Zealand followed the same path as in Australia, although Australia's rates fell more steeply each year, adding up to a sizeable cumulative advantage.[288; 289] We do not know exactly why this happened. Smoking rates seemed to be much the same – if not a little lower in New Zealand. Without systematic monitoring of the contents of the food supply it is impossible to be definite, but it appears that saturated fat was taken out of the Australian diet more quickly than in New Zealand. One reason for this was the protected place of butter in the New Zealand economy. Margarine production was strongly discouraged by statute until 1971, when polyunsaturated margarine was available, briefly, only on doctor's prescription.[290] Pressure from the National Heart Foundation led to amendments in the Margarine Act and margarine was freely available in New Zealand from 1972.[291]

Table 4 shows that fat consumption in New Zealand was consistently greater than in Australia. Butter is the biggest difference of all between the two countries – New Zealanders consumed about 9 kilograms of butter and ghee per head in 2007. This is less than half the amount that was eaten in 1961, but more than twice the Australian figure for the same year.

Cancer

Mortality caused by specific cancers is not well captured by existing data systems before 1970. However, New Zealand is fortunate to have a National Cancer Registry (NCR) that was in operation from 1948. This means we can look more closely at incidence trends and, by inference, changes in cancer mortality, from the 1950s onwards. The data are not perfect (for example, registration was not compulsory until 1994), but are satisfactory for a broad review. It is important to appreciate that the implications for mortality differ by cancer type. For instance, lung cancer has a 90–95 per cent five-year case fatality rate, meaning trends in incidence and trends in mortality tend to move together. But melanoma is usually cured nowadays, meaning that the NCR gives a fair idea of mortality trends only if survival remains fairly constant over time – which we know is not the case, due to a shift to earlier diagnosis and considerable improvements in treatment.

The Ministry of Health has recently used NCR data from 1955–57, and mortality data from 1970 onwards, to describe historical trends and project cancer rates in the future (Figure 27). Also shown is an earlier series compiled by Donovan (1970),[292] perhaps vulnerable to some error because of disease coding, but good enough to shed light on cancer mortality pre-1970s.

For all cancers combined (including melanoma, but excluding non-malignant skin cancers), incidence rates more than doubled from the mid-1950s to a peak at the turn of the century, with most of this increase occurring before 1980 (Figure 27).

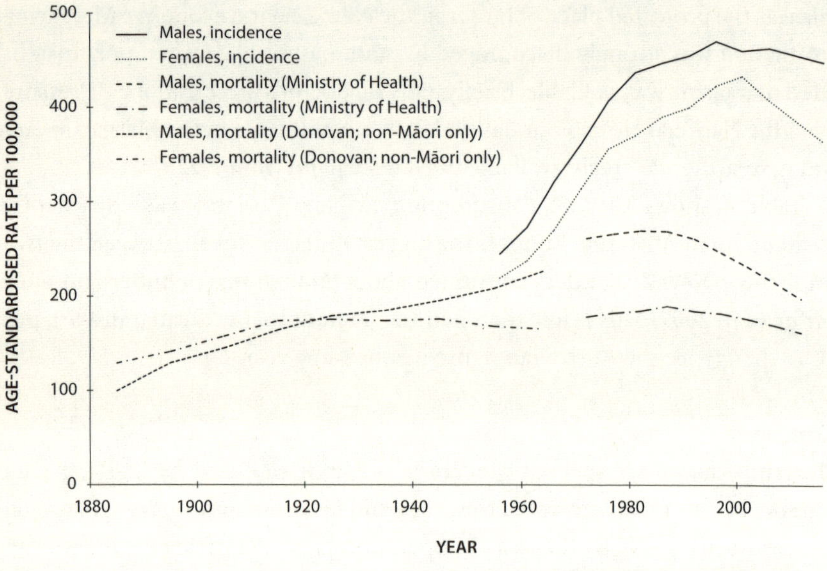

Figure 27: Trends in adult (15+ years) cancer registrations (incidence) and mortality of malignant cancer in New Zealand

Source: Ministry of Health incidence from 1956; mortality from 1970: Ministry of Health, *Cancer in New Zealand: Trends and Projections* (Wellington: Ministry of Health, 2002); and Ministry of Health, *Cancer Incidence Projections: 1999–2003 update* (Wellington: Ministry of Health, 2008). Donovan mortality from 1881–90 to 1961–68: Donovan, J. W., 'Cancer Mortality in New Zealand: 1. General' (*New Zealand Medical Journal* 72, no. 458 [1970]: 9–12); '2. Digestive System' (*NZM* 72, no. 459 [1970]: 104–110); and '4. Other Primary Sites' (*NZMJ* 75, no. 478 [1972]: 144–148). WHO world population was the 'standard' for all series. Note that the separated incidence estimate for 2016 is a projection with some uncertainty (that is not shown in graph), and likewise the separated 2006 and 2012 mortality estimates are predictions from the earlier 2002 report, *Cancer in New Zealand: Trends and Projections*.

Mortality rates for the Donovan and Ministry of Health series roughly meet each other at the 1970s transition. (Note that the Donovan series only includes non-Māori data.) What can we conclude about mortality trends?

First, that female cancer mortality rates possibly increased till about World War I for females, then remained about the same (in very rough terms) till about 1990, and have been decreasing since. A similar pattern has been reported in Australia,[190] where female cancer mortality rates varied little between 1920 and 1990. Second, it appears that New Zealand male cancer mortality rates have been steadily increasing from the late nineteenth century to about 1980, then falling. Again, this matches the trends in Australia.[190] The increase in male cancer mortality (with an early peak and then a fall amongst females) is probably due to the balance of smoking (that hit males more in the 1960s through 1980s) offsetting improvements in cancer survival across many cancers, and the increasing preponderance of cancers that have higher rates among males (e.g., colorectal cancer and leukaemia).

In Figure 27, the lines for mortality and incidence diverged in the 1990s (mortality fell, incidence continued to rise). Some of the improvement in survival from cancer is due to earlier diagnosis, some to improved treatment, and some due simply to cancers with very poor survival (e.g., stomach cancer) becoming less common while cancers with better survival (e.g., breast, melanoma and prostate) have become more common.

Mortality from cancer has not fallen as fast in relative terms as cardiovascular disease and unintentional injuries. This means that cancer is responsible for a greater proportion of deaths at each age group over time, and therefore what happens with cancer mortality rates is having a greater influence on what happens to life expectancy trends. The growing influence of all-cancer mortality is likely to increase further in the next few decades, barring a major turnaround (e.g., a resurgence of cardiovascular disease due to obesity). We will revisit what this proportionate shift to cancer mortality might mean for future life expectancy trends in the final chapter.

Underlying the 'all cancers combined' incidence trends is huge variation by cancer site (Figure 28, overleaf). Male lung cancer rates peaked about 1980, compared to a much more recent – but lesser – peak for females. Changes in tobacco consumption (including both the proportion of the population who smoked, and the amount of tobacco consumed by each smoker) explain the variations in lung cancer incidence. We will examine the effects of tobacco on the health of New Zealanders more closely later in this chapter – suffice to say here that the greatest impact on mortality and life expectancy occurred between 1940 and 1980. Pancreatic cancer – also strongly associated with smoking – follows similar trends to those for lung cancer.

Trends in the other cancer sites provide a strong hint of the changes that occurred in social and living conditions in post-World War II New Zealand. Consider breast cancer. The major risk factor for breast cancer is oestrogen exposure, which increases with earlier menarche and later menopause (both of which are strongly influenced by nutrition), and later and fewer children (functions of access to birth control, gender equity, economic circumstances and prevailing gender roles). The doubling of breast cancer incidence rates post-World War II has been a consequence of changes in these factors – higher calorie diets, increased career opportunities for women, delayed child-bearing and improved contraceptive technologies, albeit with some odd ethnic variations that we will examine more in the next chapter. What effect has increasing breast cancer incidence had on female mortality? Some, especially at older ages, but not as much as you might expect: breast cancer survival is reasonably high and has improved in recent decades due to earlier detection (e.g., screening programmes) and better treatments. Consequently, breast cancer mortality is now declining despite static or slowly rising trends in incidence, and the change is substantial: the death rate from breast cancer fell by 20 per cent between 2000 and 2010 for non-Māori;[293] rates were unstable over time for Māori.

Stomach cancer occurs among people infected with *Helicobacter pylori* at a young age. This infection is associated with household crowding, and the risk of stomach cancer is amplified by salt-cured foods, smoking, and low vegetable and fruit intake. The large reductions in stomach cancer rates in New Zealand mirror what has happened in many other countries, and reflect improvements in living conditions beginning in the early twentieth century. Refrigeration – including refrigerated transport – is likely to have played a role in reducing the need for meats and other foods to be preserved in salt. Stomach cancer is not common, but reducing the incidence of the disease will have an effect on mortality rates, especially for non-European groups who are affected more frequently than the population as a whole, because the case fatality rate for the disease is so high.

What causes colorectal cancer is perhaps less well understood than appeared a couple of decades ago. In addition to hereditary factors, rates are

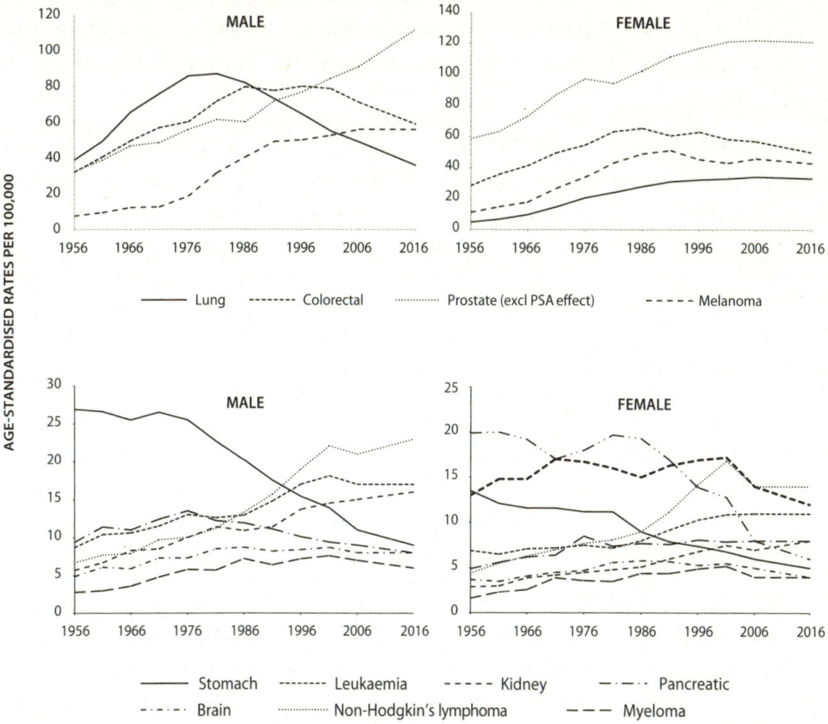

Figure 28: Trends in cancer registrations (incidence) of selected cancers, by sex

Source: Ministry of Health, *Cancer in New Zealand: Trends and Projections* (Wellington: Ministry of Health, 2002) and Ministry of Health, *Cancer Incidence Projections: 1999–2003 update* (Wellington: Ministry of Health, 2008). Note that the estimate for 2016 is a projection with some uncertainty (that is not shown in graph).

higher amongst those who eat large amounts of red or processed meats and relatively little by way of fruit, vegetables and (probably) dietary fibre.[294] Foods that are calcium-rich may be protective. Alcohol consumption and obesity increase the risk, while physical activity is protective.[295] But none of these putative associations are particularly strong. We speculate that the peak incidence of this cancer in New Zealand in the 1980s and 1990s reflects high levels of red meat consumption (lamb and beef in particular) in the middle part of the twentieth century, but other dietary changes may have been important as well. For instance, the free milk in primary schools programme provided most New Zealand children with a half pint (about 280 millilitres) of full-cream milk, every day, between 1937 and 1967, and it has been suggested that this may have contributed to the declining incidence of colorectal cancer which is evident in successive generations born from about 1938 onwards.[296; 297] As colorectal cancer is a common cancer with approximately 60 per cent five-year survival (and this figure has been improving in recent decades), changes in incidence will have some impact on trends in life expectancy.

Falls in cervical cancer incidence may be attributed to screening programmes and to some extent the reduction in smoking. There are many cancer trends, though, that we simply do not understand, such as recent increases in lymphomas, leukaemias and brain cancers.

Unintentional injury and suicide

Road traffic crash mortality rates increased until about 1970, and have fallen massively since then for 35–69-year-olds and since about 1990 for 15–34-year-olds (Figure 29). Suicide rates among 15–34-year-olds increased four-fold from about 1970 to 2000, and have fallen since. The patterns and rates in Australia were very similar over the same time period (www.mortality-trends.org).

The increase in mortality from these two causes, albeit at different times, was responsible for some of the lack of progress in non-Māori life expectancy in the post-World War II period up to 1980. The fall in mortality rates (due in large part to concerted safety and public health campaigns to reduce the road toll) has contributed to recent improvements in life expectancy.

Tobacco

Tobacco was the biggest obstacle to improvements in life expectancy in the twentieth century. At the time of writing this book, with a prevalence in New Zealand of less than 20 percentage points, up to 5000 deaths per year (out of about 30,000 overall deaths per year) would be avoided if nobody smoked. We do not know precisely what was the impact of smoking on mortality and life expectancy throughout the twentieth century, but it was large. Passive smoking contributed to sudden infant death syndrome and respiratory diseases (and presumably heightened mortality from tuberculosis, influenza and many other diseases) and slowed reductions in child mortality. Cardiovascular disease and lung cancer are the adult diseases most strongly associated with tobacco, but so are other respiratory conditions such as chronic obstructive

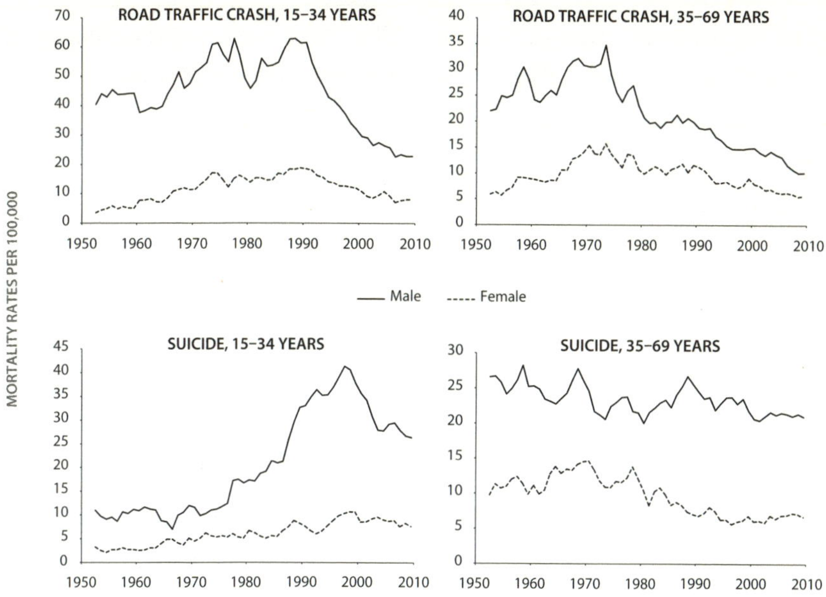

Figure 29: Road traffic crash and suicide death rates for 15–34 and 35–69-year-olds, New Zealand, from c.1950

Source: G. Whitlock, Mortality Trends website (www.mortality-trends.org).

pulmonary disease, a constantly growing list of cancers,[298] and some unintentional injuries (e.g., those caused by fire).[299]

For the year 1976, D. R. King and colleagues estimated that 15 per cent of all deaths (19 per cent of male and 8 per cent of female deaths, or 3700 deaths in total) were due to tobacco.[300] They used 1976 census data (which included a smoking question) combined with overseas estimates of the association of smoking with mortality.

We have estimated the difference in life expectancy in 1980–82 between current and never smokers, by taking the 1981–84 mortality data and linking back to the 1981 census, which included a smoking question.[301] On this basis, it is possible to calculate mortality rates by fine gradations of age, and by cross-classifications of sex, ethnicity and household income. Considering males and females overall, we estimated a four-to-five-year gap in life expectancy in the early 1980s between never and current smokers (Figure 30). (Ex-smokers are somewhere in between, although difficult to interpret as the time since quitting varies, and varies again across sex and other social groups.)

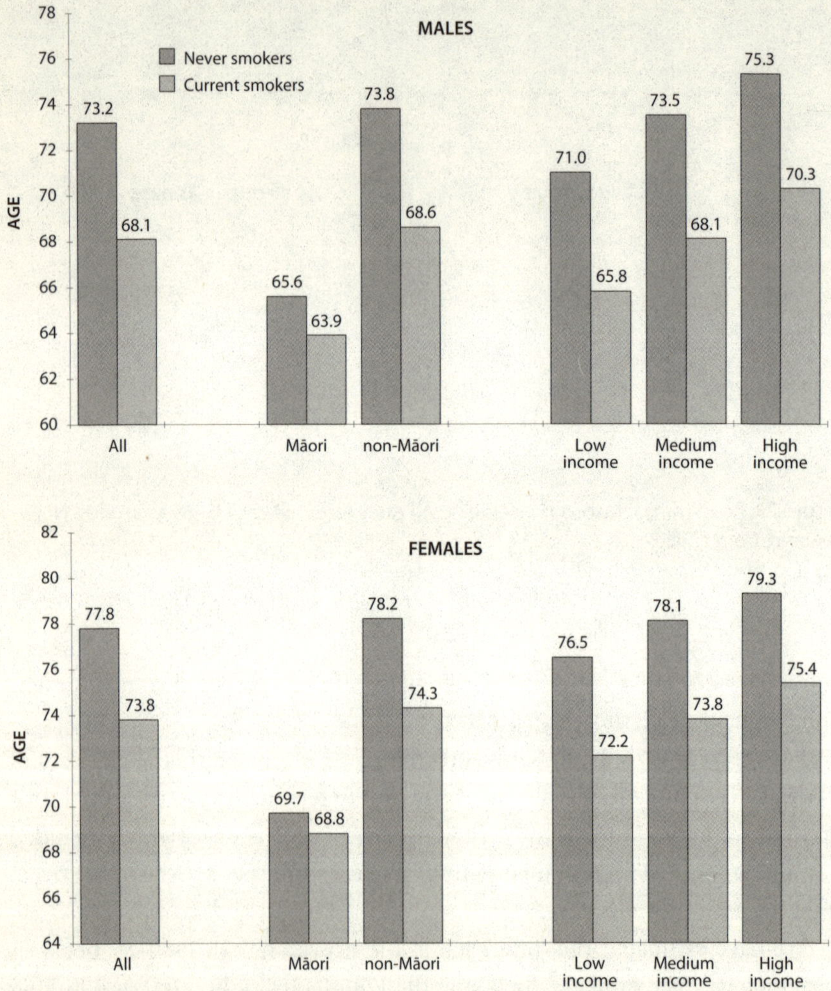

Figure 30: Life expectancy in 1981–84 for never and current smokers, for the total population and by ethnicity and household income, by sex

Source: K. N. Carter, T. Blakely, and M. Soeberg, 'Trends in Survival and Life Expectancy by Ethnicity, Income and Smoking: 1980s to 2000s' (*New Zealand Medical Journal* 123, no. 1320 [13 August 2010]): 1–13.

If Cook and subsequent explorers and settlers had never brought tobacco to New Zealand, male and female life expectancy in 1980–82 would have been close to that of never smokers shown in Figure 30, namely 73.2 and 77.8 years for males and females. Note that this estimate for males (73.2 years) is approximately the same as the life expectancy of Japanese men in the early 1980s. Japan was then number one in the world life expectancy rankings. Ironically, Japanese men at that time were heavy smokers, but they benefited also from many other health-promoting lifestyle factors and effective population-wide health care.[302]

Figure 30 also shows life expectancies in 1980–82 for never and current smokers by ethnicity and by tertiles (thirds) of equivalised household income. The gap between never and current smokers among Māori was much less than in non-Māori. Why is this? We have looked closely at this question,[303; 304; 305] and think the reasons are as follows. First, the census question about smoking will be measured with error. This error probably means that we have under-estimated the difference in mortality, or life expectancy, between smokers and never smokers across the board. If error in this census variable was greater for Māori, then we may have under-estimated the smoker/non-smoker difference in life expectancy more so among Māori than non-Māori.

Second, and more important, the background (i.e., non-tobacco-related) mortality rates for Māori are much higher than for non-Māori. Smoking causes a similar *absolute* increase in the mortality rate for Māori and non-Māori, but this means the percentage difference in mortality between current and never smokers among Māori is much less (because the baseline mortality is higher). For example, if the mortality rate among Māori never smokers is 300 per 100,000 and among non-Maori is 100 per 100,000, and being a current smoker adds an absolute increment of 100 per 100,000, then the rates among current smokers will be 400 and 200 per 100,000 for Māori and non-Māori, respectively. This equates to current:never rate ratios within ethnic group of 1.33 (400/300) and 2 (200/100) for Māori and non-Māori, respectively. When these rate ratios are plugged into the life tables used to generate life expectancies, we found a similar pattern to that seen in Figure 30 (a smaller gap between never and current smokers amongst Māori than non-Māori). Finally, in the early 1980s the age-specific mortality rates for Māori meant that fewer Māori survived (in the life table) to the ages where fatal smoking-related diseases are most common, limiting the impact of smoking on differences in life expectancy.

We will revisit this issue in the last chapter of the book when we project what life expectancy might be in 2040 if New Zealand is tobacco-free by 2020. As Māori mortality falls for reasons other than reducing tobacco consumption, the impact of smoking on life expectancy will be more evident (that is, the gap between new and current smokers will increase).

Susie Johnston examined the social history of smoking in New Zealand, from 1920 to 1962 (the date of the Royal College of Physicians, UK, report on the harms of tobacco). She commences one chapter thus:

> In March 1953 Major Spraggon, sales manager of the National Tobacco Company, visited his local Rotary Club in Napier, boasting to its members that New Zealanders were among the heaviest smokers in the world. Spraggon claimed that they smoked more tobacco than their Australian or British counterparts. In that year, New Zealanders consumed 7.4 lbs per adult head of population (over 15 years of age), where the Australians smoked only 6.8 lbs and the British 6 lbs each. New Zealanders were the fourth highest consumers, per capita, of tobacco in the world. This high consumption did not come by chance, but rather as a result of over thirty years of hard work in the development of a domestic tobacco industry.[306]

The tobacco industry 'success' is an important part of the story of New Zealand's life expectancy. In 1900 we consumed 2.31 pounds of tobacco per head of population,[307] and by 1920 5.0 pounds per year. Murray Laugesen, perhaps New Zealand's most prominent anti-tobacco campaigner in the last 40 years, has constructed a times series of 'cigarette equivalents per person 15 years and older' in New Zealand, since 1920 (Figure 31).[308] The metric assumes that each gram of loose tobacco is equivalent to one manufactured cigarette. It is also per citizen – not per smoker. The majority of tobacco sold in New Zealand till World War II was loose tobacco. The total per capita consumption per capita peaked in the 1950s, at the time of Major Spraggon's speech in Napier, and stayed at much the same heights till the mid-1970s.

There were lots of ups and downs in tobacco consumption, including a 20 per cent fall in consumption during the Great Depression. (One would not want to make having a depression a public health recommendation, but economic hard times do encourage people to give up smoking.) Most of the harmful effects of tobacco on cardiovascular disease pass within months to years of quitting, but the increased risk of cancer takes years to decades to subside. This will be part of the reason why macroeconomic indicators such as GDP per capita do not have a clearly anti-cyclical and negative association with mortality (i.e., why mortality rates do not immediately increase when GDP goes down).[18; 309; 310; 311] Rather, there may be some health gains from economic downturns, such as reduced smoking and fewer road traffic crashes, which are offset by health losses caused by austerity, such as higher suicide rates and restricted access to health services.[312]

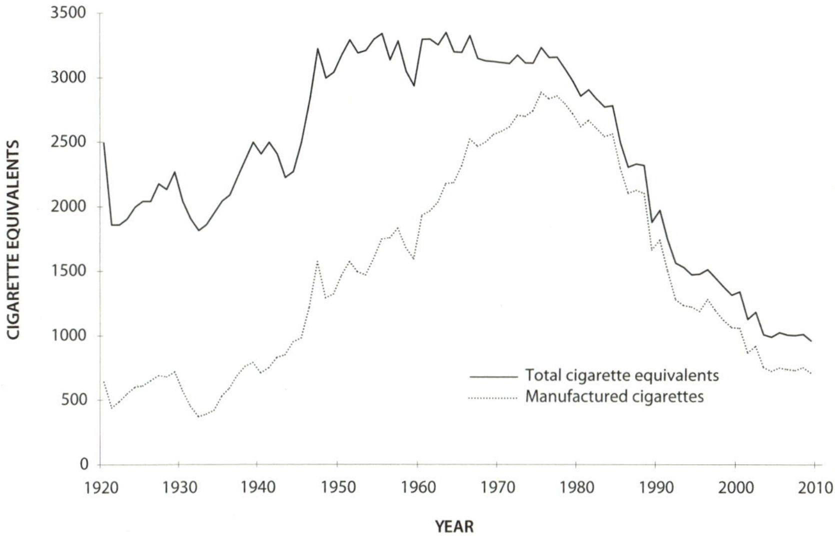

Figure 31: Cigarette equivalents (grams of loose tobacco plus number of cigarettes) per person aged 15 years and over, per year

Sources: M. Laugesen, *Tobacco Statistics 1991: Trends in Tobacco Consumption and Smoking Prevalence in New Zealand* (Wellington: Cancer Society, 1992); and yearly reports from Statistics New Zealand. The excess of total cigarette equivalents over manufactured cigarettes is that due to loose tobacco.

Tobacco consumption in New Zealand slipped during World War II, due to rationing of supplies at home, but the troops did not go short of cigarettes.[306] Nordmeyer's 'black budget' of 1958 included a 39 per cent tax rise on tobacco, and caused consumption to fall temporarily, but smoking resumed previous levels when Labour reversed many of its austerity measures. Subsequent budgets applied price increases as a public health measure (which coincidentally boosted government revenue), and the 1991, 1998 and 2000 budgets achieved, on average, a 7 per cent reduction in consumption for a 10 per cent increase in price.[313]

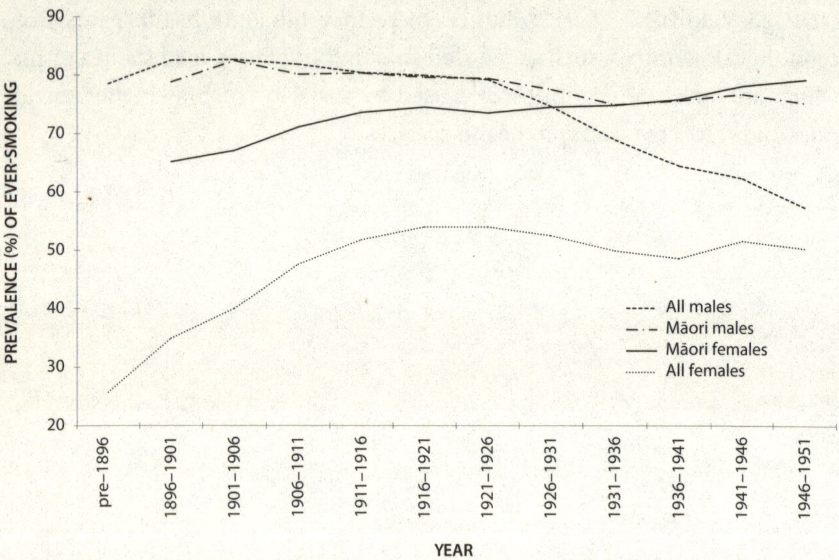

Figure 32: Prevalence of ever-smoking for entire birth cohorts (i.e., both the living and dead) by 1976 census

Source: B. Easton, 'Smoking in New Zealand: A Census Investigation' (*Australian Journal of Public Health* 19, no. 2 [1995]): 125–9.

We do not have good information on smoking prevalence throughout the twentieth century. However, it is possible to infer social patterns of tobacco consumption using census data, presenting current and ex-smoker prevalence by age group, which is equivalent to an analysis by birth cohort. Brian Easton undertook one such analysis, using information from the 1976 census – the first to include a question on smoking.[314] One problem with this analysis is that the older people, or the earliest birth cohorts, appear to have lower lifetime smoking prevalence (i.e., [current + ex-smokers] / [total birth cohort still alive]) due to smokers dying earlier! Easton attempted to overcome this using basic demographic tricks that have their limitations, but the figures provide a fair indication of lifetime smoking prevalence by year of birth (Figure 32).

The patterns for 'All' (driven essentially by non-Māori) fit with theoretical expectations about phased tobacco epidemics as seen across many developed countries.[315] That is, male smoking was (much) higher for earlier birth cohorts, but was matched by female smoking rates in more recent birth cohorts. For example, 'All males' born between 1896 and 1901 had an estimated lifetime smoking prevalence of 83 per cent, compared to 35 per cent for females, but by the 1946–51 cohort the lifetime prevalences were 57 per cent for males and 50 per cent for females.

The pattern for Māori is different. Early Māori male cohorts smoked as much as non-Māori, but rates have not come down subsequently in the same way as non-Māori. Māori females were heavy smokers from the outset, and recent cohorts have in fact overtaken Māori males.

Tobacco was an important trade commodity in the earliest exchanges between Europeans and Māori. For example, the land on which the city of Auckland was established was purchased from Ngāti Whātua in 1840 for £66 in cash and goods worth £215 (which included 50 blankets, ten waistcoats, four casks of tobacco and one box of pipes).[316] Reid and Pouwhare comment, 'During the years that followed, Māori people took up tobacco with enthusiasm.'[317] Unlike Europeans, amongst Māori both men and women used tobacco freely. The damage to Māori caused by tobacco must have been substantial from the late nineteenth century, but is difficult to quantify. Reid and Pouwhare have reflected on the massive decline in the Māori population up to 1900:

> By the turn of the century, it seemed to many that we [i.e., Māori], as a race, would not survive. Our very extinction was predicted. The main causes included introduced diseases and changes in lifestyle imposed by the laws and policies of the imperial and colonial governments. The role tobacco played in this is not clear, although it must surely have aggravated the devastation of chest infections such as tuberculosis, influenza and pneumonia.[317]

Tobacco, acting largely through cardiovascular disease, is a major reason why non-Māori life expectancy for males did not increase through the 1960s and 1970s, and why increases among females were less in this period than the long-run trends of the previous 150 years (Figure 22). The tremendous increases in Māori life expectancy from 1940 to the 1980s happened *despite* tobacco and ischaemic heart disease. That is, reductions in Māori mortality due to diminishing infectious diseases were of such magnitude that they overwhelmed the harmful effects of tobacco.

Both non-Māori and Māori life expectancy would, without doubt, have been higher throughout the 1940 to 1980 period in the absence of tobacco. Exactly how much higher is difficult to estimate – perhaps one or more years at each calendar year for Māori (perhaps more so c.1940), and up to three years for non-Māori (perhaps less so c.1940).

SOCIAL AND ECONOMIC DETERMINANTS OF CHANGES IN LIFE EXPECTANCY

Many aspects of the social environment (e.g., economic activity, trade, welfare policy) influence health status (Figure 33).[318] We have already considered how changes in individual behaviours may have affected changes in life expectancy in the post-war era. We now turn our attention to some of the upstream social determinants such as economic performance, and social and health policy.

Economic good times, and low income inequality

Post-World War II New Zealand was distinguished by high GDP (by international standards), and relatively low income inequality. One would expect, as a result, better welfare services, higher standards of living, and improved proximal determinants of health such as personal behaviours and use of health care. However, the association of macroeconomic indicators, such as GDP, with health is not straightforward. Figure 34, overleaf, shows non-Māori life expectancy and GDP per capita (log scale) in New Zealand from 1870 to 2006. We do not see an obvious connection between wealth (GDP) and health (life expectancy). Indeed, the period of strongest growth in GDP (1930s to c.1970) covers the period during which life expectancy improved least (the 1960s and 1970s). In fact, if one plots a graph of five-yearly changes in GDP with five-yearly changes in life expectancy, there appears to be an inverse association (health tends to improve following a deterioration in the economy)!

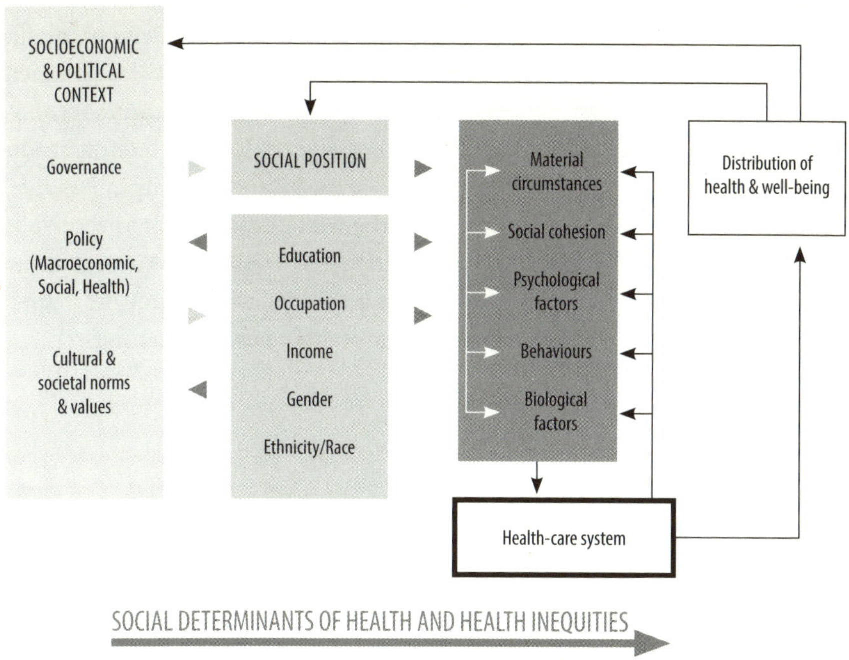

Figure 33: Framework of the influence of social determinants on health

Source: Commission on Social Determinants of Health, 'Closing the Gap in a Generation: Health Equity through Action on the Social Determinants of Health' (Geneva: The World Health Organization, 2008).

Undoubtedly, a strong economy makes it possible to invest in systems and people that may return health gains in the medium-to-long-term future. But this is not guaranteed. For example, secular trends in health behaviours (such as high fat diets and smoking) may be insensitive to macro-economic indicators, or in some instances may be spurred on in health-damaging directions by higher discretionary incomes.

Samuel Preston pointed out that measures of economic performance (such as GDP) are weak predictors of life expectancy in middle- to high-income countries.[250] He argued that diffusion of ideas and technologies is far more important, based on two important observations. One was the non-linear graph relating GDP to life expectancy (or virtually any other health statistic). Beyond a point roughly equating to the difference between medium- and high-income countries, further increases in GDP made little difference to health.

Secondly, Preston pointed out that life expectancy at any given level of wealth had improved over time (implying that a greater health output was obtained from the same economic resource). Preston argued that one country's technological breakthrough diffused quickly to other countries, and as a result health and life expectancy improved everywhere – a positive externality, if you like. Exceptions exist, which we will revisit in the next chapter, such as the 1980s to 1990s experience for Māori in New Zealand, HIV/AIDS in Africa and the breakup of the Soviet Union. The point here is that macroeconomic indicators, such as GDP, are not strong predictors of mortality rates in all settings.[312]

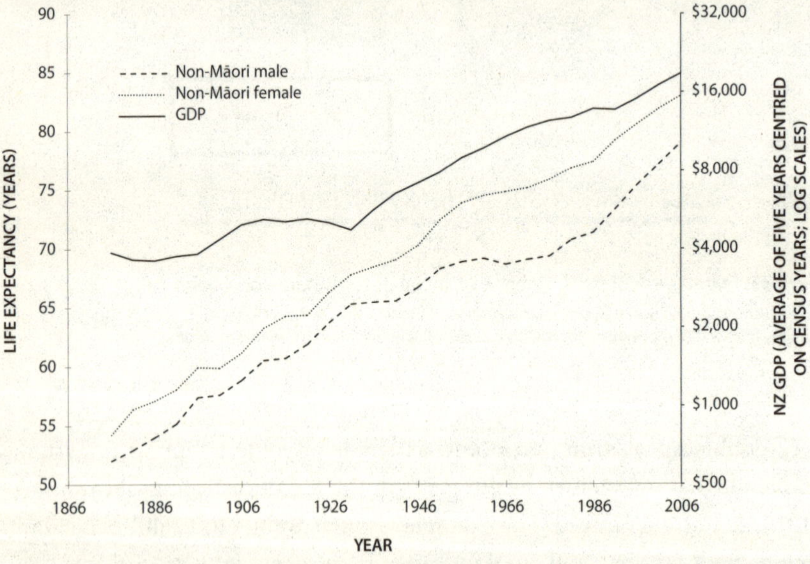

Figure 34: Non-Māori life expectancy and GDP per capita (log scale)

Source: Life expectancy series from J. Oeppen and J. Vaupel, 'Broken Limits to Life Expectancy' (*Science* 296 [2002]: 1029–31); the Human Mortality Database; and Statistics New Zealand. GDP per capita are taken from The Groningen Growth and Development Centre, University of Groningen, Netherlands (www.ggdc.net/maddison/). GDP is purchasing power parity adjusted, and in 1990 Geary–Khamis dollars.

Migration

Migration may occur between countries, and within countries – and both may influence health status. Selection processes favouring relatively healthy migration between countries was one reason for New Zealand's high life expectancy pre-World War II (see earlier chapters in this book). Post-World War II, the speed of Māori urbanisation within New Zealand was remarkable: in the 30-year period from 1936 to 1966, Māori moved from 90 per cent rural (compared with 38 per cent for non-Māori) to 56 per cent urban (compared with 77 per cent).

There were push and pull factors at work. Earlier in the century, it had been made plain to Māori that they were not welcome in the city. In 1935 the Mayor of Auckland, Ernest Davis, opined 'the Māori is a child of nature, and it is better for both him and the pakeha that he should live in the country and not in the town'.[316] The disruption of the war years, and economic growth subsequently, opened the way for Māori to migrate in large numbers to urban centres. Government policies explicitly encouraged this movement to meet post-war demands for labour. There were negative effects, caused by dislocation from whānau, hapū and iwi, and turangawaewae ('a place to stand', usually associated with tribal home or lands). However, urbanisation also led to higher incomes, educational opportunities, better housing, and access to social and health services. A health dividend resulted.

Non-Māori ranks were bolstered by post-World War II migrants from Europe, including many new arrivals from the Netherlands, but Britain was still the major source of migrants. In 1976, about 300,000 of the New Zealand population or 10 per cent were British- or Irish-born.[256]

Pacific people were a very small minority of the non-Māori population pre-World War II, but a large surge of migration from the islands began in the 1950s. In 1945 the Pacific population in New Zealand was just over 2000 people, Samoans being the largest group. In 1981, there were almost 120,000 people living in New Zealand who identified as Pacific. Extrapolating backwards from more recent data, and noting the higher mortality rates in the Pacific island countries compared to New Zealand in parallel with lower barriers to migration, without doubt mortality rates for Pacific people living in New Zealand would have been higher that European New Zealanders. There are also pockets of epidemiological research to support this contention: for instance, Pacific people in Auckland in the 1970s had coronary heart disease rates that were higher than those of European New Zealanders (although much less than Māori).[319]

Social and health policy

The 1940–80 period was launched by an ambitious and radical piece of legislation, the Social Security Act of 1938. This moved New Zealand to a Scandinavian-like model of welfare, emphasising universal cover. The benefits that were provided included superannuation, age, widows', orphans', miners', invalids', family, sickness, unemployment and emergency. The Act implemented entitlement, or a right, to a reasonable standard of living. Elements of the benefit structure survive today, and the extent and cover of the benefits was little changed until the 1980s. One would expect that these social changes preferentially advantaged the health of lower socio-economic groups, by protecting families and children from poverty and securing access to social and health services. However, empirical evidence of the health gains from these social policies is – to our knowledge – absent.

The 1935 Labour Government was responsible for the major health system changes around the time of World War II, as a consequence of the Social Security Act and, directly, through specific health policies. These included moves to extend social services and prevention – particularly infant and child health, and Māori health (most notably control of tuberculosis).[137] Many of the new policies were opposed, or at least not welcomed, by the New Zealand Branch of the British Medical Association (NZBMA). Most notably, the NZBMA opposed the provision of free primary medical care via capitated funding (i.e., bulk funding to primary care based on the patient mix, rather than payment per patient visit). Unlike in the UK, the government in New Zealand could not carry the day. The compromise was provision of free secondary hospital care, alongside state funding of a 'fee for service' for each consultation in primary care. This arrangement left open the door to medical practitioners to charge and collect co-payments – which they did. The fee for service/patient co-payment system in primary care survived until the 1999–2008 Clark Labour-led Government, when it was superseded by capitation funding of primary care – although general practitioners retained the right to charge co-payments.

We think it is reasonable to conclude that the major shift in health care from private to state funding reduced barriers to care. But did this result in improvements in life expectancy? Probably, but only modestly. The 1940s saw the advent of highly efficacious treatments such as antibiotics and anti-tuberculosis treatments. State-organised and -funded primary (partly) and secondary health care increased equitable access to, and continuity of, these treatments. However, much of medicine up to the 1970s still involved a considerable amount of 'care' and 'watching nature'.

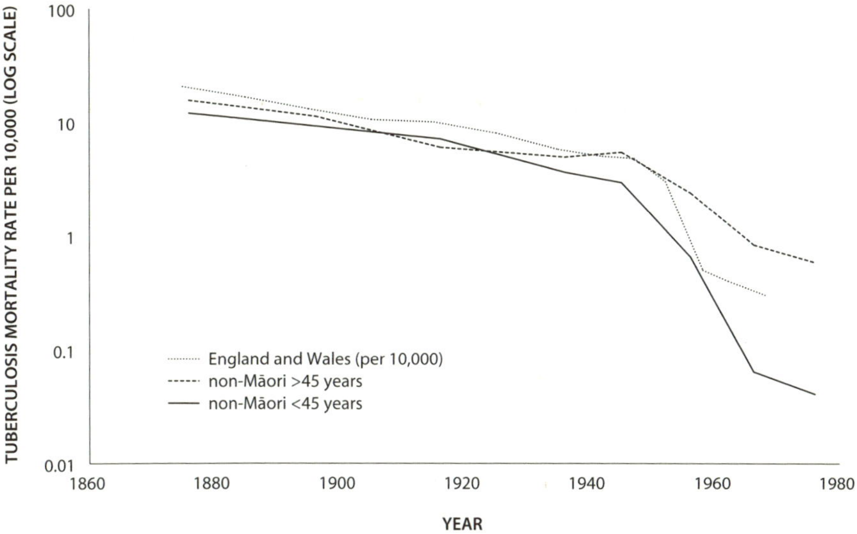

Figure 35: Tuberculosis mortality

Source: England and Wales data from T. McKeown, *The Modern Rise of Population* (New York: Academic Press, 1976); and New Zealand data from I. Pool, 'Mortality Trends and Differentials', *Country Monograph Series No. 12: Population of New Zealand*, edited by Population Division Economic and Social Commission for Asia and the Pacific (New York: United Nations, 1985: 209–42).

Thomas McKeown[320; 249] is the best known of those who have argued that medical care contributed little to increases in life expectancy up to the mid-twentieth century. McKeown argued, by a process of excluding other likely explanations, that nutrition and standards of living were primarily responsible for the decline in mortality in England and Wales since the 1850s. The McKeown thesis has been criticised, most notably by scholars such as Preston who hold that advances in technology were important, including both prevention (e.g., sanitation and hygiene) and treatment (e.g., anti-malarial drugs).[250] Moreover, a closer look at some of McKeown's own analyses suggests that health care achieved a good deal more than he gave it credit for. McKeown referred to the large reductions in tuberculosis mortality that preceded the age of effective treatment as proof of the importance of nutrition and living standards. In Figure 35 (previous page) we have taken McKeown's original graph, and have plotted the data differently, using a log scale that conveys relative reductions in mortality across time. What is apparent now is the acceleration in mortality decline in the 1940s and 1950s, evidence of the impact of anti-tuberculosis treatments such as streptomycin. We show data for New Zealand as well, and the pattern was similar in this country.

Thanks to advances such as antibiotics, medical care in the second half of the 1900s was responsible for a greater share of the improvements in life expectancy than ever before. As a result of reducing barriers to health services, we believe the first Labour Government of 1935 to 1949 made a vital contribution to long-term health gains in New Zealand.

6

Mortality Divergence

1980 to 2010

The last two decades of the twentieth century were eventful. New Zealand's economy stumbled, and the social reforms that were introduced subsequently divided the country and brought hardship to many New Zealanders. Life expectancy for non-Māori resumed its upward trajectory after a plateau in the 1960s and 1970s. On the other hand life expectancy gains for Māori slowed, and actually stalled in the 1980s and 1990s – a function in part of the structural reforms that bore down harder on Māori than non-Māori. During this time the coronary heart disease epidemic was declining fast, and significant steps were taken to control the damage caused by tobacco. Medical care improved to the point that treatment made a discernible difference to the burden of avoidable mortality. A sign of the increasing potency of health care is that, for the first time, we see inequalities in mortality attributed to differential access to services. However, by the 2000s, all social groups were enjoying strong mortality rate reductions – despite increasing rates of obesity. This period hints at what the future may hold; a growing contribution of treatment and health services to life expectancy gains (and consequent volatility in health inequalities depending on how well services meet the needs of disparate social groups); the continuing importance of population-wide preventive interventions; and the influence of the wider social context on health determinants and population mortality rates.

LIFE EXPECTANCY AND ALL-CAUSE MORTALITY TRENDS

The major features of mortality in this period were the increasing inequalities to the end of the century and then a hint of convergence since the late 1990s. The trends in life expectancy for non-Māori and Māori diverged markedly in the last two decades of the twentieth century (Figure 36). Non-Māori life expectancy improved by about four years between 1981 and 1996, compared to a gain of only one-to-two years for Māori. The pattern was the same for both males and females.

Standing back, we can see that non-Māori (males in particular) had shaken off the sluggish 1960s and 1970s and recovered the tempo of steadily improving life expectancy from earlier in the century. Indeed, it looks in the graphs as though the non-Māori curve was springing back to where it might have been if life expectancy was not held back during the 1950s to 1970s. At the same time improvements for Māori slowed to a crawl. In previous decades there had been very strong progress in life expectancy, amounting to a gain of more than half a year of extra life every calendar year. This trend did not continue in the 1980s.

Then the picture changes again from the late 1990s. Indeed, the improvements between 1996 and 2011 for Māori were greater than non-Māori (6.5 and 4.8 years respectively for males, and 5.5 and 3.1 years for females), with gaps closing between ethnic groups to 7.4 years for males and 7.2 years for females in 2011.

Putting together the entire post-World War II epoch, therefore, we have a pattern of convergence of Māori and non-Māori life expectancy between the war and 1981 (due to both non-Māori stasis and very strong gains for Māori); followed by divergence between 1981 and 1996 (due, conversely, to strong gains for non-Māori with little change for Māori); and then rapid improvements for all – Māori more so.

What explains these trends? Upfront, an important principle is to try and understand each 'line' itself, before understanding differences or 'gaps' between the lines. We will examine demographic explanations (e.g., what age groups contributed most?; what causes of death decreased most?), societal explanations (macroeconomic and structural reform), trends in risk factors (tobacco), and trends in health services (access to primary care, receipt of life-saving interventions).

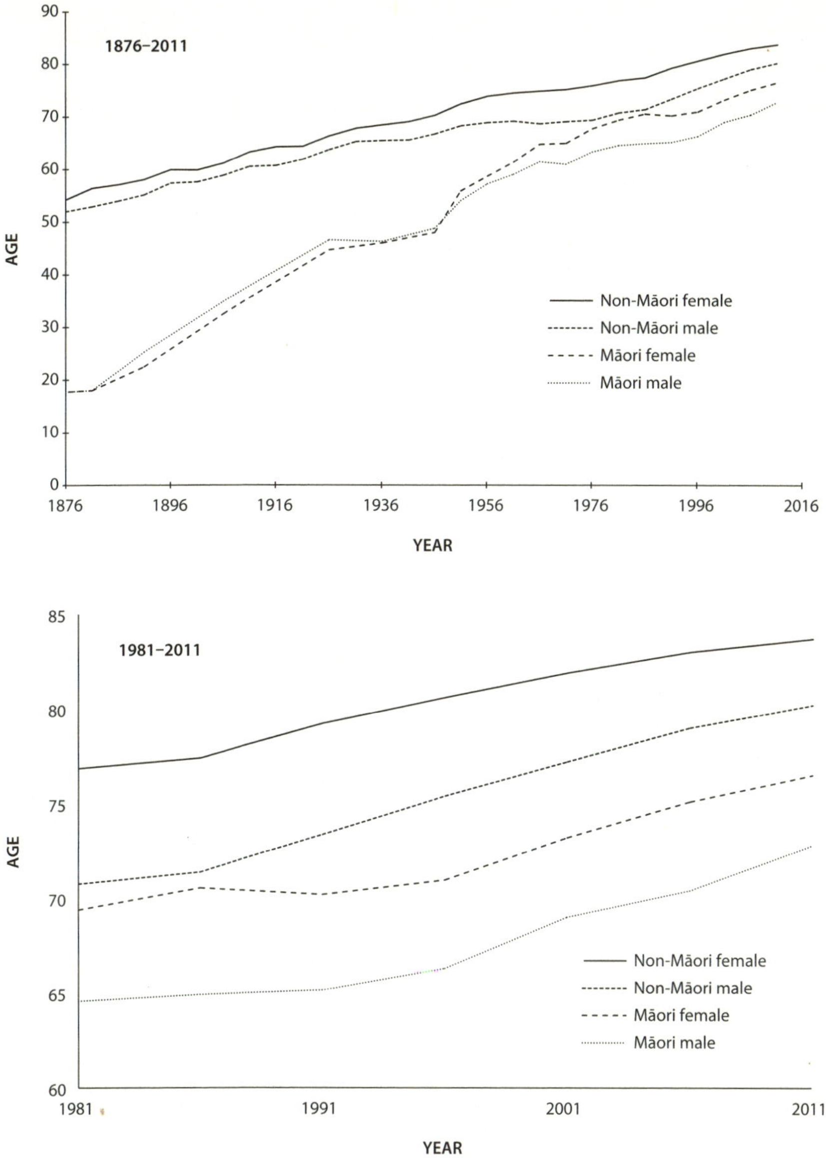

Figure 36: Life expectancy of Māori and non-Māori

Source: M. Tobias, T. Blakely, D. Matheson, K. Rasanathan, and J. Atkinson, 'Changing Trends in Indigenous Inequalities in Mortality: Lessons from New Zealand' (*International Journal of Epidemiology* 38, no. 6 [1 December 2009]: 1711–22); Statistics New Zealand.

The big demographic shift in New Zealand in the late twentieth century was the rising numbers of Pacific and Asian people, and the advent of linked census-mortality data meant their mortality rates could be calculated with more accuracy than previously possible. Figure 37 shows the age-standardised mortality rates for the four largest ethnic groups, for 1–74-year-olds combined. Consistent with the life expectancy graphs, Māori had (much) higher rates than European/Other, and there was little change in Māori mortality (especially males) in the late 1980s and 1990s. Pacific mortality rates were intermediary between Māori and European/Other, but improved little so that by the 2000s they were closer to Māori figures. Asian mortality rates were consistently lower than European/Other rates, and steadily decreased over the period.

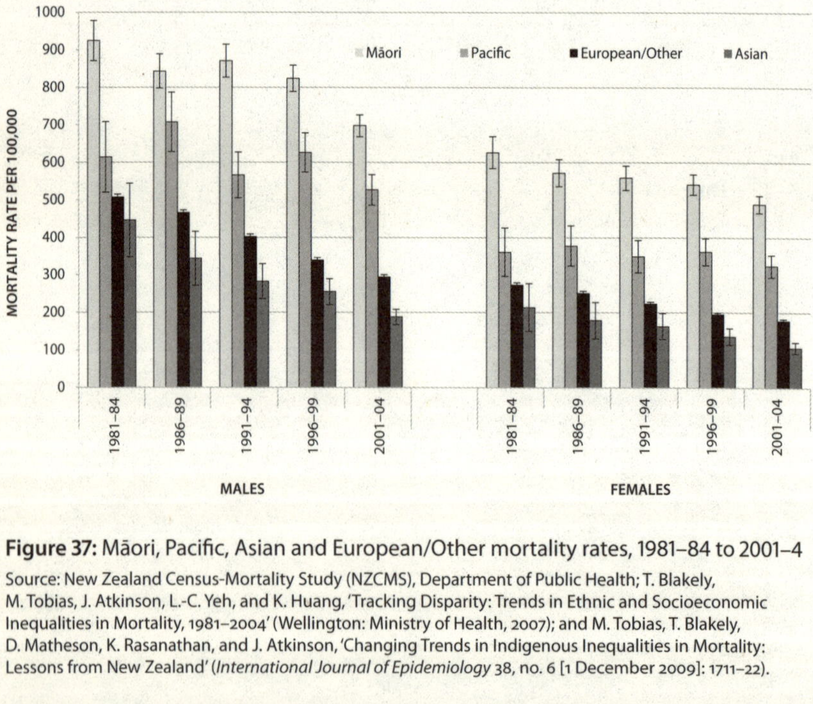

Figure 37: Māori, Pacific, Asian and European/Other mortality rates, 1981–84 to 2001–4

Source: New Zealand Census-Mortality Study (NZCMS), Department of Public Health; T. Blakely, M. Tobias, J. Atkinson, L.-C. Yeh, and K. Huang, 'Tracking Disparity: Trends in Ethnic and Socioeconomic Inequalities in Mortality, 1981–2004' (Wellington: Ministry of Health, 2007); and M. Tobias, T. Blakely, D. Matheson, K. Rasanathan, and J. Atkinson, 'Changing Trends in Indigenous Inequalities in Mortality: Lessons from New Zealand' (*International Journal of Epidemiology* 38, no. 6 [1 December 2009]: 1711–22).

Mortality rates declined for all household income groups (Figure 38), roughly in parallel such that absolute gaps in mortality rates remained much the same from 1981–84 to 2001–4. However, the flip side is that relative inequalities increased from 1.47 to 1.75 times higher mortality in low-income compared to high-income males, and from 1.32 to 1.54 among females. So were socio-economic inequalities increasing? We answer this question 'absolutely not, relatively yes'. Actually, this pattern is quite common internationally,[321] and begs the question as to what matters most – relative or absolute inequalities? One approach to take is that, in the context of reducing average mortality rates for all social groups, reductions in both absolute and relative inequalities are the ideal, with reductions in absolute inequalities but stable relative inequalities being the second best option. Figure 38 shows the third best option – stable absolute inequalities but widening relative inequalities, not as bad as both widening absolute and relative inequalities, but far from 'best' as well.[321]

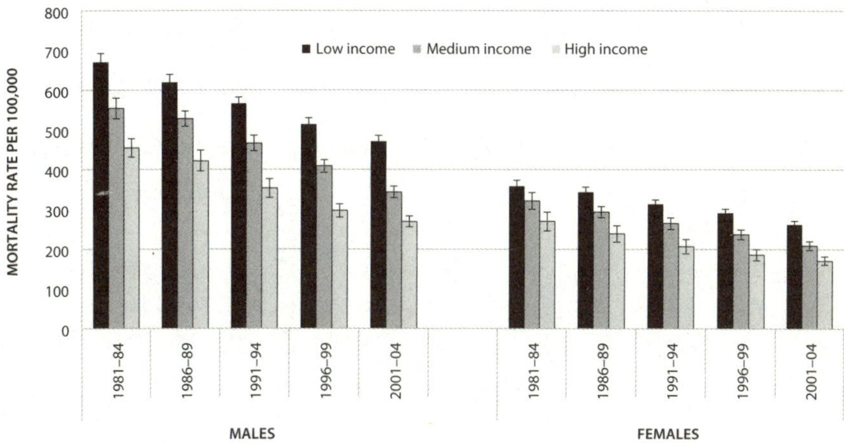

Figure 38: Mortality rates by tertile of household income, 1981–84 to 2001–4 (standardised for age and ethnic group)

Source: New Zealand Census-Mortality Study (NZCMS), Department of Public Health; T. Blakely, M. Tobias, J. Atkinson, L.-C. Yeh, and K. Huang, 'Tracking Disparity: Trends in Ethnic and Socioeconomic Inequalities in Mortality, 1981–2004' (Wellington: Ministry of Health, 2007); T. Blakely, M. Tobias, and J. Atkinson, 'Inequalities in Mortality During and after Restructuring of the New Zealand Economy: Repeated Cohort Studies' (British Medical Journal 336 [January 24, 2008]: 371–75).

What was the impact of changes in mortality rates by age group on changes in Māori and non-Māori life expectancy? Figure 39 (overleaf) builds on the analyses presented in the previous chapter, and takes us through to 2010 to 2012 (shown as just '2011' on the graph to reduce clutter). The total height of each bar is the change in the life expectancy for the denoted time period, and each bar is decomposed according to the contribution by mortality at different ages.

For example, one can see that for non-Māori males there were approximately three-year increases in life expectancy from 1934–38 to 1950–52, and 1980–82 to 1990–92. From 1960–62 to 1970–72, however, there was no improvement in non-Māori male expectancy, due to a small gain from reducing infant mortality (that component above the x-axis in Figure 39) being offset by deteriorations in middle-age mortality (that component beneath the x-axis).

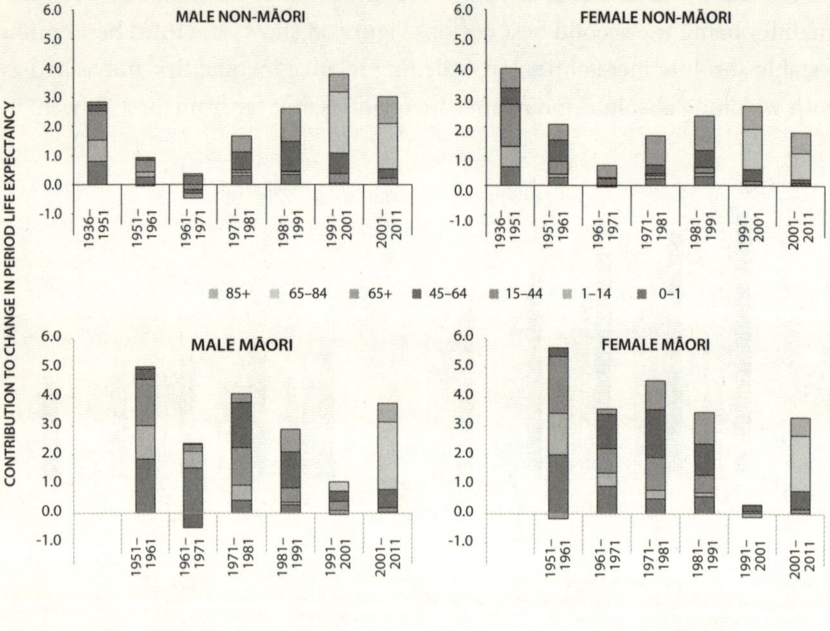

Figure 39: Contributions by age to changes in life expectancy over time, by sex by ethnic group

Source: Except for the New Zealand Census-Mortality Study (NZCMS) 81–84 to 91–94 data, all data are taken from official SNZ life tables, and provided by Kim Dunstan, Statistics New Zealand. The NZCMS data are based on modified SNZ life tables that overcome under-counting of Māori deaths on mortality data by using linked census-mortality data.[301] Caution is required in interpreting trends in age contribution among Māori pre-1980.

Considering the contribution by age to non-Māori life expectancy, falls in infant mortality (<1 year) were particularly important before World War II for both males and females, and reductions in child (1–14 years) and youth (15–44 years) mortality were particularly important from 1936 to 1961. Reductions in 45–64 and 65+-year-old mortality were important at all times for females. Among non-Māori males, improvements in 45–64 and 65+ mortality did not begin until 1971. But the most staggering recent change is among the oldest age category. We show the 65+-year-old group broken down into 65–84 and 85+ from 1991 onwards. By the latest 2001 to 2011 comparison, 30 per cent of male and 38 per cent of female non-Māori improvements in life expectancy were due to decreases in mortality among 85+-year-olds. The momentum has shifted.

The contribution by age to Māori life expectancy trends is more difficult to quantify, because of inaccuracy (known from 1981 to 1995[322; 323] and highly likely before 1981) in the recording of ethnicity on mortality data. Thus, we will not overly interpret the data but rather look for patterns. Gains in Māori life expectancy from 1950–52 to 1980–82 were initially driven by reductions in infant mortality (and perhaps reductions in child mortality), and in the 1960s and 1970s reductions in 45+ mortality became very important. The big fall in the total height of the bars for 1981 to 1991, to 1991 to 2001, is in part due to data inaccuracy. But the 2001 to 2011 comparison is not prone to bias in recording ethnicity on death records, and we can see that just as with non-Māori it is the 65+-year-olds that are driving gains – but not concentrated in the 85+-year-olds to the same extent as non-Māori.

Summarising, gains in both Māori and non-Māori life expectancy since the 1980s are largely a function of reducing middle-age and older mortality. There are still important preventable causes of death in young age groups, such as suicide. But the momentum for recent improvements in life expectancy has shifted to middle and older age-group reductions in mortality. Which prompts the question, what diseases in middle age are responsible for these falls in death rates?

CAUSE-SPECIFIC MORTALITY

Cardiovascular disease rates up to the age of 74 have fallen by nearly two-thirds between 1981–84 and 2001–4 for European/Other and by a lesser, but still impressive, 40 to 45 per cent for Māori (Figure 40, overleaf). Changes of this kind have been seen in many developed countries in the last few decades: in Australia, cardiovascular disease mortality amongst 35–69-year-olds has fallen by 80 per cent since 1970 (Figure 26).

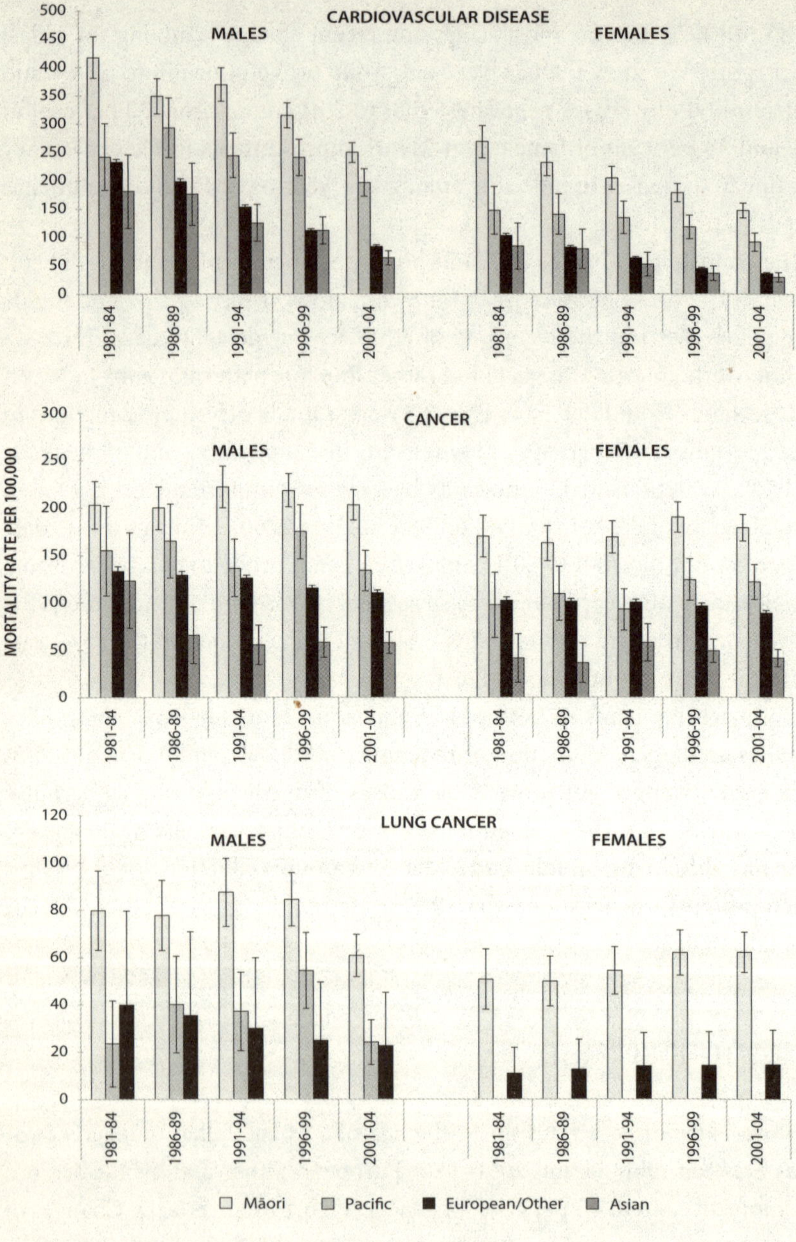

Figure 40: Cause-specific mortality from 1981–84 to 2001–4, by ethnicity

Source: T. Blakely, M. Tobias, J. Atkinson, L.-C. Yeh, and K. Huang, 'Tracking Disparity: Trends in Ethnic and Socioeconomic Inequalities in Mortality, 1981–2004' (Wellington: Ministry of Health, 2007); and M. Tobias, T. Blakely, D. Matheson, K. Rasanathan, and J. Atkinson, 'Changing Trends in Indigenous Inequalities in Mortality: Lessons from New Zealand' (*International Journal of Epidemiology* 38, no. 6 [1 December 2009]: 1711–22).

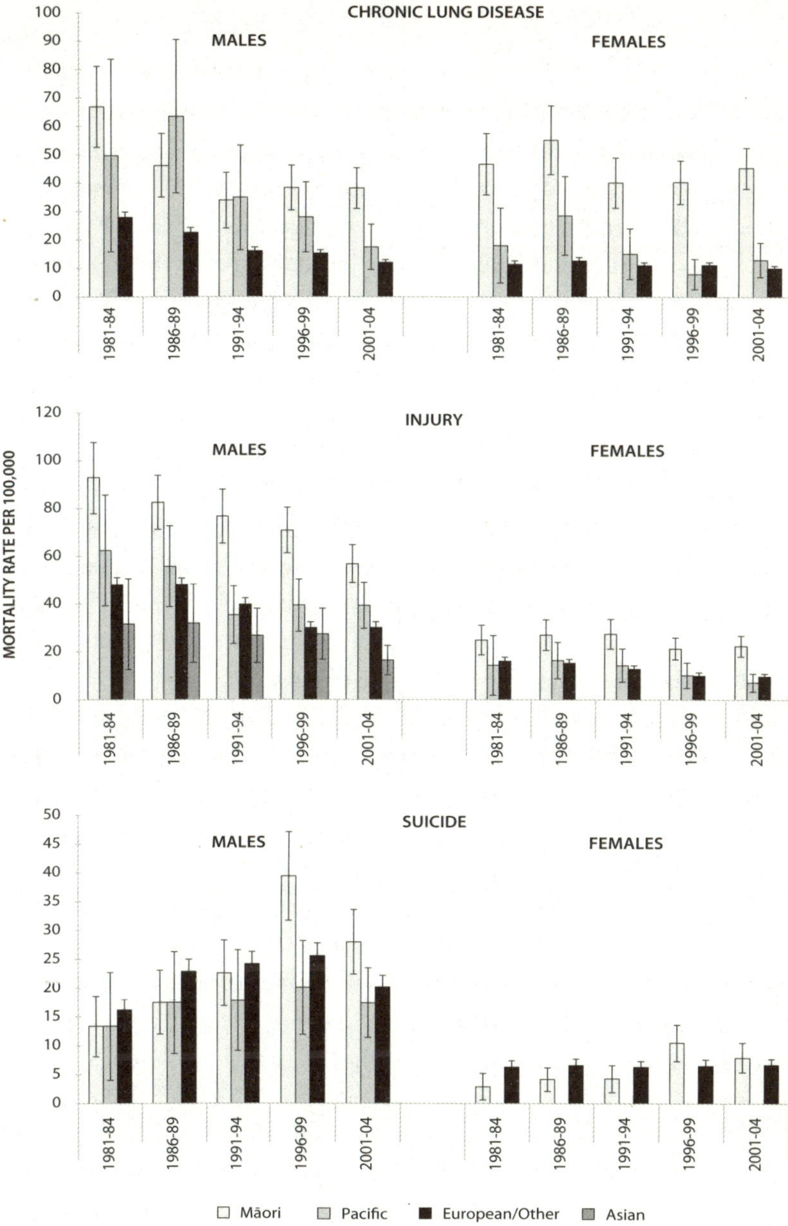
CHRONIC LUNG DISEASE
MALES
FEMALES
INJURY
MALES
FEMALES
SUICIDE
MALES
FEMALES
MORTALITY RATE PER 100,000
1981-84
1986-89
1991-94
1996-99
2001-04
Māori
Pacific
European/Other
Asian

There remain large inequalities between Māori and Pacific and European/Other. Higher cardiovascular disease rates among Māori were reported by community-based epidemiological surveys in the 1960s and 1970s,[282; 324; 325] with special note made of hypertensive disease and particularly high rates for Māori women compared to European women. By 1981–84, Māori females had a mortality rate 2.6 times greater than their European/Other female counterparts, and Māori males had a rate that was 1.8 times greater than European/Other males. The absolute gap in death rates between Māori and European/Other has not changed greatly since the early 1980s, and may have decreased a little for females. But the difference in relative terms has increased since the reference value (European/Other mortality) has diminished considerably. In 2001–4, Māori males had three times, and Māori females four times, the cardiovascular disease mortality of their European/Other counterparts.[326; 327]

Inequalities in cardiovascular disease mortality also exist by socio-economic position. For example, males in the lowest third of equivalised household income had a 1.5 times greater cardiovascular mortality than their high income counterparts in 1981–84, a gap that widened to 1.8 times in 2001–4. Likewise, the female gap widened from 1.4 to 1.7 times.

As cardiovascular disease mortality rates decline, the contribution of cancer to overall mortality rates and life expectancy proportionately increases. Mortality rates from cancer now exceed mortality rates from CVD at most ages, but since CVD is a common cause of death amongst the very old, the total number of CVD deaths is greater than that from cancer.

Mortality rates for 1–74-year-olds for all cancers combined have come down by 17 per cent and 13 per cent for European/Other males and females, respectively, since 1981, but stayed the same for Māori males and possibly increased for Māori females (Figure 40). As a consequence, the gap widened and Māori mortality from cancer was roughly twice that for European/Other by 2001–4. Pacific cancer rates were intermediary, but closer to European/Other than Māori rates. Asian rates were consistently lower than European/Other rates – an observation we shall return to later in this chapter.

Lung cancer, the cancer most strongly associated with tobacco smoking, has very large inequalities between ethnic groups – Māori rates are nearly three times greater than European/Other rates for males, and over four times greater among females. Pointing to historic patterns in tobacco consumption a couple of decades prior, European/Other male rates fell steadily in the 1980s and 1990s, Māori male rates began to fall in the 2000s, but both Māori and European/Other females rates have continued to increase.

Chronic lung disease rates show large inequalities similar to lung cancer, but rates appear to have been steadily reducing among both Māori and European/ Other. Unintentional injury mortality has steadily fallen for all ethnicities by sex groups, with the possible exception of Māori females, but moderate to large Māori–European/Other inequalities exist at all points in time.

Suicide mortality is high by international standards among <44-year-olds, but not high enough to have a major impact on life expectancy. However, the large increase in male rates, particularly among Māori males, at least puts a brake on life expectancy improvements.

The groupings of cause of death shown here make up the majority of all deaths. The big one that is missing is diabetes, which is not well captured as a cause of death in mortality records. In the future, diabetes will become more important in its own right, partly because of the obesity epidemic and also because other diseases are receding so quickly.

RISK FACTOR TRENDS

Nutrition and physical activity

It is surprisingly difficult to find good historical data on what New Zealanders eat. The United Nation's Food and Agricultural Organization (FAO; faostat.fao.org) provides information on what was happening at a country level from the 1960s onwards. The trends nationally were increasing consumption of vegetable oils (including olive oil) and poultry, and reducing consumption of animal fats and butter.

But what about individual diets? Figure 41 (overleaf) traces percentage fat in the diet, and total energy intake, by ethnicity from 1989, 1997 and 2008–9, using the Life in New Zealand survey and the two National Nutrition Surveys (NNS). We are not aware of any other (semi-) reliable data back to or prior to the 1980s. The trends over time in all four sex-by-ethnic (Māori, non-Māori) groups are the same: rapid increases in body mass index (BMI); increase then fall in total energy intake (such that 2008–9 levels roughly equate to 1989

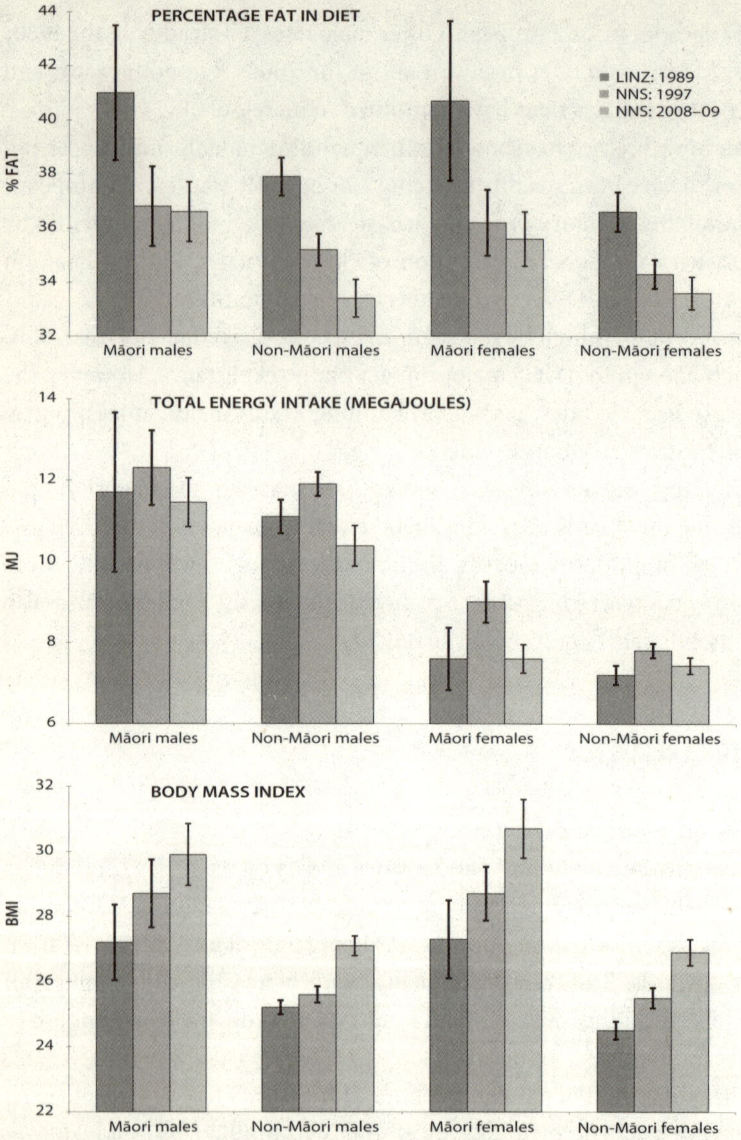

Figure 41: Body mass index (BMI), total energy intake (megajoules, MJ) and percentage fat in the diet, by sex and ethnicity, from the 1989 Life in New Zealand survey (LINZ) and the 1997 and 2008–9 National Nutrition Surveys (NNS)

Source: N. Wilson and D. Russell, 'Life in New Zealand Survey', *Commission Report Volume II: Survey Protocol* (Wellington: Hillary Commission, 1991); D. Russell, W. Parnell and N. Wilson, *NZ Food: NZ People. Key Results of the 1997 National Nutrition Survey* (Wellington: Ministry of Health, 1999); University of Otago and Ministry of Health, *A Focus on Nutrition: Key Findings of the 2008/09 New Zealand Adult Nutrition Survey* (Wellington: Ministry of Health, 2011).The figures from the NNS 2008–9 for non-Māori are actually those for European/Other. Error bars are 95 per cent confidence intervals.

levels); and steady, substantial falls in fat as a percentage of total energy intake. At every point in time Māori have higher BMI, higher energy intake and (usually) higher percentage energy intake from fat.

We must be wary about the apparent paradox of decreasing energy intake in the presence of increasing BMI. Energy intake is notoriously under-estimated in nutrition surveys, and what appears to be a decline may be due simply to the reporting bias being more pronounced in 2008–9 than in 1997. Another explanation might be that New Zealanders have become less physically active, so that they tend to put on weight despite eating less.

Measuring physical activity reliably is as difficult as measuring diets! You have to consider (and measure) leisure, work-related and transport-related activity. And to reliably determine trends over time, the same instrument has to be used. The 2002–3, 2006–7 and 2011–12 New Zealand Health Surveys do this,[122] and there is really no sign of change in physical activity over this decade. Focusing on differences in physical activity between social groups at any one point in time, though, Māori have equivalent or better levels than European/Other, and Pacific people have lower levels than either. Regarding physical *in*activity – which is not just the flipside of physical activity – levels appear to have reduced if anything since the 1996–97 Health Survey, although they bounce around a bit (pun intended).

Nutrition surveys in 1997 and 2008–9 include a wide range of nutritional markers.[328; 329] Saturated fat intake – traditionally regarded as the 'bad' component of total fat – is falling steeply for all New Zealanders, as is cholesterol intake, and these two dietary trends are thought to be the major reason for reductions in total cholesterol levels in the blood. Fruit consumption is increasing over time, but vegetable consumption has not changed.[122] Māori tend to have higher saturated fat intake and lower fruit intake, but there has been little if any difference in blood pressure across ethnic and deprivation groupings in the past. Data from the 1989 Life in New Zealand survey – whilst having few Māori – also suggests little if any difference in blood pressure between Māori and non-Māori.[330] However, in the recent adult nutrition survey (2008–9) significantly higher blood pressure was found for Māori.[331]

The changes aren't all positive. A growing proportion of the New Zealand population is food insecure, meaning they cannot routinely afford sufficient and healthy food. This group, concentrated among Māori, Pacific and deprived populations,[329] is likely to consume cheap, high-density fatty food. The implications are more diabetes, obesity and cardiovascular disease, increased risk of some cancers, and greater wear and tear on bones and joints.

Overall, apart from BMI and food security, nutrition indicators have been heading in a pro-health direction. There is plenty of room for improvement; for example, New Zealanders have high saturated fat intake compared to other countries. Gaps between social groups exist. The favourable trends in (most) risk factors match the fall in cardiovascular disease mortality. Without the rise in bodyweights, mortality might have fallen even faster. We will pick up the obesity issue again in the final chapter.

Tobacco

Tobacco is an important cause of cardiovascular disease, many cancers (lung most notably, but also oral, upper airways, oesophageal, pancreatic, bladder, cervical and others)[332; 333; 334] and respiratory diseases (chronic obstructive respiratory disease and emphysema, and increases the likelihood of death from pneumonia following respiratory infection).[299] The time between initiating smoking and increased risk of disease occurrence is less than five years for cardiovascular and respiratory disease and less than ten years for cancers.[299] The effects of quitting smoking are apparent rapidly: this is most evident for cardiovascular diseases, with reductions observed within a year of reducing exposures to tobacco smoke, but the first downturns in cancer are also seen quite early, for example, within five years.[299]

The total burden of mortality in a population that is attributable to tobacco is a function of the amount of tobacco smoked over time, and increases exponentially with duration and intensity of tobacco use. To understand the impact of changing tobacco use on mortality trends from 1980 requires data on tobacco consumption back to the 1960s and 1970s. Overall, per capita consumption of tobacco in New Zealand has fallen by two-thirds since the 1970s, as illustrated in the previous chapter (Figure 31), but the decline stalled in the 2000s. Differences in smoking within New Zealand are now larger than they have ever been, with high socio-economic and European (and Asian) populations having the lowest smoking rates. Until recently there was mixed evidence whether smoking rates are continuing to fall among both Māori and European – census and health survey data suggest 'yes',[335] but other sources 'no'.[336] The most recent 2011/12 Health Survey put the adult prevalence of current smoking at 18 per cent, down from 20 per cent in 2006/7, and youth down from 14 per cent to 6 per cent over the same five-year period.[122] Worryingly, the same survey suggested Māori smoking was unchanged at 41 per cent despite an increasing focus in media and quit campaigns. Pacific smoking prevalence was 27 per cent and Asian 10 per cent – both pretty much unchanged from five years earlier. European/Other has a statistically significant fall from 19 per cent to 17 per cent.

More encouragingly, and probably more reliably as well, the 2013 census smoking rates show very promising progress since the 2006 census: a fall in smoking prevalence from 20.7 per cent to 15.1 per cent for all adults aged 15 years and older; and a nearly 10 percentage point fall for Māori from 42.2 per cent to 32.7 per cent. Assuming the census is a more reliable monitor of trends, and we do believe it is more reliable, this is very good news. It seems likely that some, but not all, of these falls are attributable to annual 10 per cent increases in excise tax since 2010.

We return in the final chapter to these trends, and consider what changes will be necessary to achieve the Smokefree Aotearoa goal of less than 5 per cent prevalence by the year 2025.

Because 80 to 90 per cent of lung cancer is attributable to tobacco, incidence rates provide an excellent marker of the long-run tobacco disease burden. Figure 42 (overleaf) shows lung cancer incidence by ethnicity and income, from the CancerTrends study that links census and cancer registrations.[337] Several patterns over time are notable. European/Other male lung cancer incidence has been steadily falling since the early 1980s, indicating that peak tobacco consumption among European/Other males must have occurred before 1960 (positing an average time lag of 20 years). European/Other females have experienced a steady increase in lung cancer since 1980, although this appears to have now plateaued and the rate is expected to fall in the immediate future. We deduce that smoking by European/Other females peaked in the 1970s and early 1980s.

Lung cancer rates for Māori men have been stable, and possibly falling, through the 1980s to 2000s, reflecting a high smoking prevalence back to at least the 1970s and a relatively slow downward trajectory in smoking in the 1970s and 1980s. The trend for Māori women is different. Female lung cancer rates have steadily increased during the 1980s to 2000s, are now overtaking the Māori male rates, and are at least three times as high as European/Other females.

Pacific female lung cancer rates have increased, consistent with an unrelenting rise in tobacco consumption since the 1960s. Pacific male rates are higher than for Pacific females, though less than Māori, and perhaps peaked in the late 1980s and 1990s. The indications are that Pacific male smoking (be it in New Zealand or country of origin) was at a maximum in the 1960s and 1970s.

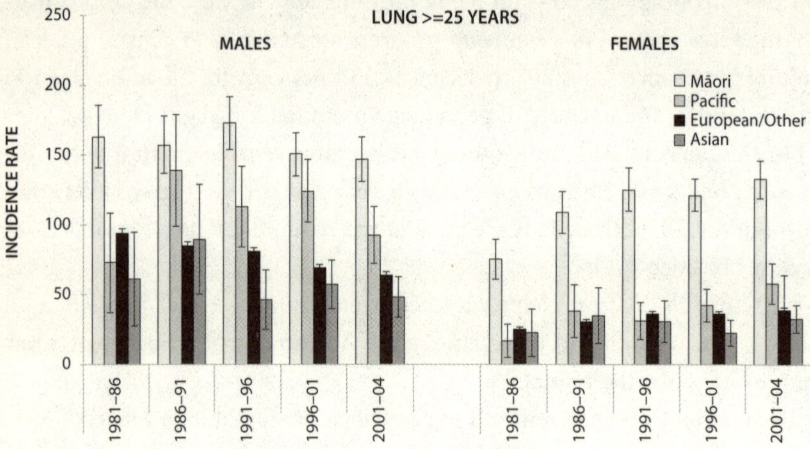

Figure 42: Lung cancer incidence for the 1980s to 2000s

Source: The record linkage study of census and cancer registry data: T. Blakely, C. Shaw, et al., *CancerTrends: Trends in Cancer Incidence by Ethnic and Socioeconomic Group, New Zealand 1981–2004* (Wellington: University of Otago and Ministry of Health, 2010). Ethnic rates are standardised by age, and income rates by both age and ethnicity, ensuring comparability over time.

Tobacco is the biggest single preventable cause of death in New Zealand, causing 4500 to 5000 deaths per year.[336] This amounts to 15–20 per cent of all deaths, and a greater proportion of 'premature' mortality (that is, deaths before age 65). Tobacco smoking is also responsible for 10–20 per cent of the gap in mortality between Māori and European/Other 45–74-year-olds.[304; 305] So it is not surprising that changes in the consumption of tobacco (an increase in the proportion of smokers quitting, or a decrease in number of cigarettes smoked per day among those still smoking, or reduced exposure to passive smoking) make a very important contribution to the rate of mortality decline.

At least half of the fall in cardiovascular disease mortality in developed countries (including New Zealand) in the late twentieth century has been attributed to changes in risk factors such as high fat diets and smoking.[338; 279; 339] The exact contribution of smoking, though, is trickier to pin down. In one New Zealand analysis by Capewell and colleagues from 1982 to 1992, 30 per cent of the fall in coronary heart disease mortality was attributed to falls in smoking, compared to 12 per cent for falls in cholesterol and 8 per cent for falls in blood pressure in the same time period.[279] However, things change over time. A more recent analysis by Martin Tobias and colleagues covering the period 1980 to 2004 for ages 35 to 64 years estimated that 80 per cent of the fall in death rates could be attributed to falls in blood pressure, cholesterol and smoking.[278] Considered separately, falls in blood pressure were estimated to contribute to 42 per cent of the fall, cholesterol 36 per cent and tobacco 22 per cent. (Note that the sum of these three percentages is greater than 80 per cent, because when considered together you need to allow for their interactions and 'joint effects'.) Smoking made its major contribution to the reduction in heart disease in the 1980s but cholesterol reductions were important throughout this period, and blood pressure only recently. Importantly, there remains huge potential to reduce coronary heart disease rates by radical cuts in smoking, and ongoing improvements in diet and physical activity.

What about the contribution of changes in smoking prevalence to changes in life expectancy itself? We are not aware of previously published work looking directly at this in New Zealand. However, with the aid of life tables by smoking status based on the returns from the 1981 and 1996 censuses,[301] we calculated the life expectancies that would have applied in 1996 had smoking prevalence remained at the levels of 1981, and vice versa (life expectancies in 1981 had the 1996 prevalence figures applied). For *males*, we estimated that between 10 per cent (applying 1996 prevalence to 1981 mortality rates) and 20 per cent (applying 1981 prevalence of smoking to 1996 mortality rates) of the increase in life expectancy over this time period was due to falls in smoking prevalence. These somewhat crude analyses may under-estimate the total impact of tobacco due to errors in the figures we used for smoking prevalence and mortality. Furthermore, we did not account for effects of passive smoking. For *females*, the contribution of smoking to increases in life expectancy in this period (1981–96) was negligible. The proportion of female never smokers did not change, and the fall in current smokers was balanced by an increase in ex-smokers. The modest decline in smoking rates among females in this period probably contributed to falls in CVD mortality, given the very short lag between smoking cessation and reduced disease risk. But this was balanced by the longer run impact of smoking-related cancers (see the lung cancer graphs, Figure 42).

Alcohol

Alcohol is a cause of injury mortality, some cancers (e.g., liver, breast, oesophageal), cardiovascular disease at high average dose (e.g., hypertensive heart disease and haemorrhagic stroke) and repeated binge drinking (e.g., heart rhythm disturbances), liver cirrhosis, and other miscellaneous causes of, or contributors to, death. It is also a cause of many other social harms. It is, of course, also a pleasure enjoyed by many and may protect against cardiovascular disease in 'moderate doses' – although much of this apparent protective association may be due to moderate drinkers doing many other things moderately, and not the alcohol itself.

Alcohol is deeply rooted in New Zealand culture.[340] So too other countries, and when it comes to consumption, New Zealand is 'middle of the pack' compared with other OECD countries (Figure 43). Robert Scragg estimated that in the late 1980s alcohol actually prevented more deaths than it caused.[341] But the deaths averted were at older ages (i.e., cardiovascular disease), whereas the deaths caused by alcohol (i.e., injury such as road traffic crash) were at younger ages, meaning that the years of life lost due to alcohol (compared to averted) were much greater. Put another way, alcohol causes death and disability at young ages, which means it will be a 'drag' on life expectancy which is more sensitive to deaths at younger ages.

Recently, Jennie Connor and colleagues have provided the latest update in 'burden of disease' estimates for alcohol.[342] They incorporate latest epidemiological data for best estimates of the causal association of alcohol consumption with mortality, e.g., including some beneficial effects of moderate consumption for diabetes, ischaemic stroke and ischaemic heart disease, but deleterious effects for many cancers and – of course – injury. They also tried to allow for binge-drinking consequences. Unlike Scragg two decades earlier, they find that the total number of deaths due to alcohol exceeds deaths averted by alcohol – and consequently a much larger impact in terms of years of life lost due to the younger age (on average) of deaths attributed to alcohol. About 5.4 per cent of all deaths under the age of 80 were attributed to alcohol, with a higher percentage among Māori, i.e., there are large ethnic inequalities in alcohol-related death rates. In addition to the well-known diseases of alcohol such as injury, liver disease and cardiovascular disease (in net, due to some beneficial effects on cardiovascular disease in middle age offset by harm from injury and cancers), the biggest percentage of deaths due to alcohol among both Māori and non-Māori women was due to breast cancer.

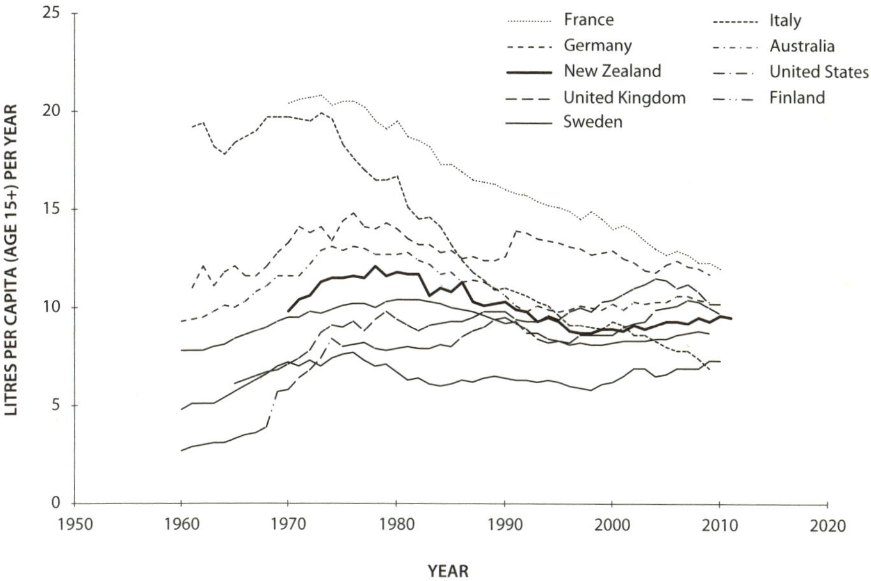

Figure 43: Alcohol consumption for New Zealand and selected OECD countries
Source: Data extracted from Organisation for Economic Co-operation and Development statistics (www.oecd.org).

Thus, the net effect of alcohol is harm. Work in Australia has found that interventions to reduce alcohol consumption across the population (e.g., through tax, marketing restrictions) have some of the biggest impacts of any public health measures on increasing the number of years people live.[343; 344] The same is likely true in New Zealand. We do not know how the changing drinking patterns over time in New Zealand (be it average consumption as in Figure 43, or binge drinking and differences by age) impacted on trends in life expectancy – we only know that life expectancy could have been improved at any point in time by 'better' patterns of alcohol consumption.

SOCIAL AND ECONOMIC DETERMINANTS

Migration and demographic change

As we pointed out in earlier chapters, new migrants are often healthier than the resident population, but this will not always be the case. Some migrants come from countries with such poor health that the 'healthy migrant effect' still leaves them at a disadvantage in their new home. Furthermore, some of those who move, including refugees and those who come as part of family reunions, bypass many of the checks that tend to select against individuals with health problems. Did migration influence trends in life expectancy in New Zealand from the 1980s till present?

In earlier times migration to New Zealand was predominantly from Europe. The United Kingdom and Australia were still the dominant sources from 1980 onwards, between them contributing a third to 60 per cent of migrants in any year. There was a surge of Asian migration, particularly from China, in the early 2000s which for a brief period matched the flow from Australia (but was still less than the UK). Permanent migrants have come also from India, Japan, the Philippines and Korea, and together with arrivals from China made up about a quarter of new settlers in New Zealand in the 2000s. The proportion of the New Zealand population of Asian ethnicity rose from less than 2 per cent in the 1980s to 9 per cent in the 2006 census. In Figure 44 we display mortality rates for Asian, Pacific and European/Other by years of usual residence in New Zealand.

Several important points emerge. First, there is a steep gradient of increasing mortality within both Asian and European/Other ethnic groups with increasing duration of residency in New Zealand. Second, within categories of New Zealand-born or years of usual residence (and sex), there is little difference between Asian and European/Other. For example, the mortality rate of male New Zealand-born European/Other (4561 per 100,000) is little different from that for New Zealand-born Asian (5083 per 100,000). In other words, it is recent migration that explains the mortality advantage of Asian people in New Zealand (see Figure 37), rather than enduring social and cultural characteristics associated with being Asian. Such a convergence of migrant and host statistics is not always the case. For instance, as we mentioned in the introduction to this book, Greek migrants to Australia in the 1980s enjoyed mortality rates that were lower than those for Australians overall, and the gap was much the same whatever the length of residence.[345]

Amongst Pacific people we see no convincing association of years of residence with mortality. This might be due to a lack of health selection (given that migration to and from the Pacific islands is easy and relatively open), or because people with poor health living in the Pacific selectively migrate to New Zealand to be with family and have access to better health services. Another explanation might be that health gains for Pacific people moving to New Zealand (due to better access to health services, for instance) are balanced by new risks to health (such as alcohol and mental health problems).

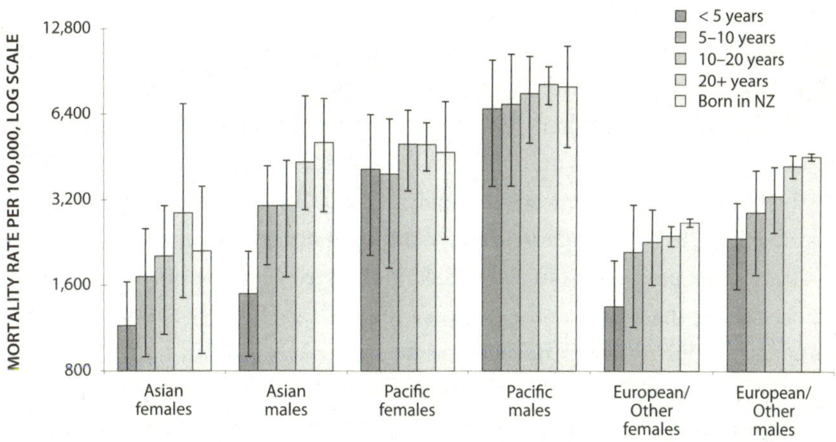

Figure 44: Mortality rate per 100,000 for 25–74-year-olds, by years of usual residence in New Zealand, for the 1996–99 and 2001–4 New Zealand Census-Mortality Study cohorts combined

Source: A. Hajat, T. Blakely, S. Dayal, and S. Jatrana, 'Do New Zealand's Immigrants Have a Mortality Advantage? Evidence from the New Zealand Census-Mortality Study' (*Ethnicity & Health* 15, no. 5 [2010]: 531–47).

Is the influx of Asian migrants a cause of the rapid increase in non-Māori life expectancy in the latter part of the twentieth century? Yes, but we suggest its contribution was minor.

Statistics New Zealand does not separate Asian and European/Other life expectancy trends, and because of the small numbers of deaths in some age categories, Asian rates are too unstable in the NZCMS to generate accurate life tables. However, if in very rough terms we assume that the Asian mortality rates were two-thirds of European/Other at every single year of age (which is consistent with the pattern across coarsely specified age groups), that this was purely due to a healthy migrant effect, and that about 8 per cent of the non-Māori population was Asian in 2001, then we can estimate that non-Māori mortality rates would have been 2.7 per cent higher if there had been no migration from Asia (i.e., 8% × 0.33 = 2.7%). Applied to 2001 non-Māori life tables, this small increment in mortality results in a decrease of 0.26 years (for females) and 0.29 years (males) in life expectancy at birth. As the Asian population made up less than 8 per cent of the population for most of this period, we estimate that no more than 0.20 to 0.25 years of the gain in non-Māori life expectancy in the 1980s to 2000s might be due to a healthy migrant effect from Asian migration. (Interestingly, this is similar to our estimate of the contribution of Southern European migrants to the lift in Australian life expectancy between 1940 and 1990.[290]) If these figures are approximately right, the healthy Asian migrant effect explains about 3 per cent of the eight-year improvement in New Zealand life expectancy at birth between 1980 and 2000.

The Pacific population in New Zealand doubled as a proportion of all non-Māori during the 1980s, and aged, meaning that their higher mortality rates compared to European/Other would have tended to restrain increases in life expectancy overall – perhaps offsetting the effect of Asian in-migration.

Migration of European/Other may have an impact, if the proportion of recent migrants increased during the 1980s to 2000s. However, much of European/Other migration is cross-Tasman, and the degree of health selection may vary depending on the relative economic performance of the two countries. We note that the proportion of the Australian workforce in 2008 that was New Zealand-born was considerably higher for unskilled trades than amongst skilled workers.[346] This trend would tend to minimise the difference in life expectancy between Australia and New Zealand.

Māori migration to and from Australia is common. It is plausible that flows to Australia in the late 1980s and 1990s increased as economic conditions in New Zealand deteriorated, and Māori unemployment climbed to 25 per cent. (It is not possible to check this proposition directly as ethnicity is not collected on arrival and departure data.) If Māori migrating to Australia in the late 1980s and early 1990s were healthier than Māori who did not migrate, then this may be one reason for the levelling off in Māori life expectancy that was observed on this side of the Tasman. In the late 1990s, when the New Zealand economy improved and job prospects were brighter, one might speculate that healthier Māori returned to New Zealand, and gave a leg-up to the increase in Māori life expectancy. On the other hand, it is conceivable that migration to Australia in the 1980s and 1990s was predominantly unemployed Māori whose health status was less favourable on the whole than Māori with ongoing employment in New Zealand. On balance, we believe there probably were health selection effects associated with cross-Tasman migration, but these are unlikely to have been strong enough to alter life expectancy trends appreciably for Māori in New Zealand.

Physical environment

In the last quarter of the twentieth century there was overall a reduction in household crowding in New Zealand,[347] although this was not true for some groups (most notably Pacific children).[348] Poor housing conditions for many Pacific and Māori families has been a factor for many infectious diseases which, contrary to the trends in non-communicable diseases and injury (described above), have increased in recent decades.[349] Crowding certainly played a big part in determining the location and magnitude of the epidemic of meningococcal disease in the 1990s and early 2000s.[350] The effect of household conditions on chronic disease mortality and life expectancy is more muted and difficult to identify. A reduced exposure to infectious agents at young ages may manifest in a reduction of certain life-threatening chronic diseases many years later, for example, liver failure (Hepatitis B) and stomach cancer (*H. pylori*).

There were improvements in other aspects of the physical environment that may have assisted mortality decline. Outdoor air pollution, caused by the emissions from motor vehicles, home fires and industrial processes, contributes to respiratory diseases, cardiovascular conditions, and stroke.[351] In most high-income countries, levels of air pollution have declined considerably in the last 30 years. In the United States, a study of metropolitan areas from the late 1970s to the mid-1990s found that improvements in air quality were linked with rising life expectancy, after adjustment for factors such as regional prosperity and smoking rates.[453] A fall of 10 μg/m^3 in fine particle levels was associated with an improvement of 0.6 years in life expectancy at birth.

In New Zealand air pollution has been less of a problem, historically, than in North America or in Europe. The major issues have been smoke from home heating (particularly when coal is used), and traffic emissions. Restrictions on the use of coal for home heating, introduction of more efficient wood-burners, the removal of lead from petrol (1996), reductions in the sulphur content of diesel and more stringent emission standards for motor vehicles have all contributed to improvements in air quality (though balanced to some extent by the multiplication of vehicle traffic). In Auckland, total suspended particulate levels came down from about 80 μg/m^3 in the early 1960s, when systematic monitoring was instituted, to less than 20 μg/m^3 in 2005.[352] (See Figure 45.) It is not known how much of this reduction occurred in the fine particle fraction (less than 2.5 microns in diameter) nor how representative the change was of conditions in the population at large (because of the lack of comprehensive monitoring).

While considerable improvement has been made, there is opportunity to reduce the health impacts of air pollution further. Gerda Kuschel and colleagues have estimated that anthropogenic (man-made) pollutants were responsible in 2011 for about 1100 premature deaths a year in New Zealand, 600 hospital admissions and 1.5 million restricted activity days. The social costs of air pollution were attributed to household fires (56 per cent), vehicle emissions (22 per cent), open burning (12 per cent) and industry (10 per cent).[353]

Between 1981–4 and 2001–4 the rate of deaths from injury fell by almost 50 per cent (Figure 40). Road crash injury (which contributes just over a quarter of all injury deaths) caused close to 600 deaths a year in the early 1980s (around 20 deaths per 100,000 population), but in 2010 the road toll was 375 deaths (a rate of 8 per 100,000).[354] What was responsible for this improvement? With road crash injury, important factors have been safer vehicle design, less drinking and driving, speed limits, driver licensing changes, road improvements and better trauma care. There have also been, recently, injury-saving changes in transport patterns in New Zealand and in other countries (including fewer vehicle kilometres travelled and more public transport use).[355; 356]

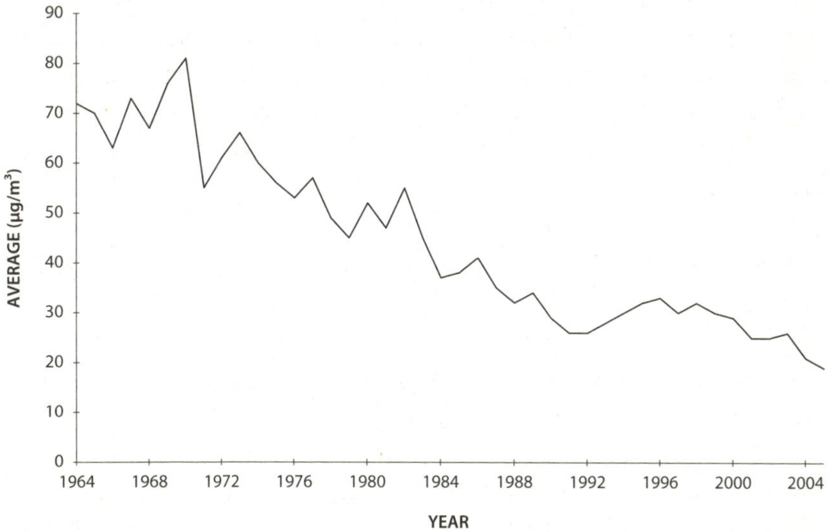

Figure 45: Air pollution measured as total suspended particulate matter, Auckland, 1964–2005

Note: µg/m³ = micrograms per cubic metre.
Source: Auckland Regional Council, *Air Quality Data CD* (Auckland: Auckland Regional Council, 2006).

PERSONAL HEALTH CARE AND PUBLIC HEALTH INTERVENTIONS

The good news first – both public health interventions and personal health care save lives. Building on the technological revolution in health-care treatments since World War II, the life-saving and life-prolonging effect of health care has never been more important than now.

The cardiovascular disease story is a powerful one to demonstrate the joint importance of personal health care and public health interventions. Cardiovascular disease rates have risen and fallen in phase with rises and falls (some would say epidemics) of risk factors. The steep increases in heart disease and stroke in the early-to-mid twentieth century were due principally to changes in diet (higher fat and energy intakes) and smoking (increased consumption of machine-made cigarettes). These behavioural changes did not occur in a vacuum. They took place in a world of business and consumer pressures (New Zealand, after all, earns a considerable portion of its income from the export of saturated fat), and the influences of international trade (e.g., the blandishments of tobacco companies). For a multitude of reasons, heart disease mortality peaked in the 1960s – perhaps a little later for Māori and low socio-economic groups. The important point is that we are now enjoying the downhill ride on the far side of the epidemic curve. The steepness of the decline is influenced by what we do as a society, both in preventing disease occurrence and treating people who are affected. It is estimated that about half of the reduction in cardiovascular disease mortality since about 1980 can be attributed to reduced disease incidence due to changes such as fewer cigarettes being smoked and less consumption of saturated fat, and the other half can be attributed to improvements in medical treatments.[338; 279; 339]

We do not know for sure if the roughly 50:50 contribution of prevention/treatment to cardiovascular disease mortality applies to all ethnic and socio-economic groups, but it seems a reasonable default assumption. The proportion attributable to secondary prevention could be gifted to either the treatment or prevention camps since interventions to slow progression of disease may be behavioural or medical treatment. The relative contributions of prevention and treatment will vary by context and time. For example, in a country that invests heavily in treatment services but achieves no change in risk factor trends, then the decline in CVD mortality would be attributable entirely to treatment. Exact ratios aside, the key points here are that both prevention and treatment matter, and as treatments become more and more efficacious (as they most certainly have for CVD) then the influence of health care services on life expectancy becomes more important. However, prevention is – as a general rule, and if using population-wide approaches – much more cost-effective.[344]

Improvements in smoking, dietary fat and exercise may occur without deliberate public health interventions. Sometimes these changes are more akin to movements in fashion. Kunitz[1] describes the process whereby ischaemic heart disease rates fell first among the middle classes, as they took up behaviours such as running and ceasing smoking during the 1970s. Such secular trends in lifestyle, however, are not completely independent of health considerations. The middle classes respond early to expert advice, such as the Surgeon General's warnings about the harm of tobacco in 1964,[357] which is rapidly translated into the opinion and behaviour of fashion leaders. Stopping smoking becomes the 'new black', with one of its triggers being public health pronouncements.

A theme throughout this book is of long-run trends, and short-run perturbations. We suggest that the organised efforts of society act on both the long-run and short-term causes of mortality. Perhaps a useful metaphor is a track on which society walks (or bicycles) to good health. We, society, make a concerted effort to avoid interruptions on the journey, which means clearing away barriers and avoiding diversions. But public health also plays a part in building the track, ensuring there are well-defined edges, a low-friction surface and a helpful gradient, and in this way adds momentum to the long-term improvement in conditions. Regulations, social capacity building and education all contribute to smoothing the way to lower mortality. A good example is working with the food industry, to remove salt from manufactured food,[358] thereby contributing to reduced blood pressure in the population and lower stroke incidence and mortality. This public health activity can happen imperceptibly behind the scenes, and slowly shifts the public's 'taste' for salt. Of course it is not always behind the scenes. On occasions public health would not have progressed without political engagement, challenge and advocacy.

Tobacco is a good example of hands-on public health. The Smokefree Environment Act 1990 halted sponsorship of sporting and cultural activities by the tobacco industry, and prohibited smoking from public buildings (e.g., office space, but not pubs and hotels). Subsequent amendments have extended the law to include pubs and hotels, and all workplaces. Accompanied by the Health Sponsorship Council taking over sponsorship of sports and cultural events and undertaking widespread health education and social marketing about the risks of active and passive smoking, and the combined activities of many other public health agencies and actors, the social norms regarding tobacco smoking have shifted in New Zealand society. Tobacco tax as a fiscal disincentive has added to the mix, as has subsidised access to cessation services and nicotine replacement therapy through the Quit group. The prevalence of smoking has fallen (as shown earlier in this chapter). More radical action to end the tobacco epidemic is now required – a subject we will visit in the next chapter.

On the treatment half of the cardiovascular disease story, there have been many advances in life-saving treatments. Building on coronary artery bypass grafting (CABG), angioplasty (insertion of a catheter into a blocked coronary artery, followed by balloon dilation to open blockages) was a novel treatment in the 1980s, increasingly routine in the 1990s, and in the 2000s increasingly accompanied by stenting (the placement and leaving of a plastic tube in the coronary artery to physically keep it open).

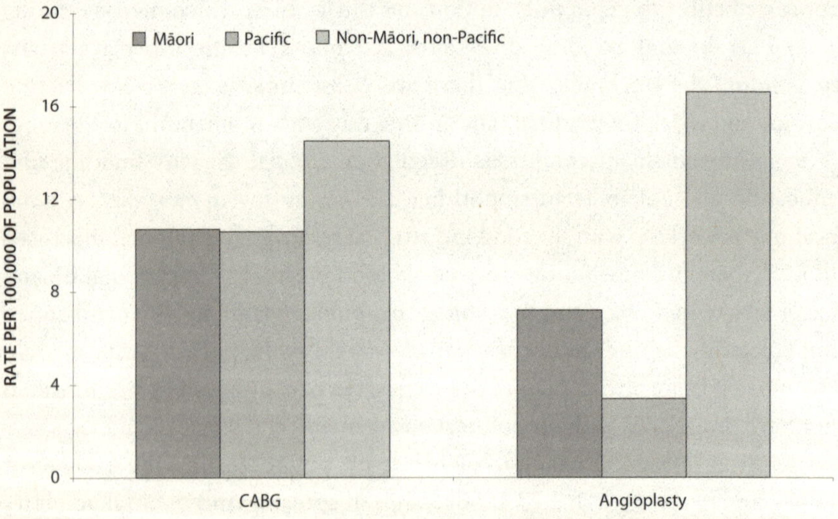

Figure 46: Rates of receipt of coronary artery bypass grafting (CABG) and angioplasty for females from 1990 to 1999, by ethnicity

Note: Rates are age-standardised.
Source: C. Tukuitonga and A. Bindman, 'Ethnic and gender differences in the use of coronary artery revascularisation procedures in New Zealand' (*New Zealand Medical Journal* 115 [2002]: 179–182).

Figure 46 shows the rates of these two interventions by ethnicity for females in the 1990s. (The pattern for males is very similar.) This graph does not inform us what the rate of receipt should have been based on rates of presenting ischaemic heart disease, best practice guidelines and prioritisation based on cost-effectiveness compared to all other publicly funded health care interventions in the 1990s. But it does show the relative receipt of these two interventions from which two important findings are evident. Despite higher ischaemic heart mortality among Māori and Pacific compared to European/Other in this time period,[326; 327] Māori and Pacific peoples receive lower rates of the two life-saving treatments of CABG and angioplasty. There may be some appropriate reasons why the relative receipt of these treatments does not exactly mirror relative rates of ischaemic heart disease mortality, e.g., higher co-morbidity among Māori (particularly respiratory conditions) may rule out general anaesthesia necessary for CABG. But it is not plausible that these differences explain entirely the bias in treatment patterns. There appear to be inequities in the delivery of life-saving health treatments that need to be corrected, if average life expectancy is to be maximised and ethnic inequalities reduced.

Just as fashion is often led by the more socially powerful (but not always, as in the case of hip hop and baseball-cap reversal), so too is the diffusion of new innovations. César Victora has merged this concept of diffusion with Tudor Hart's long-established 'inverse care law' (those with the least need receive the most treatment),[359] to hypothesise the 'inverse equity law'.[360] A new technology is commonly taken up first by the socially privileged, followed by the less privileged. The privileged reach saturation first, followed by the less privileged at some point in time well after the treatment is considered routine care. (The particularly marked inequality in angioplasty treatments between Māori or Pacific and European/Other might be due to the greater novelty of this intervention during the 1990s.)

There are other examples of rapid changes in the social patterns of disease. Meningococcal disease rates in the 1990s steadily rose (perhaps fuelled by increased household crowding during the 1990s),[350] then fell concomitant with an immunisation campaign. Road traffic fatality rates continue to fall with concerted efforts of multiple agencies and stakeholders, with changes in engineering (e.g., safety bags in cars, road design), enforcement (random driver stops) and education ('If you drink and drive, you are a bloody idiot').

Cancer mortality tends to change more slowly – understanding of disease aetiology and prevention is sometimes limited (although we do know how to prevent perhaps a third of cancers), and treatments are partially effective. That all said, there is change occurring. The data for breast cancer incidence and mortality trends illustrate interplays of prevention and treatment that are similar to those observed with cardiovascular disease – but you have to look a little more closely.

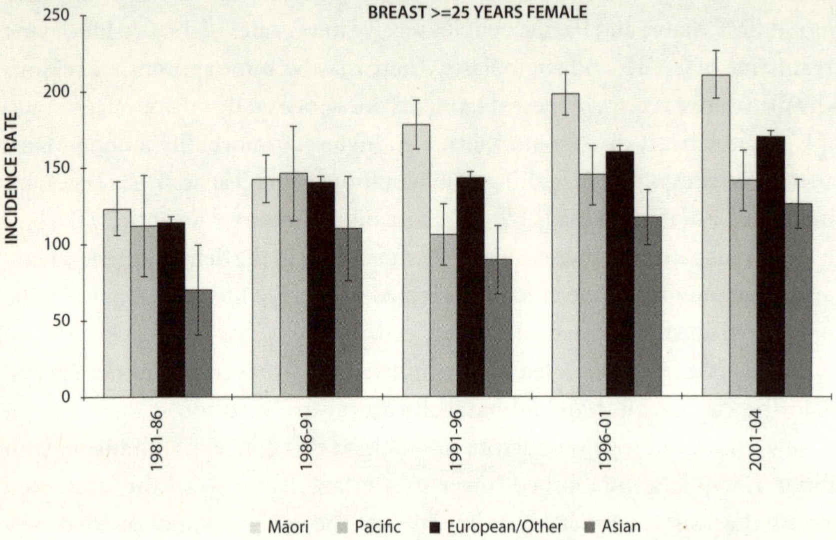

Figure 47: Breast cancer incidence and mortality by ethnicity for the 1980s to 2000s

Blakely, T., C. Shaw, J. Atkinson, R. Cunningham, and D. Sarfati. 'Social Inequalities or Inequities in Cancer Incidence? Repeated Census-Cancer Cohort Studies, New Zealand 1981–1986 to 2001–2004.' *Cancer Causes and Control* 22, no. 9 (2011): 1307–18.

Risk factors for the development of breast cancer include having fewer children, older age at first child, not breast-feeding, earlier menarche and older age at menopause, higher alcohol consumption, less exercise and post-menopausal obesity.[361; 362] Family history, or genetics, matters too, but cannot explain the substantial increases in breast cancer incidence in the twentieth century. Figure 47 shows that incidence since the 1980s is increasing among all groups, but more rapidly among Māori. This may be explained by large reductions in fertility among Māori women some decades ago, allowing for time lags. (However, the higher rates overall among Māori are difficult to explain – all the risk factors suggest European/Other should have higher rates.) Also shown in Figure 47 are breast cancer mortality trends over the same time period. Whilst acknowledging that time from diagnosis to death may be ten or many more years, it is intriguing to note that mortality for Māori increases less rapidly than incidence, and mortality even falls for European/Other. Survival is improving over time, but why? Possible explanations include earlier diagnosis, at a less advanced stage of disease, due to organised screening (mammography was introduced in the 1990s), and greater awareness among women and their primary care providers. Treatments have improved, be it surgical techniques, radiation therapy, or pharmaceuticals such as tamoxifen (used for advanced oestrogen receptor positive breast cancer since about 1980, and since the 1990s for early stage) and trastuzumab (Herceptin, available for HER receptor positive tumours since the 2000s). As with cardiovascular disease, it appears that both personal health care and public health interventions make a difference. And again similar to cardiovascular disease, the gap in breast cancer mortality between Māori and European/Other seems to be widening faster than the gap in incidence, suggesting that European/Other have better access to life-saving treatments.

In this book, we have noted ethnic inequalities in New Zealand. A common question is 'how much of these inequalities are due to differing socio-economic position?' The answer is 'some, but far from all'. For example, gaps in cancer survival are greater between Māori and non-Māori than between socio-economic groups, with socio-economic position explaining a small part of the ethnic gap.[363; 364; 365] Ethnic gaps in mortality rates are greater than those by socio-economic position,[321; 327] and we speculate that if it was possible to measure socio-economic position without error across the lifecourse, then perhaps two-thirds of ethnic gaps in mortality might be 'explained by' socio-economic inequality.[304] Nevertheless, it is the ethnic inequalities in health that are most 'stark' in New Zealand.

In the 1960s and 1970s, McKeown argued that personal health care had not had and did not have a major impact on mortality trends.[320; 249] He might have been right then. But the same argument is not correct now – health care is an increasingly important driver of reductions in mortality in modern societies, adding to the mortality impacts from longer running successes of public health interventions. It would appear that medical care may be both responsible for more people living longer with disability, and also responsible for people living with less functional limitation from their disability due to better supportive care.[160]

SOCIAL AND MACRO-ECONOMIC FACTORS

Changes in risk factors and health do not occur in a vacuum. It takes a concerted and deliberate effort of society to establish a sophisticated comprehensive health system. More fundamentally, one's ability to live a healthy lifestyle is contingent on socio-economic factors which are a function of higher order variables such as politics, trade and power relationships.[366; 367]

Were there significant upstream social changes that influenced health from the 1980s? Absolutely. Did mortality decline alter its trajectory as a result? Almost certainly for Māori, and probably for lower socio-economic non-Māori.

The first two decades after 1980 were dominated by structural macro-economic changes following the election of a Labour government in 1984, and these policies continued through the first term of the National government elected in 1990. They were the years of Rogernomics (named after Roger Douglas, Minister of Finance from 1984 to 1988) and Ruthanasia (named after Ruth Richardson, Minister of Finance from 1990 to 1993). These two represent the sharp swing to a neo-liberal and deregulated policy agenda in New Zealand during the 1980s and 1990s. They were each influential by force of personality and position, but did not stand alone. The prevailing mood of the time, internationally, was pro-market and anti-state intervention (reflected in, for example, International Monetary Fund policies and the Washington Consensus). Douglas and Richardson administered to New Zealand a bitter pill that they thought would make everyone better off in the future, often accompanied by the argument 'there is no alternative' and justified by the prospect of 'trickle-down' benefits in the future that would make everyone richer.

Much has been written about this turbulent period (e.g., Belich's '1984 and all that…' chapter in his second volume of New Zealand history,[256] and many other studies[368; 369]). Here, we will provide a brief overview of the political and economic debates of the time, and look more closely at how social factors may have affected rates of mortality (and morbidity) decline.

As seen in the last chapter, New Zealand society fared well in the 1950s and 1960s and enjoyed one of the highest living standards in the world. The country's economy was strong, in large part due to New Zealand's privileged position as supplier of butter, meat and wool to Britain, and this continued until Britain entered the European Economic Community in 1973.[256] The country could afford a strong welfare society with reasonably good access to health and other services. But governments were slow to adapt to the changing times after 1973, leading to intense economic pressures (falling terms of trade and double-digit inflation) and the incoming Labour government in 1984 faced a crisis. In response, from 1984 to the early 1990s, New Zealand experienced major social and economic changes. In short order, governments introduced a substantially flattened income tax system; fully targeted income support; a regressive consumption tax; market rentals for housing; privatisation of major utilities; user charges for health, education and other government services; and a restructured labour market designed to facilitate 'flexibility'.[368; 369; 256]

Disruptive change weighed particularly heavily on Māori and Pacific people, with inequalities between Māori and non-Māori widening in employment status, education, income, and housing.[370; 371; 372; 373] The manual occupations that were commonly filled by Māori dominated the workplaces that were hit hardest by the structural reforms, with large layoffs, privatisation and a shift to offshore sources of labour.

Unemployment rose in the late 1980s, and peaked in 1991 at 9 per cent. Among Māori and Pacific people, unemployment rates were as high as 25 to 30 per cent – and remained above 15 per cent till the end of the 1990s (Figure 48, overleaf).

As a consequence of unemployment, benefit cuts and other, external, forces (e.g., global changes in the economy and trade), income inequality increased. The New Zealand Gini coefficient, an economic measure of the shares of income across the population, went from being below the OECD average to well above it.[370; 374] In parallel, rates of poverty (income less than 60 per cent of median net of housing costs) rose from less than 10 per cent in the 1980s to nearly 25 per cent around 1994, then improved to about 15 per cent in 2008.[375] Again, Māori and Pacific were more severely impacted than European/Other. Child poverty was more common, affecting about a third of New Zealand children in the early 1990s and 20 per cent in 2008 (using a threshold 60 per cent of median household costs after housing).[376; 377]

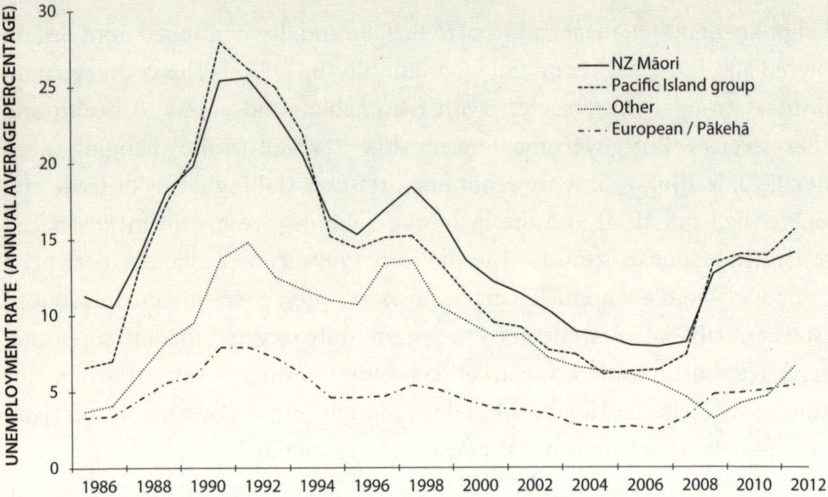

Figure 48: Unemployment rate in New Zealand from 1986 to 2012

Source: Household Labour Force Survey, Statistics New Zealand; and Ministry of Social Policy, *The Social Report: Te Purongo Oranga Tangata 2009* (Wellington, Ministry of Social Policy).

Improvements in social inequality since the mid-1990s can be explained partly by cyclical fluctuations in national and international economics. But there were also important, deliberate changes in policy, influenced by public concerns that a large section of the New Zealand population was not being treated fairly. The neo-liberal approach was softened from the mid-1990s onwards, a change that accelerated after the election of a centre-left government in 1999. There was a commitment made to 'closing the gaps' between Māori and other ethnic groups and between the economically privileged and disadvantaged. Policies included greater regulation of the labour and housing markets and increased social assistance.

What does this mean for life expectancy?

There is a long-running debate in public health, epidemiology and economics about how population health is affected by economic changes. Internationally, downward trends in mortality have continued in the face of economic recession,[18; 378] and sometimes mortality declines are actually accelerated in economically difficult times.[309] On the other hand, the collapse of the former Soviet states caused social upheaval and a crash in life expectancy.[379; 380; 381]

A study of 26 European countries investigated the effects of rapid rises in unemployment between 1970 and 2007.[248] A 1 per cent rise in unemployment was associated with a 0.79 per cent (95 per cent confidence interval 0.16 to 1.42) increase in suicide rates in those aged less than 65 years, a 0.79 per cent (0.06 to 1.52) rise in homicide deaths, a 1.39 per cent (0.62 to 2.14 per cent) *decrease* in road traffic crash deaths, and there was no discernible impact on overall mortality. Of particular importance, this study found that the association of changes in unemployment rates with suicide was less marked in countries that invested more in active labour market programmes (e.g., labour market training, special youth programmes, transition from school to work programmes). It appeared that social policy could provide a buffer, to some extent, against the harmful effects of rising unemployment.

Regarding the personal experience of unemployment, a well-designed Swedish study that thoroughly adjusted for confounding factors (e.g., previous mental health status) found a 50 per cent increase in mortality rates for the four years following unemployment (for a period of three or more months) during the 1992–94 recession.[382] In New Zealand, we observed increases in suicide among those unemployed at the 1991 census in the three years subsequent to the census,[383] and increased rates of self-harm among those made unemployed during freezing work factory closures.[384] A meta-analysis of 87 longitudinal studies found a moderately strong association between being made unemployed and deteriorating mental health, and re-employment was found to be associated with improvements in mental health.[385]

What does this all mean for life expectancy trends in New Zealand? We cannot assume that 'averaged' experiences in other countries at other times and with different social policy mixes and cultural predispositions will apply to New Zealand. Local factors make a difference. For example, non-Māori life expectancy improved by very little in the 1960s and 1970s (particularly for males), *despite* New Zealand having one of the highest GDPs per person in the world. This was due to the force of the ischaemic heart disease epidemic, driven by tobacco and a long history of a diet rich in saturated fat. Put another way, had New Zealand not had times of relative economic prosperity in the 1960s, maybe non-Māori life expectancy would have levelled off, or even gone backwards.

During the 1980s and 1990s, non-Māori life expectancy increased rapidly – despite widening income inequality and increasing unemployment rates (that affected non-Māori as well as Māori, albeit less so). Why was this? Possible explanations include the turning of the tobacco epidemic, a reduction in consumption of saturated fat, the advent of effective medical treatments, and hence a decline in non-Māori cardiovascular disease that outweighed deleterious effects of social and economic change. Here we strike the concept of 'fungibility'– non-Māori benefited from the structural and macro-economic reforms, but the social costs were borne predominantly by Māori. We speculate that there may also be cohort effects, whereby health stocks accrued by non-Māori in previous decades lead to lower mortality from the 1980s onwards, and these more than balance any deleterious effects of that period. Finally, it may be that the rapid improvements in public health and personal health care were more thoroughly captured and capitalised on by non-Māori.

As is evident, the *rate* of mortality decline is the net effect of many factors, and we do not understand them sufficiently well to mathematically add and subtract all the component variables. Rather, we have to piece together those parts of the tapestry that are accessible, and construct an interpretation that is 'likely correct'.

Exhibit 1: Stasis in Māori life expectancy during the 1980s and 1990s, and take-off subsequent

The minimal improvements in Māori life expectancy in the 1980s and 1990s stand out – see Figure 36. The most common explanation we hear from the many students and colleagues to whom we have shown this figure is 'Rogernomics'. Is this a coherent explanation? We argue 'yes', at least for Māori and in the context of New Zealand at the time. As has already been shown above, the impact of unemployment and worsening poverty was particularly severe for Māori. It was not just the individual experience of unemployment; there were also far-reaching effects on communities, for example, when local factories and freezing works closed. Overall, Māori were affected more commonly than non-Māori, and the coping capacities of families, friends and whānau were tested. The withdrawal of social welfare services, and the shake up that took place in the health system, added to the risks for isolated individuals. For example, high co-payments in primary (and for a while secondary) care may have acted as a barrier to early diagnosis and prompt treatment of common, modifiable conditions such as ischaemic heart disease and diabetes.

Māori rates of cardiovascular disease mortality did not come down as rapidly as they did for European/Other, and indeed went up (statistically significantly so) for Māori males from 1986–89 to 1991–94 (Figure 40).[327] The pattern for male suicides (Figure 40) is another example of widening social inequalities.

Trends in cancer mortality may be influenced by socially patterned environmental exposures and differential access to early detection and treatment. However, it is difficult to pick out the component causes with confidence, because of the long time lags that apply with cancer. Changes in incidence of smoking-related cancers, for example, are affected by exposures 20–30 years previously.

Exhibit 2: Stasis in mortality declines among low socio-economic 25–44-year-olds, and widening relative inequalities in mortality by income

Figure 38 showed 1–74-year-old all-cause mortality from 1981–84 to 2001–4, by thirds of household income. Rates tended to fall for all income groups in parallel, meaning that the absolute gap in mortality was relatively constant over time – except from 1996–99 to 2001–4 where the gap possibly decreased.[321] On a relative scale, the percentage by which the low-income population's mortality exceeds that of the high-income population widens over time, from 47 per cent to 75 per cent for males, and from 32 per cent to 54 per cent for females. A similar pattern is seen in many high-income countries in recent decades – death rates for different social groups declining in parallel, in absolute terms, and this means, due to the force of arithmetic necessity, that relative inequalities increase. When New Zealand is compared with countries that did not experience radical structural change (e.g., Norway, Finland and Denmark), the trends in social inequalities in mortality are much the same.[386]

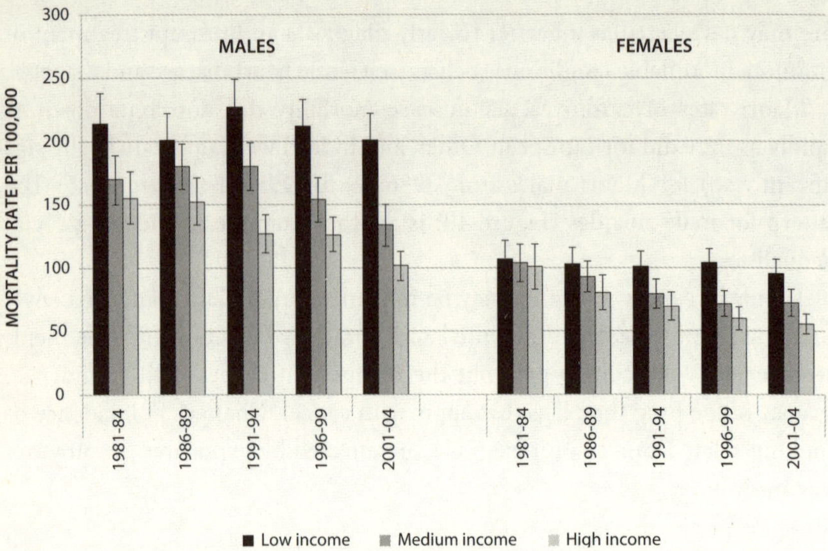

Figure 49: All-cause mortality by income tertile for 25–44-year-olds

Source: New Zealand Census-Mortality Study (NZCMS), Department of Public Health; T. Blakely, M. Tobias, J. Atkinson, L.-C. Yeh, and K. Huang, 'Tracking Disparity: Trends in Ethnic and Socioeconomic Inequalities in Mortality, 1981–2004' (Wellington: Ministry of Health, 2007); T. Blakely, M. Tobias, and J. Atkinson, 'Inequalities in Mortality During and after Restructuring of the New Zealand Economy: Repeated Cohort Studies' (*British Medical Journal* 336 [24 January 2008]: 371–75).

Considering 25–44-year-olds (Figure 49), however, the contrasts are more marked. Here, there is no improvement in low-income mortality rates over time, but marked improvements for high-income groups. The causes of death responsible for this divergence in mortality trends are largely suicide and unintentional injury (within which road traffic crash deaths dominate), but other diseases also contribute.[326; 321] It may be that the lag between 'cause' and 'effect' is short, for both suicide and unintentional injury, and therefore the impacts of social adversity are easier to pick up in socially disadvantaged young adults than in older age groups.

7

Summing Up, Looking Forward

In this chapter we return to the main themes of the book, and sum up the central findings. New Zealand non-Māori were top of the longevity league table from 1870 to 1940 due to the wealth of natural resources, health selection of migrants, lack of crowding, and progressive social policies. Maori were excluded from, and in some ways paid for, the demographic success of European settlers. During the twentieth century, mortality decline for Māori followed the standard epidemiological transition, with falling infant and infectious disease mortality replaced by non-communicable disease – in particular, cardiovascular disease – as the major impediment to low mortality. After World War II New Zealand did not keep up with the gains in child and youth mortality that were achieved elsewhere, and New Zealand was slow to control cardiovascular disease compared with other high-income countries. Māori life expectancy steadily gained on non-Māori life expectancy – except during the 1980s and 1990s. At the beginning of the twenty-first century, we have returned to rapid gains in life expectancy, but this is due now to falls in death rates among 65-and-older people – and increasingly among those 85 years and older.

These observations raise many questions: 'How much longer can this rate of increase in longevity go on for?' 'Is it ethical?' 'Should we worry more about quality of life and reducing inequalities?' 'Can we sustain longer lives?' Biologically, it is plausible that mortality decline will continue – but not indefinitely. There will be strains on society over the next 50 years as more elderly people require support, but the prospects are not necessarily gloomy. As life expectancy increases, so too will healthy life expectancy, and this means more years of independent and productive 'retirement'. Sustainability refers not just to budgets and health services – there are also environmental costs to growing populations on the present patterns of consumption.

We anticipate that the increases in life expectancy and healthy life expectancy will continue. To cope with this, the age of retirement will need to rise, workforce expectations must change to make better use of what older people can provide, and modes of living (for all ages) must adapt to a much smaller environmental footprint.

MORTALITY DECLINE: MAIN FINDINGS, EXPLANATIONS AND IMPLICATIONS – THE NEW ZEALAND STORY

Ever since first landing, non-Māori living in New Zealand have experienced relatively low mortality. Why? We think it was a mix of good luck and deliberate choices. Good luck came in the form of rich natural resources, an advantaged place in the British Empire, the timing of European settlement and the momentum of the settler boom. Deliberate interventions that sustained decline in mortality include almost a century of egalitarian social policy, a relatively efficient health-care system, strong child-health programmes and effective public health regulation.

After European contact, Māori life expectancy crashed. This was caused initially by infectious disease and – to some extent – warfare. Then, after annexation, the major vectors of poor health and high mortality included loss of land, loss of culture and poverty. Within a hundred years the Māori population was reduced to perhaps a sixth of the number of people who were present when Cook landed. However, recovery at the end of the nineteenth century was even more rapid than the fall. In part, we believe it was the passage of time and biological and social adaptations to the infectious diseases that had caused heavy loss of life. General improvements in living conditions were important and so were the public health advances of the early 1900s. There was defining leadership provided by Māori politicians and health professionals who represented new ways of thinking about illness, medicine and disease prevention. According to Belich, Māori resistance and recovery were marked by 'eager, adaptive and innovative engagement with the things and thoughts of Europe'.[78] Ngata, Carroll, Pōmare, Buck and others enabled Māori to benefit from twentieth-century developments in organised health care.

Over the course of New Zealand's history the major causes of improvement in life expectancy have varied from one period to another. Diet (adequate caloric intake), standard of living and family size had the greatest effects in the nineteenth century; organised public health programmes and regulations and improved socio-economic conditions contributed in the first half of the twentieth century; and reductions in smoking, better diets and life-saving treatments added to the gains from public health prevention in the second half of the twentieth century.

Non-Māori life expectancy increased by two years every decade in the last century, and Māori life expectancy increased by three to four every decade – on average. If this long-run trend is maintained, the gap in life expectancy between Māori and non-Māori will be closed by 2040, the 200th anniversary of the Treaty of Waitangi. On this projection, the female period life expectancy would be 90 years, and the life expectancy for males would be close to 85 years. However, this is very much a glass-half-full interpretation: since 1991, the Māori and non-Māori lines in the New Zealand life expectancy graph (see the beginning of the last chapter) have been converging much more slowly. Based on what has happened in the last 20 years, it will take to calendar year 2200 before Māori reach non-Māori male life expectancy (at what seems a highly improbable 144 years of life expectancy) and until 2080 before females converge (at a more comprehensible average lifespan of 99 years).

Life expectancy is increasingly driven by mortality at older ages

As we saw in the last chapter, it is reduction in older-age mortality that is now responsible for increases in life expectancy. In New Zealand, between 1960–62 and 2010–12, the expectation of life if you reach the age of 80 has risen from 5.5 to 8.5 years for men, and from 6.4 to 9.8 years for women, according to the period life tables from Statistics New Zealand. This corresponds roughly to a 2.5-fold increase in the chance of living from 80 to 90 (from about 14 per cent to 37 per cent for males, and from 21 per cent to 47 per cent for females). The number of persons aged 100 years and over increased roughly ten-fold between 1960 and 2010, although the absolute numbers are still small (Statistics New Zealand estimate there were 400–500 New Zealanders aged 100 years or more in 2011).[387]

Overseas the picture is similar. Mortality among 80- and 90-year-olds is falling in most high-income countries, although Denmark, the Netherlands and the United States were exceptions in the early 2000s.[388] But the levelling off in the long-term decline in death rates in these three countries was temporary, and most likely due to the tobacco epidemic passing through those populations. Projections based on present-day life expectancy fail to take account of the steep decline that has occurred in smoking rates in younger birth cohorts (particularly, men born since 1950). When these groups move into the ranks of the elderly, we expect that mortality amongst persons aged 80+ will resume its long-term decline, tempered possibly by the rise of obesity. Because peak smoking rates occurred later for women than for men in the US, mortality in older men will decline more quickly than for women of the same age in the near future, and the gender gap in life expectancy in the US will shrink.[389]

According to projections released by Statistics New Zealand in 2012, period life expectancy for males is forecast to rise to 84.3 years in 2036 and 88.1 years in 2061 (median mortality assumption, 90 per cent uncertainty interval in 2061 85.2–90.5). For females, the projected increase is to 87.3 years (2036) and 90.5 years (2061), 90 per cent interval in 2061 88.2–92.4.[390] But there is good reason to believe average life expectancy for men and women born in the twenty-first century will in fact be greater than this.

The numbers we have used refer to the average years of life for a group if it experienced the age-specific death rates that apply at one point in time. We pointed out at the start of the book that this is an artificial measure, simply a convenient way of summarising rates in a given calendar year (see text box, page 3). The actual life expectancy of a group of children born in, say, 2000, depends not on the death rates of young adults and the elderly that apply in the year 2000, but on the mortality rates that are experienced in the future, i.e., based on the whole-of-life experience of a generation (cohort) of people. This measure, the cohort life expectancy, will be greater than the period life expectancy if mortality decreases over time; the opposite applies obviously if chances of survival in the future decline.

In the early 1930s, the life expectancy at birth for non-Māori New Zealanders was calculated (using the period approach) to be about 65 for men and 68 for women. In fact, the average life expectancy of males and females born at that time is close to 69 and 75 years, respectively. The explanation for these differences is the improvements that took place in the second half of the twentieth century in mortality rates for the middle-aged and elderly.[168]

If the improvements in mortality rates continue in the future, then we know that period life expectancy will continue to under-estimate actual survival. What is less certain is how big the gap between period and cohort life expectancies will be. If the force of mortality decreases over time at a constant rate, there will be a straight-line improvement in period life expectancy, and improvement in cohort life expectancy will also be linear, although increasing at a faster rate.[391] This is consistent with what has been observed. Between 1870 and 1920, 'best practice' period life expectancy across the world for females increased by 2.8 years per decade, compared with an increase of 4.3 years per decade for cohort life expectancy.[392] Based on trends in age-specific mortality since 1977, Statistics New Zealand has estimated that a male born in 2011 will live on average 90.2 years (90 per cent confidence interval 86.3–94.0), and a female 92.9 years (90 per cent confidence interval 89.3–96.2).[392]

A widely cited paper claims that if the fall in death rates in middle-to-old age continues on its present trajectory, more than half the babies born since 2000 in low mortality countries are likely to celebrate their 100th birthdays.[160] Note that this figure refers to the median age of death, which is greater than the mean when the distribution of age at death is skewed towards younger ages. But it is important also to reflect on whether the present trajectory can really be sustained, since the reduction in mortality rates in middle and older age groups will need to accelerate through this century if a straight-line improvement in life expectancy is to continue. This is not impossible, but is perhaps improbable. A more restrained estimate (but one that is still outside the range of the Statistics New Zealand projections) from the UK Office for National Statistics is that about a third of babies born in 2012 in that country will survive to age 100 years.[393]

Period effects and the life course

The New Zealand history includes numerous examples of rapid turnaround in mortality: deterioration in Māori mortality after European settlement, reversal of this trend at the end of the 1800s, and the rise and fall in deaths due to cardiovascular disease in the twentieth century, for instance. What does this common pattern, in which large changes occur across the population in a short period of time, tell us about likely causes, including the timing of critical exposures and the mechanisms linking environment and disease?

Note that big shifts in disease rates, observed at one time in all age groups, and both men and women, are most unlikely to be caused by exposures in early life. By way of illustration, the prevalence of obesity in the United States almost doubled between 1975 and 1995 and the upturn in rates occurred at about the same calendar time (the late 1970s) for all ages.[394] If intra-uterine exposures or factors in early childhood played a major role in causing the epidemic, one would have to hypothesise a lag time of 70 years for babies born around 1900, of 60 years for babies born around 1910, 50 years for individuals born in 1920, and so on. This is not plausible – it is difficult to think of any mechanism of differential effect by year of birth. The epidemic in ischaemic heart disease in New Zealand followed the same pattern. We described this in chapter 6: there was a rise in all age groups for both men and women from the mid-1950s, with a peak in 1966–70, and then rates fell, in parallel, in all age groups.[271]

There are lots of other examples: obesity rates in New Zealand[395] and Australia,[396] the decline in coronary heart disease in the United States[271; 397] and the rise of coronary heart disease in China.[398] These are all instances of strong 'period effects', which, for the reasons outlined above, must have been caused by factors that acted relatively quickly and impinged on everyone.

These observations are relevant to the debate over the best points for intervention in the life course. Should public health concentrate on early life, for instance, when infants and children are developing rapidly, and may be physiologically and behaviourally programmed for high disease risk in adulthood? Is adolescence and the young adult period the key, given this is the time when life-long patterns are established in education, family formation and career? Or will disease prevention and health promotion achieve the biggest gains if they concentrate on the group with highest disease rates, middle- and older-age adults, where individuals (and the population) have the most to gain (or lose)?

We showed in chapter 5 that it is not difficult to distinguish conceptually between cohort and period effects, but in practice the margins are often blurred. Cohort effects may lay the ground for period effects later on, for example. We would expect well-nourished and educated children to grow into adults more likely to invest in their future health, and to be able to respond effectively to whatever challenges and opportunities arise in the future. However, the empirical evidence for preventive activity is strongest for interventions that improve the health status of many age groups over the short run – that is, period effects.

Indeed, rapid success in population health is essentially the creation of strong period effects. This does not mean it will be simple or easy to identify the causes and then to apply them to create health gain or to block health losses. Nor should one forget that immediate benefits can accrue from dealing with factors that affect disease rates both in the short and long run – for example, giving up smoking reduces cardiovascular disease risks almost immediately, as well as preventing cancer decades down the track.

The big gains in life expectancy in recent decades have come about as a result of changes in adult mortality rates, and this is where the potential lies for further improvements. Because mortality rates for children and young adults are already very low, reductions in these age groups will not gain much in the way of extended life expectancy. If society makes it a priority to lengthen life expectancy further, then it makes sense to concentrate on what determines mortality in the adult years. There are other grounds for a strong policy focus on child health, but if the goal is to increase life expectancy then adult mortality must be the focus.

When we talk about 'the causes of disease', it is necessary to distinguish between the reasons an individual falls ill, and what explains the rates of disease in a population. The famous British epidemiologist Geoffrey Rose wrote in 1985 that 'aetiology confronts two distinct issues: the determinants of individual cases and the determinants of incidence'.[399] Rose's point has been missed in much that has been written subsequently on the origins of chronic disease, where there has been a tendency to confuse causes of individual cases with the 'uber-causes' of population epidemics. To return to our earlier example: genes are a cause of obesity, in the sense that a person's genetic makeup helps explain where they are placed in the overall distribution of body mass index.[400] But genes do not explain why the whole distribution of body mass has shifted upwards so rapidly in so many countries.

Epidemics are caused, with few exceptions, by mass exposures that are widely distributed. Examples of 'mass exposures' that act on obesity include larger food portion sizes;[401] accelerated marketing; availability and affordability of energy-dense foods;[402] and widespread introduction of cheap, potent sweetening agents such as high fructose corn syrup.[403] In a similar fashion, low birth weight may be described as a cause of individual cases of coronary heart disease, since being born light is associated in some studies, independently of other risk factors, with the probability of dying from the disease.[404] But low birth weight does not explain heart disease as a mass phenomenon. The great epidemic of coronary heart disease has come and (largely) gone, with very little variation in average birth weights.[405; 99] What caused incidence to decline in New Zealand, Australia, the US and the United Kingdom were widespread changes in behaviour and health services, with rapid effect: namely, a drop in smoking, less saturated fat in the diet and better control of high blood pressure.[397]

Fungibility

An important lesson we draw from the New Zealand experience is that human longevity is fungible. What this means is that long life requires trade-offs, exchanges and transfers. The conditions necessary for low mortality do not appear out of thin air: if resources are sequestered for this purpose, then they are not available elsewhere. This principle applies at the biological level – organisms trade off maintenance and repair (the processes that secure longevity) for reproduction. There is a social dimension as well. Historically, gains for the powerful and privileged have often come at the expense of the less powerful. Access to fertile land was an important basis for the good health of non-Māori in the second half of the nineteenth century. Māori paid for this, economically, socially and with their own health. On a broader scale, countries like New Zealand that used empire as a springboard cornered the lion's share of many natural resources globally, and prospered at the expense of developing countries that were slower off the mark.

Fungibility has a larger perspective. The twentieth century leaped ahead thanks to the products of industrial revolution – life expectancy doubled, globally, in a hundred years, in parallel with exponential increases in consumption of natural resources and production of material goods. We have noted, earlier in this book, that very high levels of consumption are not absolutely necessary for low mortality. However, the industrial revolution was the basis for progress in many areas such as food production, housing, public health services and medical care. There was a downside, evident in health-damaging levels of pollution and social disruption. But on balance, it is difficult to argue against the proposition that open-ended use of fossil fuels, fresh water and forests (just as examples) supported the twentieth-century expansion in human populations. The question is: can open-ended consumption be sustained? If not, what are the consequences of drawing down on natural resources that would otherwise be available for future generations? We return to this question later in the chapter.

Choosing our future

It is clear that humans have the capacity to influence mortality trends, through technology, policy, welfare and medical care, even if we fully understand neither the nature of ageing nor the causal mechanisms that link environmental exposures with the length of the average lifespan. Therefore the question arises: should we strive to increase life expectancy? and if so, how important is this goal compared with other social objectives?

It is conceivable that society may choose not to pursue longer lives, and instead focus on other goals such as environmental protection. But even if this is not the case, there are choices to be made. Do we focus on the fundamental biological science of ageing, or retain a disease orientation in research and service provision? What priority should be given to 'upstream' prevention strategies, such as better urban design to promote social well-being and physical activity, compared with unimpeded and equitable access to effective treatments? Do we primarily focus on mortality, or shift efforts to reducing morbidity? Or do we try and do bits of everything?

These questions point us in the direction of the ethics of longevity, since choices involve trade-offs and resolution requires value judgements as well as accurate information about gains and losses.

ETHICS OF LIVING LONGER

As doctors, public health medicine specialists and epidemiologists, we have been trained to give first priority to activities that postpone death. It is so fundamental to what we do, we do not question it. We never say to colleagues, or to the public: 'Actually, it would be a good thing for social, economic and environmental sustainability if we abandoned efforts to extend life expectancy. Therefore, let's leave tobacco smoking alone, and cut funding to health services.' We never even think to say this – the imperatives are health first, which in its simplest terms means avoiding (or, in reality, postponing) death. But there is good reason to pause, and ask the question: should we seek to extend life expectancy without reservation?

Increased longevity may be a benefit to the individual whose life is extended, but society at large will carry the burden of these extra years of life if they are not spent in good health and if the individual in question is not a productive contributor to society. The social burden includes more than the costs of formal health care and informal family support. Longer lives may cause loss of opportunities for younger members of the population; social stasis in a conservative, elder-dominated society; and greater depletion of the environment due to a more numerous population.

Existing public health ethical frameworks are not particularly helpful on the fundamental matter of increasing longevity.[406; 407; 408; 409; 410] They are pitched at the level of populations and, while acknowledging the challenge of trade-offs, they assume the goal of ever increasing improvement of health – by which we mean longevity. The same is true of protocols and guides to the prioritisation of health services, i.e., who gets what, given scarce resources.[411] The ethical principle of utilitarianism is often invoked, with the aim of maximising utility across the (current) population. But still the implicit goal is to increase health, both in quantity and quality.

There are, embedded in these frameworks, principles that apply to the big question of how long life should be. The Nuffield Council on Bioethics invokes the Stewardship Model, which although still mostly focused on the 'here and now' does draw in considerations of future generations, inter-generational equity and environmental concerns.[408] The US Public Health Leadership Society stresses the interdependence of individuals on each other – 'rightful concern for the physical individuality of humans and one's right to make decisions for oneself must be balanced against the fact that each person's actions affect other people'. Principles of distributive justice that apply to inequalities, and 'proportionality' of actions are relevant to how much effort society invests in further increasing longevity.[406]

Our position? We are inclined to be pragmatic for now, focusing on mitigation (i.e., avoiding where possible loss of healthy life-years), without any assumptions about upper bounds of survival, or the precise length of a 'fair innings'.[412] Acknowledging the primordial human desire to live longer, however bleak the circumstances, we must strive nevertheless to live better. 'Living better' means taking seriously the challenge of population growth; it implies also living within the planet's carrying capacity, and sharing around a high standard of living with billions in middle- and low-income countries. The notion of a 'fair innings' means that increases in the length and quality of life are shared equally between social groups, across countries and from one generation to the next.

HOW HIGH CAN LIFE EXPECTANCY GO?

At the beginning of chapter 3 we referred to the paper in *Science* in 2002 that reviewed maximum life expectancy from 1840 to 2000.[159] The principal finding was that the improvement over these 160 years was steadily linear, without sign of diminishing speed of advance. A later paper written by some of the same authors reported that the linear extension of highest reported population life expectancy continued in the first decade of the twenty-first century.[160]

Can New Zealand keep up the pace? Will we soon face a time of diminishing returns, a period when the rise in life expectancy simply has to flatten out, because there are no more opportunities to squeeze mortality further? No, we say, there is plenty of room for improvement. In New Zealand there are substantial and avoidable inequalities between different groups, to the detriment of the whole population. Note that if there are two-fold differences in mortality rates across socio-economic groups, and if everyone in the future achieved the mortality rate of the highest socio-economic group, then one-third of deaths would be avoided (or more strictly speaking 'delayed'; see Figure 50, overleaf).

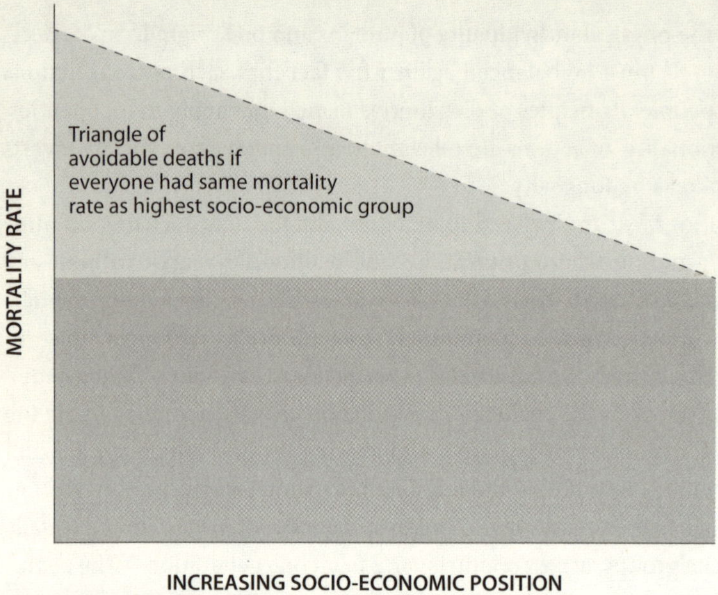

Figure 50: Effect of equalising mortality rates across socio-economic categories

Note: If the mortality rate of the lowest socio-economic group is twice that of the highest socio-economic group (as it often is), and if rates are distributed as a gradient across socio-economic position, then a third of all deaths are avoided if everyone achieves the mortality rate of the highest socio-economic group.

It makes sense, intuitively, that the long history of life expectancy will follow a sigmoid curve. There were slow improvements initially with the accumulation of resources and knowledge, and now we are in the midst of a time of rapid improvement as social change washes through successive generations. But eventually there must be a levelling out as the potential for improvement is exhausted.

However, the year-on-year declines in mortality that we see in the longest-lived countries are a sign that if there is a plateau, a flat stretch on the sigmoid curve, it has not yet come over the horizon. Japanese women, the world record-holders, now live to 86 years on average, about three years more than New Zealand women, and improvements in that country (for women) are not slowing down.[270] Japanese mortality rates have been falling steadily, by about 3 per cent per year, for more than 30 years, even amongst men and women in their 80s and 90s.[413]

There are two parts to the improvement in average life expectancy. One is reduction in premature mortality, meaning that most deaths are delayed until old age. This has been described as mortality compression, or the 'rectangularisation' of survival, since the proportion of the population surviving is little changed until an advanced age, and then falls abruptly (Figure 51). The other way in which life expectancy can be increased is to increase the maximum age at death. This might be called 'extension of longevity', and entails shifting the whole survival curve to the right. If gains have been made historically by compressing mortality (or reducing mortality rates at young ages only) without much of a shift in the maximum age at death, then a ceiling or limit on life expectancy seems more likely. But if mortality reduces across all ages (by half initially, then 80 per cent as shown in Figure 51), an upper limit on human longevity seems less likely, in the short-to-medium term at least. We note that gains in life expectancy in recent decades have occurred primarily due to falling mortality in older ages. This pattern fits with 'shifting the curve to the right', and suggests we will see the increase in life expectancy continue.

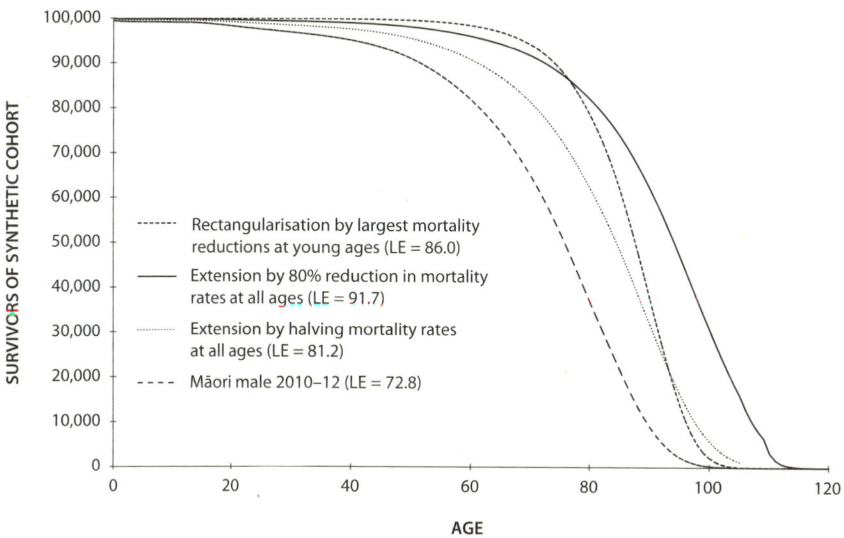

Figure 51: Rectangularisation and extension of survival, using Māori male 2010–12 life table as baseline

Source: Statistics New Zealand period life tables.

Analysis of nine European studies has teased out the contributions of mortality compression and longevity extension to increasing life expectancies at age 50 from 1922–2006.[414] (The authors chose 50 as the starting point since roughly 95 per cent of newborns in high-income countries successfully complete a half-century, and it is mortality beyond 50 that now has the strongest influence on life expectancy trends.) Overall, more life-years were gained from longevity extension than from the 'rectangularisation' of survival, and this applied in the most recent decades as well as earlier periods. For example, in Switzerland an increase of 13.8 years lived beyond 50, on average, was made up of 8.2 years due to longevity extension and 5.6 years attributed to mortality compression. This finding was not affected by vagaries in the death registrations of extremely old people. (The investigators deleted the 10 per cent highest ages at death, to avoid problems with a small number of deaths at very advanced ages with possibly inaccurate coding.) The authors concluded that the waxing and waning of the tobacco epidemic in European populations is likely to be the biggest single factor acting on mortality compression. What is pushing out the maximum age at death is more difficult to explain.

Much of the speculation about the future (limits to) life expectancy gains has this flavour – teasing apart the mortality rates, forecasting trends and other mathematical extrapolations. But what can we learn by examining the question from the perspective of mechanistic processes that may limit future gains? That is the objective of the sections below, before we return to risk factors and diseases and explore opportunities for further mortality decline.

Biological limits

Ageing has been likened to the running down of a biological clock, or the inevitable outcome of accumulated wear and tear in the genome. Although the biological changes that accompany ageing are very well described, this knowledge cannot (yet) be translated into explanations for the observed trends in human mortality.[415] For example, in laboratory animals it is possible to extend lifespans by about 20 per cent by blocking the release of specific transmitter chemicals in the hypothalamus, but it is too soon to tell what significance, if any, this has for humans.[416] Dietary restriction, as a means of reducing metabolic traffic and cutting down on genetic wear and tear, might explain why mice can live longer if they eat less, and recent attempts to replicate the finding with larger animals have reported some success.[417; 418] For example, R. J. Colman et al. reported a statistically significant ($p=0.03$) three-fold decreased rate of ageing-related mortality in caloric-restricted rhesus monkeys. Total mortality rates were not statistically significantly different (but trending that way).[419] Historically, there is no evidence yet from human populations that dietary restriction boosts life expectancy – in fact, one could argue that the association runs the other way. A doubling in life expectancy in many countries in the last hundred years has been associated with a 20–30 per cent increase in average body mass.

Oxidative stress may be one mechanism by which the effects of ageing are manifest, but treating people with antioxidants does not alter mortality. The view of ageing as accumulation of damage has a strong basis, but it is difficult to identify precisely how and where the critical changes occur. For instance, the plaques and fibrous tangles that are associated with Alzheimer's disease are present also in the brains of older people who die with cognition more or less intact.

The idea of programmed ageing is appealing, in its simplicity, but does not fit with the huge advance in longevity that has occurred in a short space of time. Nor does the 'ticking clock' metaphor sit comfortably with what is known about the inner workings of the cell. Thomas Kirkwood points out that the genes that influence ageing act 'by adjusting hundreds of mechanisms for maintenance and repair', and he concludes, 'If ageing was programmed, this would be a clumsy way to do it.'[415]

In the absence of an obvious mechanism to determine lifespans, Arthur Caplan asks: 'is death unnatural?'[420] He argues that even if mortality is inevitable, it does not follow that death is 'natural' in the sense of being biologically ordained. Genetic inheritance has an influence, but falls some way short of determining longevity. Overall, known genetic markers explain about a quarter of the variation in life expectancy.[421] In general, deaths in early life are a function of nurture not nature – they are rarely correlated with genetic factors, which are much more important in deaths at 60 years and over.[422]

The biological machinery of life does not necessarily run down with advancing years – germ cells, passed on from one generation to another, are potentially immortal (in the absence of a chance mutation), for instance.

It was thought in the past that mortality increased exponentially with age, but this relation is not fixed. At advanced ages, in a number of species (including humans), it has been observed that mortality rates stabilise and may even reduce.[423] Furthermore, some species (admittedly, very simple organisms) have no discernible limit on lifespan. The freshwater *Hydra* is an example.[424]

In the first chapter we referred to the growing interest in the science of telomeres.[425; 426; 427; 428] To recap, telomeres are repetitive capping sequences at the ends of chromosomes that shorten (in somatic or non-germ cells) with each cell division because the very ends of chromosomes are intrinsically difficult to replicate faithfully. Telomeres that are very short trigger cell senescence, perhaps to protect the integrity of chromosomes. The length of the telomere depends on the number of cell divisions a cell has gone through and on activity of the enzyme telomerase. Telomerase is a repair agent that replaces the lost sequences, and levels of the enzyme vary widely depending on factors such as inheritance, exposure to mutagens in the environment, diet, psychological stress and early life environments. As a result telomeres offer a tantalising biological pivot point on which to focus research into ageing. Telomere shortening is associated with numerous degenerative diseases (e.g., diabetes,[429] respiratory disease,[430] and dementia[431; 432]). And there is some interesting experimental evidence. For example, Sheldon Cohen and colleagues are renowned for locking up volunteers in hotel rooms, exposing them to cold viruses and watching to see who is affected. In one experiment, a one standard deviation shortening in telomere length was associated with a 71 per cent (95 per cent confidence interval, 8 per cent to 172 per cent) increased odds of developing a cold.[433]

There are some hints that telomere length varies by social position, which would accord with the notion of more rapid ageing among lower socio-economic groups, but the pattern is not consistent. For example, telomeres were shorter on average among less educated people in the UK Whitehall study,[434] but this difference did not apply between income groups. In the west of Scotland, where life expectancy varies more than 13 years between the richest and poorest areas, a large survey found no relation between socio-economic status and telomere length.[435] In the United States, where there are also substantial inequalities in health by race and social standing, telomere length was once again positively related to education, but not at all to income, and (contrary to what might be predicted) was greater for African-Americans than other racial groups.[436]

Before we get carried away about telomeres being the biological key to delaying ageing, two caveats. First, association is not causation. Telomere shortening may be as much a biomarker of 'wear and tear' as the conduit from environmental insults to ageing. (In all probability, it is probably a bit of both.) Second, telomere shortening serves a good purpose! It stops cells replicating, which is very handy for preventing cancer cells proliferating. Indeed, telomere shortening has been likened to tumour suppression activity. So it is possible that boosting telomerase levels (e.g., with some new anti-ageing drug) might reduce the incidence or progression of degenerative disease, but increase cancer incidence. We repeat, this is speculative – but interesting.

If death is not pre-determined, is it 'natural' in another sense, which is that death has a purpose? For example, it is often argued that death makes way for the new – it is not a benefit to the individual, but death serves the greater good, ensuring resources are shared and there is room for development and improvement. But if this is the case, Arthur Caplan claims, the argument cannot be made on the basis of evolution. In evolution, selection acts on traits that give an immediate return (not one delayed to subsequent generations), and moreover, evolution is driven principally by the individual phenotype, not the characteristics of groups. In social animals, population-level variables (such as extent of cooperation) will have an influence on the likelihood that the genes of individuals are propagated. But the effect is indirect, and subject to perturbations of many kinds (such as the 'free-rider' phenomenon, in which selfish individuals prosper at the expense of those who put the interests of the group first). In general, between-individual differences act much more powerfully on gene frequencies than do between-group variations.[43]

Another explanation for ageing is that it is simply an accidental by-product of pressures that favoured reproduction over maintenance. This continues the theme of trade-offs ('life expectancy is a fungible quality'), based on the observation that long-lived species reproduce late and infrequently. Within the organism, the machinery for cell repair requires energy; if energy is diverted into reproduction, then maintenance is deferred.[437] According to this view, selective pressures act on reproductive performance, and longevity trails behind. Humans fall in the 'relatively late and infrequent' category for reproduction. The offspring of *Homo sapiens* require a prolonged period of oversight and training so the new individual can make the most of her or his large brain: for our species, a long life might be thought of as a by-product of a long youth.[438] But the empirical evidence that a woman's fertility is related to her longevity is weak and inconsistent[439] – it is not apparent that the metabolic demands of child-bearing and child-rearing shorten lifespans.

So the biological basis of ageing is not easily understood. But there are strong hints that there are some modifiable processes (e.g., the 20 per cent increase in life expectancy found by Guo Zhang et al.[416] in mice described above). And we know that every time a cell reproduces itself (mitosis), there is a risk of a mutation somewhere in the genetic code. These mutations occur infrequently and in a chance or stochastic manner. But 'chance' does not mean 'regardless of the environment'. A cigarette smoker may have a one in a million chance of a genetic mutation each time a cell divides, compared to one in a billion for a non-smoker. Given that some mutations result in unrestrained cell division (i.e., neoplasia or cancer), and assuming that the probability of mutation never reaches zero no matter how 'good' the environmental context is, then there must be some biological limit below which disease rates can fall no further. And assuming we never achieve 100 per cent cure rates for all these diseases, there must be a lower limit to mortality rates and therefore a ceiling on life expectancy. We just do not know what those limits are!

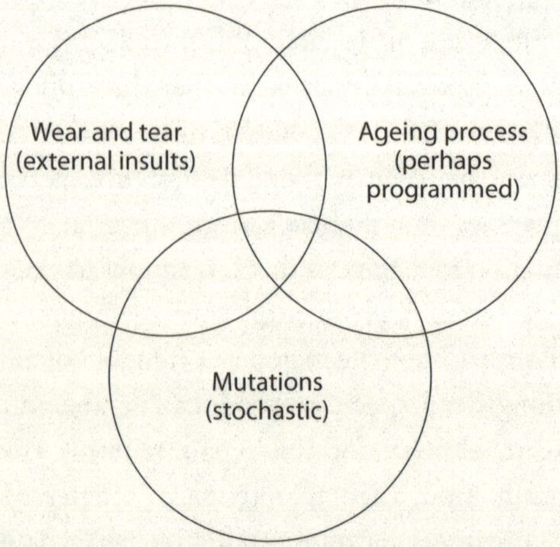

Figure 52: An indication of the forces that may be involved in ageing

In addition to random mutations, and environmental carcinogens acting on DNA to increase the frequency of errors during cell division, it is necessary to take account of epigenetic processes, that is, how genes express themselves. Figure 52 is a simple schematic or heuristic. Wear and tear caused by the interaction between the organism and environment, the ageing processes that may have an element of programming about them (e.g., the trade-off of reproduction and repair, telomere shortening) and mutations (and, more widely, genetic processes) are all at play, but highly overlapping. For example, heavy alcohol consumption stresses liver cells and causes increased cell division resulting in cirrhotic nodules and scars. But alcohol also has a toxic effect directly on the genome, increasing the rate of mutations. Together, the wear and tear and mutation effects multiply the incidence of liver cancer.

Environmental limits

Present patterns of consumption carry high risks. Not just the problems of pollution ('business as usual' use of fossil fuels might heat the world by more than 4 degrees in less than a hundred years), but many resources are being used far more rapidly than they are being replaced. Oil deposits, for instance, are depleted approximately a million times faster than they are created. Unless other energy sources are tapped, and more sustainable technologies developed, present generations are effectively 'eating the future'.[440] The risk is that our present well-being (including record low mortality) may have been achieved only by impoverishing future generations. That is fungibility in an ecological sense – good health is achieved by transferring ecological resource from the future to the present.

Most reviews of limits on life expectancy have focused on features of human biology, and some attention has been paid to the economic costs and social strains of supporting an increasingly aged population. Few have explored the possibility of environmental restraints. Indeed, improvements in life expectancy have been interpreted by some as evidence that what were once environmental limits (supplies of food and energy, for instance) have now been overcome by and large.[441] Others argue that life expectancy is a backward-looking view of human achievement, because it is built on historic drawing down of natural resources and there can be no guarantee that what was available in the past will continue in the future.[43]

Chris Murray and Lincoln Chen suggest that the causes of long-term mortality decline could be divided into flows (acute influences) and stocks (factors that slowly accumulate, are not rapidly depleted and provide momentum to long-term trends).[18] The tendency for better nourished, taller parents to bear taller, healthier children[242] is one example of a long-term force for low mortality. Is it possible that exploitation of environmental resources has provided much of the impetus for mortality decline, and therefore the environment, broadly defined, might also be described as one of the vital 'stocks'? There is certainly a temporal relation between the relatively recent plunge in mortality (as described in chapter 1, life expectancy at birth probably hovered around 30 years for millennia prior to 1800) and ramped-up consumption of environmental resources, whether the latter is measured in tonnes of coal burnt, hectares of land cleared or the proportion of river flows diverted to human use.[442]

It is not difficult to identify ways in which the 'bank' of natural resources has under-written mortality decline. Improved nutrition has undoubtedly been an important force in the last two hundred years for better population health, for example.[443] But providing more food to more people has incurred substantial environmental costs, including 'mining' of soil nutrients, reduced biodiversity, contamination of land and waterways with agricultural chemicals, and the depletion of fossil fuels required to manufacture and distribute food.

Water is fundamental to good health, whether it be water for drinking, washing, sanitation, irrigation or production. Between 1900 and 2000 there was a more than seven-fold increase in use of freshwater, and in many parts of the world, supplies have been depleted more rapidly than they can be replenished.[444] At-risk catchments include the Yellow River basin in North China, the Oglala Aquifer in the North American Midwest, the Murray/Darling system in Australia, the Amu Darya and Syr Darya basins in Central Asia, and much of the Indian subcontinent.[445]

Oil-based technologies and pharmacological products derived from intact eco-systems have been a foundation for modern medicine, which has been responsible for perhaps a third to a half of the decline in heart disease deaths in high-income countries in the last 20 years,[397] and is increasingly important as a factor in declining mortality among the elderly.[446] Most populations depend on carbon-intense transport for access to social services, facilities and employment (all factors that are important for health and, arguably, are required for continuing low mortality).

We might think of mortality gains as equivalent to dividends that have been drawn on environmental stocks. But have we been spending too far ahead? Environmental over-draws may take centuries to recover, or (the North Sea cod fishery, for example) may never be reversed.

In the future there will be intense pressures on the environment. Increasing numbers of people will be one cause, since the world population, currently more than 7 billion, is likely to grow to half as much again within the next hundred years. Also important will be urbanisation – the growth of resource-hungry super cities, and increasing levels of consumption within developing countries.

In May 2013, the concentration of CO_2 in the atmosphere exceeded 400 parts per million. The last time there was this much CO_2 in the atmosphere was probably in the mid-Pliocene era, 2–4 million years ago, and if emissions of greenhouse gases continue on their present path (2–3 per cent increase each year), levels may reach 500 ppm around the middle of the twenty-first century. This trajectory is right at the top end of the climate scenarios developed by the Intergovernmental Panel on Climate Change, and suggest we may be heading for warming of 4–6 degrees C (on average) above pre-industrial temperatures by 2100.[447] Averages don't tell the full story. Heating of 4–6 degrees would mean that the most extreme summers on recent record (e.g., 2003 and 2010 in the northern hemisphere) would become the new norm; much of south-eastern Australia would be facing catastrophic fire risk one year in two; and the chance of abrupt, irreversible changes in Earth systems (e.g., stalling or reversal of deep ocean currents) would be much increased.

What will be the effects on human health in a +4-degree world? It is impossible to foresee the feedbacks, thresholds and modifying factors that apply in the climate system, and likewise, we don't know how quickly or effectively humans will be able to respond. The amount of heating is important because there may be thresholds or tipping points, but in general, it is the rate of change that matters most. Adaptation in natural and human systems is speed-limited, whether we are talking about species mobility, behavioural coping mechanisms or evolution of heat-tolerance. And the rate of warming that is projected in the next 100 years is unprecedented. There have been two occasions previously in geological records of the Earth heating by 4–5 degrees, but these events did not occur in the course of a century, they occurred over thousands or millions of years.[448]

Agriculture will be seriously threatened, especially in the tropics and subtropics where it is already too hot for optimal growth of many crops, where poverty is common, and where population growth in the next half century will be most rapid.[449] Parts of the world will be too hot for outdoor work for much of the year, and by 2200, global labour productivity may be reduced by as much as 60 per cent in the warmest months.[450] Warming in higher latitude regions will be much greater than the global average, and will provide new opportunities for infectious diseases. It is difficult to forecast the effects on health of more severe floods, storms, droughts and wild-fires, though these changes are expected to be part and parcel of a greenhouse-charged climate. Population displacement, migration and increasing social conflict are all higher-level consequences of climate change, and are also associated with heavy risks to health.[451]

The picture is not altogether bleak. The correlation between consumption of energy (one of the fundamental environmental stocks) and life expectancy is close only at low levels of energy use, and there are countries (such as Sri Lanka and Cuba) that have achieved low mortality with a relatively shallow ecological footprint.[452] There are signs in the high-income countries of increasing efficiency in energy use, and substantial improvements in health-damaging local pollution. (Pope et al. argue that reductions in fine particle levels in the air in United States cities since 1980 could be responsible for 15 per cent of the improvement in life expectancy in the last 20 years.[453]) However, high-income, high-consuming countries such as the United States (and New Zealand) have not yet shown willingness to reduce the amount of energy they sequester, or to make radical changes to energy sources.

Optimists point out that past patterns of consumption do not fix future trends: there are alternative, low-consumption trajectories that might be more health-promoting than an extension of 'business as usual.'[454] For example, diets in rich countries might include less ruminant meat, and transport systems world-wide encourage walking and cycling in place of short car trips. However, the scale of the problem is daunting. Holding global heating to no more than 2 degrees will probably require countries like New Zealand to reduce their greenhouse emissions by about 80 per cent by 2050, and rapidly growing countries such as China and India must shift quickly to low-carbon development routes.[455] At present, it is not evident that there is public willingness, or political leadership, to achieve such demanding goals.

Down-sizing to lower-energy patterns of consumption is one way of bypassing (at least temporarily) environmental limits. But there are also stocks for good health that are renewable. Education, communications and urbanism (which have positive as well as negative aspects) are forces for good health that tend to accumulate over time, pass from one generation to another and are likely to push the mortality curve further along its present trajectory.

WHAT ABOUT QUALITY OF LIFE?

Compression of morbidity: this phrase is particularly associated with a 1980 paper by James Fries.[456] Fries envisaged a future in which people are living longer, in good health, with frailty and disease compressed into a shorter period. In the 35 years since the paper was published, the first of Fries' projections (people living longer) has come to pass. What about the 'compression' of frailty and disease?

There seem to be two forces at work. One increases the total number of years that people live, on average. At the same time, there is another force acting on the incidence and severity of disease, which means that people of the same age are, on average, more active and are less likely to be unwell than previous cohorts. For instance, a study of US national surveys found that 80 years ago men aged 50 to 74 were twice as likely to have functional limitations such as difficulty walking and impaired vision.[457] When life expectancy advances more quickly than morbidity reduction, then the years of life lived in poor health increase. When the incidence and severity of disease reduces more quickly than the increase in total life expectancy, then morbidity is compressed.

Figure 53 shows that in the United States, the number of years lived with disability increased between 1935 and 1999, but the proportion of all years lived past 65 with disability declined.[458] In absolute terms, one could argue that morbidity has expanded. But in relation to overall life expectancy, a smaller proportion of people's lives is affected – thus morbidity has compressed in relative terms. The answer to the question 'Has morbidity expanded?' may depend on whether you are thinking in absolute or relative terms.

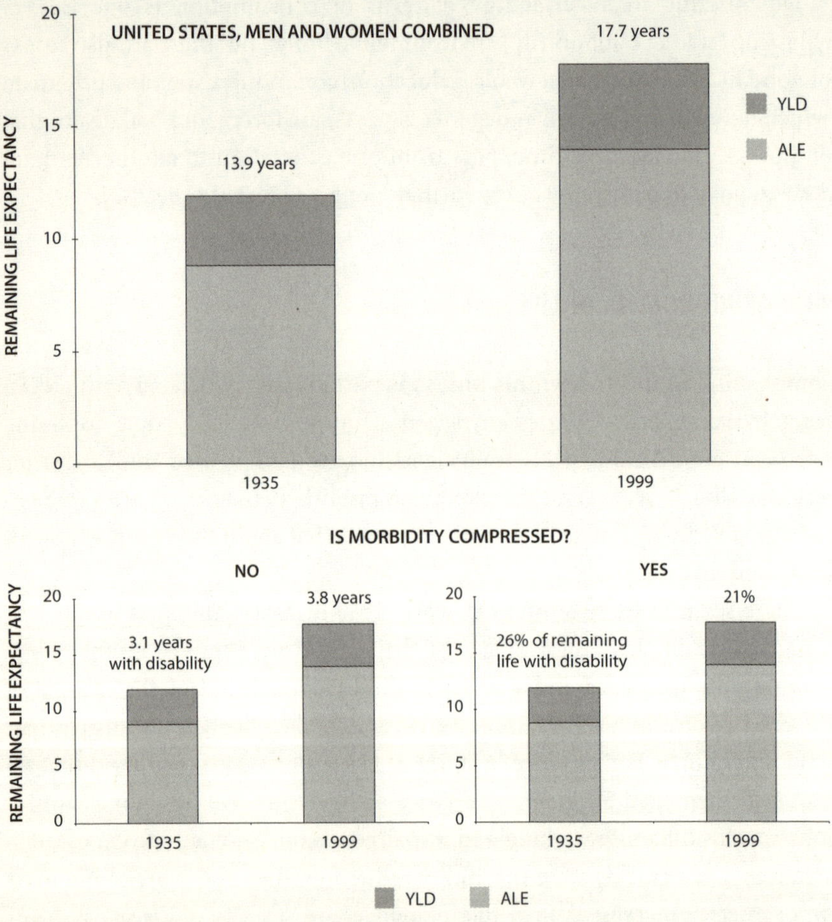

Figure 53: Years lived with disability, United States, 1935 and 1999

Source: K. G. Manton, 'Recent Declines in Chronic Disability in the Elderly U.S. Population: Risk Factors and Future Dynamics' (*Annual Review of Public Health* 29 [2008]: 91–113). Life expectancy past age 65 is here made up of years lived without disability (active life expectancy, ALE) and years lived with disability (YLD). In absolute terms, morbidity is not reduced, but the proportion of years lived with disability has fallen.

In New Zealand, an analysis of health-adjusted life expectancy (calculated by merging life tables and post-census disability surveys of functional limitation) suggests there was a modest expansion in morbidity from 1996 to 2006.[459] We need a longer time series to be certain that this change is taking place.

Prospects for quality of life

In Switzerland the number of people aged 100 and over has been doubling each decade, since 1950, mostly as a result of declining mortality in the over-80-year-olds.[460] Many other countries will experience the same phenomenon, of a radical expansion in the numbers of very old individuals. What will be the consequences for the quality of life? An ageing population, without any changes in the incidence or progression of disease, guarantees that the numbers of people with debilitating age-related disability will rise. However, the prevalence of many diseases amongst older people has increased due to better detection and more complete recording of conditions that were commonly unnoticed in the past. Added to this, more effective treatments may mean living longer with disease, but less impairment than in the past. That is what is sometimes referred to as 'dynamic equilibrium', whereby the amount of less severe morbidity expands but the amount of severe morbidity contracts. These trends have been observed in New Zealand.[461]

In many respects, the health of older people is improving. Within ten years, for example, there were improvements of 16–17 per cent in mobility of Japanese aged 66 and over.[462] In the US, in percentage terms at least, morbidity is decreasing (Figure 53).[458] A similar pattern is apparent elsewhere, as years lived with disabilities are increasing, but years lived in good health are increasing more rapidly.[160] This is not true in every country, nor with every measure of disability: Crimmins and colleagues claim the length of life with *mobility* loss has increased, on average, in the last ten years in the US, as increased longevity has outpaced reductions in this particular aspect of disability.[463] More generally, acknowledging how difficult it is to measure morbidity consistently over time,[464] we suggest that 'dynamic equilibrium' (i.e., less severe morbidity, more moderate morbidity) is the most common pattern.[160]

The link between longer life and increased cost of care is not carved in stone, even at what we currently regard as very advanced ages. In a Danish report, the proportion of individuals living independently remained constant between 90 and 100. It may be partly a survivor effect, as the frail and disabled die earlier than the more robust members of the cohort.[465] But this and other research[466] on quality of life among the most aged tells us that living into the 11th or 12th decades does not necessarily bring great frailty. Perhaps life-extending health promotion does not necessarily increase health expenditure, even when it engages those who are already old. A review of international trends suggests that improvements in healthy ageing are, on the whole, keeping pace with the increase in lifespan, so the rise in the prevalence of disability is slower than many have forecast.[160]

A study tracking residents in aged care facilities in Auckland found the proportion in aged care is falling (40 per cent of those over 85 in 1988, only 27 per cent in 2008), but those in care tend to be older and frailer than in the past.[467] Looking ahead, mortality and disability at a given age are both set to fall, but the steep rise in the number of people living to very old age groups may mean that absolute numbers of some disabling health conditions will rise. In New Zealand, it has been projected that the number of people living with Alzheimer's disease will increase 2.5-fold in the next 25 years.[468] However, age-related cognitive decline is not fixed. A comparison of two Danish cohorts of 90-year-olds (the first born in 1905, the other in 1915) found that the 1915 cohort had substantially better cognitive function, on average.[469] Others have compared the incidence of dementia in older adults (60–90-year-olds) in 1990 and 2000, and reported a reduction of 25 per cent at the second assessment.[470] These are positive indications – maybe longer lives do not necessarily bring with them greater disability.

WHAT SHOULD BE THE ORGANISED EFFORTS OF SOCIETY IN THE TWENTY-FIRST CENTURY?

The question is: in the twenty-first century, where do we start? Just maintaining the health gains that have been achieved will be a challenge; but the goal is to do better, to extend the improvements in length and quality of life. In this section we review the choices in front of researchers, service providers and policy-makers. They include a focus on the biological aspects of ageing, reversing the risk factors that cause the burden of disease to mount up, and investing in health-care services to treat disease and injury.

Slow the ageing process

Some believe we should desist from the current dominant paradigm of tackling one disease at a time, or one risk factor at time.[471] The argument runs that little is to be gained in life expectancy from targeting single diseases. (Although moderate gains on lots of diseases and risk factors will be productive – witness the last century.) Rather, a fully fledged research assault on the determinants of the biological process of ageing is needed (e.g., getting to the bottom of the story on telomere shortening), and translation of this new knowledge to population-level interventions. Presumably some as yet undiscovered neuro-chemical modulator or inhibitor, or perhaps a cocktail of known compounds, could be administered en masse to the population to slow ageing. So expressed, it sounds fanciful – and we believe such interventions probably are unrealistic, at least for the next few decades.

Tackle risk factors

By risk factors we mean those things that cause disease and injury, and are modifiable, such as smoking, obesity (resulting from excessive energy intake and physical inactivity), high blood pressure, dietary fat and bottle-feeding of infants.

We propose three steps to take before forming a view on which interventions we should focus on in coming decades. First, understand how much of the current burden of disease and injury can be attributed to each risk factor. Second, understand how life expectancy will change in the next few decades for projected risk-factor trends – including projections of 'business as usual'. Third, consider what interventions we could use to alter levels of risk factors in the future: are the interventions effective? what do they cost? and are they cost-effective?

In previous chapters we have examined trends in risk factors, and have attempted to connect them with alterations in life expectancy. Because of data limitations, this was far from a precise undertaking. In the last couple of decades an approach called 'burden of disease studies' has been developed to estimate in a more reliable fashion the links between environment and behaviour on the one hand, and disease incidence and mortality on the other. The work has been led by Chris Murray and Alan Lopez, and led recently to the Global Burden of Disease 2010 study (GBD2010).[472]

At the heart of the burden of disease method is the Disability Adjusted Life Year (DALY), a composite measure of mortality and morbidity. The mortality part counts up how many life-years were lost in a given year for all deaths in a country, assuming individuals would have lived otherwise to the age of some 'idealised population' (e.g., a life table formed by taking the best mortality rates at each age from around the world, as in the GBD2010). The morbidity part counts up the total health-related quality of life loss for all diseases prevalent in a given year, by 'awarding' each person with a disease or injury a disability weight for that condition[473] and then summing up the disability-adjusted person-years. A New Zealand burden of disease study for the year 2006 was published in 2013, championed by Martin Tobias at the Ministry of Health.[474]

The beauty of the burden of disease approach is that it takes a range of epidemiological variables (including risk-factor prevalence, and the relative risks associating these risk factors with disease incidence and mortality) and applies standard equations to work out how much of the burden of disease and injury (i.e., DALYs) can be attributed to the specified risk factors. The calculation depends on some important assumptions, such as what the 'theoretical minimum' of each risk factor is. This is easy for tobacco – the reference point is no tobacco. But for something like blood pressure, it is not immediately obvious, and what is usually applied is a counterfactual distribution (e.g., of blood pressures) that is lower and less variable than what we currently have in New Zealand – but not unheard of anywhere else in the world. Deciding on the outputs of burden of disease studies is useful in many ways. Knowing how many of the DALYs are attributable to a particular risk factor makes it possible (as we will see later in this chapter) to determine how much (healthy) life expectancy will increase for specified interventions.

In the New Zealand 2006 BDS, about a third of all the DALYs could be attributed to modifiable risk factors.[474] Not surprisingly, tobacco topped the rankings, causing 9.2 per cent of all DALYs. (However, the BDS also estimates that by 2011 obesity will have overtaken smoking in its contribution to total disease burden, a consequence of shrinking smoking rates and expanding bodyweights.) Alcohol generated about 5.6 per cent of DALYs, but also prevented about 1.4 per cent (due to moderate consumption preventing heart disease, stroke and diabetes), resulting in a net loss of 4 per cent. High blood pressure contributed 6.4 per cent of DALYs (some of which will be due to upstream factors such as salt intake and overweight/obesity that act through an increase in blood pressure), high blood glucose 4.7 per cent (in this analysis, 'diabetes' is considered as a disorder across a spectrum of blood sugar readings), and high blood cholesterol 3.2 per cent. Low physical activity contributed 4.2 per cent and overweight/obesity (or, more specifically, 'high body mass index') contributed 7.7 per cent. Contributors of between 1 and 2 per cent of DALYs included salt (which is important, as it is theoretically at least very easy to intervene on salt and reduce strokes and heart disease), low fruit and vegetable intake, and high saturated fat.[474]

It is important to appreciate that these percentages are not independent of each other. For example, physical activity and overweight and obesity all influence blood pressure, and high BMI accounted for about 60 per cent of the osteoarthritis and diabetes burdens. Due to these and many other interactions, the attributable fractions are not additive.

Demonstrating the potency of modern health care, it is estimated that adverse events in hospitals and primary care caused 3.2 per cent of all DALYs in 2006, over half of which were the consequence of premature mortality. Perhaps only a third of the impact of adverse events in the health system can be readily avoided, but this category deserves particularly close attention because of concerns about the duty of care.

The total cluster of risk factors for injury accounted for 7.3 per cent of DALYs, with transportation, self-inflicted violence (especially amongst younger adults) and falls (especially the elderly) standing out as the three biggest specific risk factors.

Future life expectancy if New Zealand goes tobacco-free

Last century, among British doctors, if you smoked you had at least a 50 per cent chance of dying from tobacco, and these deaths occurred (on average) at least ten years earlier than deaths among non-smokers.[475] In the twenty-first century smoking remains the single largest preventable cause of premature death, but the magnitude of its impact changes with the context. For example, because the background or baseline rate of cardiovascular disease has fallen, the ratio of the risk amongst smokers to the risk for non-smokers has increased.[303] On the other hand, people smoke fewer cigarettes per day now than at the time of the British doctors study, so the risks due to smoking are less than they used to be.

In New Zealand there are about 5000 deaths per year that are due to tobacco – or about a fifth of all deaths. Remember, these figures are not fixed, and will vary over time as the prevalence of smoking rises and falls, and disease risks among non-smokers fluctuate also.

We attempted to distinguish the effects of smoking on future life expectancy by modelling the marginal gains from 2006 to 2040 in two scenarios. First we assumed that smoking prevalence stays the same as that reported in the 2006 census. The alternative was that New Zealand becomes 'tobacco-free'. We picked 2040 to allow roughly 20 years for (nearly) all the adverse effects of tobacco smoking to wash out of the population, assuming that New Zealand would become tobacco-free in 2020. (The New Zealand Parliament now has 2025 as a target date by which New Zealand should be tobacco-free.)[476; 477]

We estimated that a tobacco-free New Zealand, compared to one with 2006 smoking rates continuing into the future, would see an additional five-year gain in life expectancy for Māori by 2040, three years for non-Māori and therefore a two-year closing in the life-expectancy gap.[478]

It is hard to imagine any other intervention that could achieve so much, and we believe the tobacco-free goal is eminently do-able. In principle, the options are to wind down tobacco imports, or increase tax, or both. Public health aims to influence both initiation of smoking and cessation, or quitting, but it is cessation that matters most in the short to medium term. To reach the 2025 'tobacco-free' goal we will need to double or triple the quit rates observed for non-Māori from 2001 to 2011, and increase ten-fold Māori cessation rates. In preliminary disease modelling we estimate that increasing the tobacco excise tax by 10 per cent each year till 2025 would shift the non-Māori prevalence in 2025 from about 8 per cent projected without tax to 7 per cent with tax. (This would be equivalent to increasing the price of a pack of cigarettes from $14 to $41 in 2025, in 2011 dollars.) The same tax might achieve a 2 percentage point reduction for Māori, from 20 per cent to 18 per cent. Thus, while tax increases are important, more than just tax increases will be needed to achieve a 5 per cent prevalence by 2025.[504]

The impact of the obesity epidemic on future life expectancy

In New Zealand there is one risk factor for chronic disease that is persistently heading in the wrong direction. This is bodyweight. Since the 1980s average bodyweight has increased, for all groups in the population, and consequently the proportions who fall in the categories of 'overweight' and 'obese' have also increased. Heavier people are more likely to suffer from a host of health problems, including cardiovascular disease, diabetes, high blood pressure, high blood cholesterol, osteoarthritis, asthma and sleep disorders.[479; 480; 481] In the Framingham study in the United States, 40-year-olds with obesity (defined as a BMI≥30) lived on average six–seven years less than their contemporaries who were not obese, and this gap widened to almost 13 years if obesity was combined with smoking.[482] In the United States, the first country to put on weight in epidemic proportions, and a notoriously poor performer in health statistics given its huge investments in health care, obesity explains a fifth to a third of the shortfall in life expectancy compared with other high-income countries.[483]

If people continue to put on weight, will this put a brake on improvements in life expectancy in the future? Some believe that this will happen,[32] even to the point that future generations will, for the first time, live shorter lives than their parents. But this seems an extreme position. Recent regular and uninterrupted improvements in life expectancy have occurred despite rapid increases in the prevalence of bodyweight. Moreover, it is not certain that the health risks associated with obesity in the past will apply in the same way to future generations. For example, the original Framingham study ran from 1947 to 1970, and later cohorts followed through the 1990s show more modest associations between overweight and obesity and all-cause mortality, although reanalysis of multiple studies combined suggest that overweight (not just obesity) is associated with a substantial mortality risk.[484; 485; 481] Other studies have found that risk factors for cardiovascular disease, such as high blood pressure, are less strongly linked with obesity in modern cohorts than they were 30–40 years ago.[486]

Why should being obese matter less for longevity now (and therefore, we speculate, in the future) than in earlier times? How you become fat may be as important as how fat you are. Current populations are exposed to all-round food excess and a deficiency in opportunities for exercise; in earlier times obesity resulted from a different constellation of causes (high intakes of saturated fats, for example). Improvements in treatment may have blunted some of the effects of being overweight. For instance, modern treatments can control raised blood pressure more effectively than was once the case. In other words, both the underlying causes of increasing bodyweight (e.g., the proportion of energy excess from saturated fat) and the modifiers of bodyweight's impact on mortality (e.g., access to blood pressure medication) are changing over time, and this means we cannot assume that the past associations of bodyweight with mortality apply unaltered into the future. Finally, the impact of obesity is not the same in absolute terms, because high bodyweight tends to magnify the risks of diseases such as heart disease and stroke, and these conditions are less common (in New Zealand) than in the past.

Obesity aside, future cohorts of elderly will in many ways be in much better shape than their predecessors. Younger generations are smoking less than their parents and grandparents. Fewer suffer severe infectious diseases early in life. More students complete high school and enter post-secondary education. These and other social changes mean that cohorts reaching old age in the middle of the twenty-first century are likely to be more resilient than the present-day elderly.

Net effect of future trends in tobacco and bodyweight on mortality

The co-occurrence of the waning of the smoking epidemic and the peaking of the obesity epidemic raises the interesting question of what will be the net effect of these two important trends. Such an analysis – or 'structured quantitative speculation' – has not been undertaken in New Zealand. However, at least two attempts have occurred in the United States. First, Stewart and colleagues extrapolated trends in obesity and smoking, and assumed the relative increase in mortality remained as it is now.[487] Their analyses were at the margin, in that life expectancy gains were still assumed to occur for a range of reasons other than smoking and obesity. They found that falling smoking rates would bring a 0.3 to 0.4 year increase in life expectancy at age 18, between 2005 and 2020. At the same time, increasing obesity would incur a –0.6 to –1.3 year penalty over the same period, meaning the net effect was a holding back of life expectancy (from these two factors alone; life expectancy overall will probably still increase due to improvements elsewhere). The second study, by Preston and colleagues, projected a different future. They concluded that the gains to 2040 from reducing smoking would outweigh losses due to increased obesity, and the net positive contribution to life expectancy at age 40 was 0.9 years for males and 0.3 years for females.[488]

Why did these two studies arrive at contradictory findings? Preston and colleagues use a more sophisticated future projection of obesity rates based on transition matrices, and these generate a more positive scenario (i.e., lower rates on obesity and overweight) than assumed by Stewart et al. Preston also allowed for the excess risk from smoking and obesity to diminish with age, and used a method that captures cohort effects of smoking – particularly important for females where the smoking penalty is still peaking due to later phasing of the tobacco epidemic. And let's not forget that these projections are of the net effect, meaning the difference in two projections, making them difficult and unstable to estimate in the first place.

Our interpretation? First, calculations of this kind are challenging to make because of the assumptions that must be incorporated. And they are based on projected risk-factor trends in the first place – without doubt, increases in life expectancy would be profound if there was no smoking and everyone had a 'normal' bodyweight. However, we do side with Preston and colleagues and conclude that the impacts of the obesity epidemic may not be as dire as some suggest. The reasons are the changing makeup of the obese population and the ability to mitigate its effects with treatments – although excessive weight gain will hold back future gains in healthy life-years. Thus there remains a strong case for policy action to curb obesity, so long as we can identify interventions that are effective and feasible – more of that later.

Net effect of future trends in tobacco and bodyweight on morbidity

We argued at the beginning of this chapter that we should be paying more attention to the quality of life – not just quantity. What will be the effects of smoking and bodyweight on other measures than mortality? Will morbidity expand or compress? We anticipate that the net effect of a shift from tobacco to bodyweight epidemics will cause morbidity to *expand* (that is, improvements in life expectancy may be accompanied by an increase in years lived with disability). (We do not consider here what the overall effect will be of obesity, tobacco and all other drivers of morbidity.)

Van Baal and colleagues in 2006 used a burden of disease platform to estimate life expectancy and health-adjusted life expectancy (HALE, a measure that subtracts from life expectancy years lived in poor health) for three groups: normal weight, non-smoker; normal weight, smoker; obese, non-smoker.[489] Life expectancy varied greatly between groups as expected, and so too did the HALEs. But the gap between life expectancy and HALEs was much the same, and it is this gap that represents years lived with poor health. In other words, current trends in smoking and bodyweight will lead to improved life expectancy but neither compress nor expand morbidity. The model includes disease states such as arthritis of hip and knee, back pain and diabetes, all of which are strongly related to obesity. But the loss in quality of life from simply having a high bodyweight (but not in a recognised disease state) is not captured, which means the figures under-estimate the full impact. The same is true for smoking (e.g., shortness of breath affects quality of life, but is not captured in a disease state).

Stewart and colleagues, in addition to the life expectancy modelling we described above, directly estimated and modelled quality of life for combinations of bodyweight and obesity.[487] That is, they went about it differently from van Baal, and rather than disease states they used peoples' responses to a brief, five-item questionnaire on quality of life called the EQ5D. It measures mobility, self-care, usual activities, pain/discomfort and anxiety/depression. Figure 54 shows how quality of life varied by all of age, smoking and bodyweight groupings together. Quality of life obviously decreases with age. Within groupings of age and smoking, obese people had a 0.04 decrement in quality of life compared to normal weight, and there was a reduction of 0.09 to 0.1 for persons who were morbidly obese. (There was no difference for normal weight and overweight.) Within groupings of age and bodyweight there was a 0.06 decrement in quality of life for smokers versus non-smokers.

So will we see a compression, or expansion, of morbidity as societies swap smoking for the obesity epidemic? Stewart and colleagues found that if the US magically became either tobacco-free or the population was all a normal weight, gains in quality-adjusted life expectancy would exceed gains in life expectancy in both cases – that is, morbidity compresses. And it compresses more in absolute terms for the bodyweight thought experiment (8 per cent) than the tobacco-free option (4 per cent). Thinking about it the other way around, that means the 2005 distributions of bodyweight and smoking (compared to counterfactuals of all normal weight, or all never smokers) expand morbidity, but overweight and obesity more so than smoking. So it is not surprising that the models of what will happen in the US up to 2020 with changing bodyweight and smoking patterns projected a modest (2 per cent) *expansion* of morbidity.

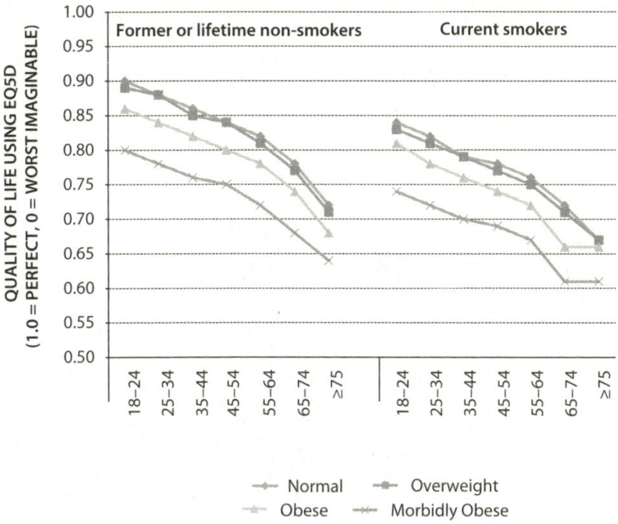

Figure 54: Health-related quality of life by age, smoking status and bodyweight

Source: 2003 US Medical Expenditure Panel, as given in S. T. Stewart, D. M. Cutler, et al, 'Forecasting the Effects of Obesity and Smoking on U.S. Life Expectancy' (*New England Journal of Medicine* 361, no. 23 [2009]: 2252–2260).

Last we consider a Dutch study, by Kligs, Mackenbach and Kunst in 2011. Using a survey that directly assessed respondents' ability to complete a range of activities of daily living, merged with mortality risks, they found virtually no difference in morbidity by smoking level (although mortality obviously varied substantially), but there was a two-to-three-year difference in life-years lived with disability from the age of 55 between obese and normal-weight people.[490] Thus, other things being equal, a shift from smoking to obesity epidemics would be associated with expansion of morbidity.

Drawing all these threads together, we conclude that if the obesity epidemic continues unabated it will contribute to an expansion of morbidity. (The overall effect, though, will be a balance of many other drivers in addition to obesity and tobacco.) The business-as-usual scenario for obesity will restrain increases in life expectancy, but not completely ablate them. We expect that treatments will do more to keep overweight and obese people alive, and so increase the proportion of people in the population living with morbidity. It is possible (though perhaps not very likely) that treatment will advance to the extent that it not only prolongs life among overweight and obese people, but also substantially improves quality of life as well. For example, eliminating joint pain and overcoming absolutely all mobility impairments would substantially increase health-adjusted life expectancy.

Treat disease

Does better access to treatments save lives and increase life expectancy? We believe the answer is 'yes', and there are plenty of examples. There is no mega-analysis that determines what the contribution of health care has been to life expectancy increases in one country since (say) World War II. It would be very challenging to carry out an analysis of this kind, since it would require data on the effects of many treatments applied to many diseases over many years. Instead, we examine what is known about the effects of treatment on the two most common causes of death in New Zealand: cardiovascular disease and cancer.

In New Zealand, as we mentioned in an earlier chapter, about half of the reduction in coronary heart disease mortality from the 1980s to 1990s is attributed to treatment, and half due to improvements in risk factors (e.g., blood pressure and tobacco).[279] The proportions are not the same in every country, nor for every period; the figures differ depending on what stage of the tobacco epidemic a country has reached. However, across a large number of high-income countries it is estimated that roughly 25 per cent to 50 per cent of the fall in coronary heart disease deaths has been attributable to treatment.[491; 397; 492; 493] There is ample room for further reduction in risk factors (such as tobacco) to lower cardiovascular disease mortality further, and opportunity also for improved coverage of mortality-lowering treatments. For example, Daniel Exeter, Rod Jackson and colleagues have determined the proportion of people in New Zealand with ischaemic cardiovascular disease who are consistently dispensed triple therapy (aspirin, statin and blood pressure lowering agent) as of 2011. The results (60 per cent nationally, varying by District Health Board from 54 per cent to 66 per cent) are published as a series of interactive maps (www.hqsc.govt.nz/assets/Health-Quality-Evaluation/CVD_standard/atlas.html). The gains that could be made from better treatment of pre-existing cardiovascular disease in each age group will decrease in the future if disease incidence continues to fall, but as we live longer there will be substantial benefits from treating cardiovascular disease at older (and older) ages. Moreover, many of the pharmacological treatments for cardiovascular disease are very cheap, and represent extremely good value for money.[344]

Cancer is more complicated, since it comprises many different disease entities. Nevertheless, gains in survival in the last 20 years have been most impressive. Across all cancers, the excess death rate has decreased by 26 per cent per decade, with particularly strong improvements for breast cancer (52 per cent decrease), leukaemia (60 per cent) and non-Hodgkin's lymphoma (44 per cent).[365] Some of this improvement is attributable to earlier stage at diagnosis and fewer co-morbidities (e.g., less chronic respiratory disease as smoking wanes). But mostly the improvement in cancer prognosis is due to better treatment, ranging from more effective surgical approaches for rectal cancer to chemotherapy for leukaemia, tamoxifen for breast cancer and multidisciplinary team management for a wide range of diseases. We expect these gains will continue in the future, even if they are restrained frequently by the cost of new treatments.

Cost-effectiveness of health care

The cost of providing health care is increasing more quickly than that of any other sector (Figure 55, overleaf). Since 1970, the percentage of GDP spent on health in New Zealand has doubled, rising from 5.2 per cent to 10.1 per cent in 2010. In the future, anticipated changes in the age structure of the population, rising public expectations and supply-side pressures will all contribute to the competition for resources.

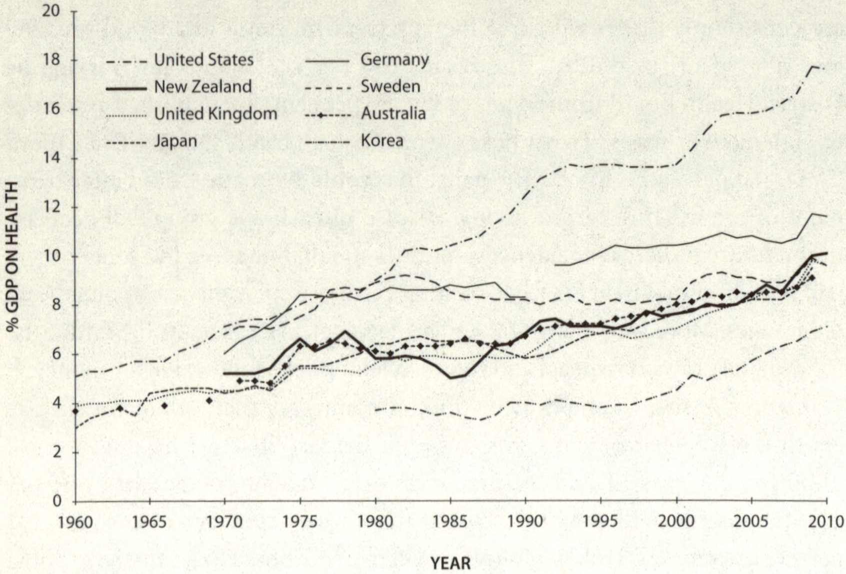

Figure 55: Percentage of GDP spent on health for selected OECD countries since 1960
Source: Data extracted from Organisation for Economic Co-operation and Development statistics (www.oecd.org).

We offer two examples of how the competition for resources might be managed by a deliberate process of priority-setting. First, New Zealand has a national agency, PHARMAC, responsible for buying pharmaceuticals (and now medical devices as well). PHARMAC has been very effective at constraining government spending by means such as preferred supplier agreements, purchasing generics, negotiated deals with the pharmaceutical industry and extensive use of cost-effectiveness analyses. Critics argue the choice of drugs is restricted in New Zealand. Supporters of PHARMAC reply that most of the 'bang' is achieved for much less 'buck' and the drugs on PHARMAC's list include all those that are known to make a big difference to common problems and fall within a generously defined range of what is affordable. In 2012 the New Zealand budget for medical drugs was $777 million; it has been estimated (by PHARMAC) that the bill would have otherwise been at least three times as much ($2,236 million).[494] By these calculations, about $1.5 billion was freed in 2011–12 to be spent on other health-care activity (or 10.6 per cent of all Government Vote:Health spending). If this arrangement continues, and succeeds in prioritising services that are both life-prolonging and life-enhancing – be they prevention or treatment – then New Zealand will be well-placed to extend its average life expectancy.

The second example comprises a body of work from across the Tasman, the Australian Cost Effectiveness (ACE) studies. These included 150 preventive and treatment interventions,[344] ranging from taxes on unhealthy foods to diuretics for heart disease, from salt reduction in the food chain to laparoscopic banding for morbid obesity (which was cost-effective per treatment, but very expensive if provided to the total population).[495] The goal was to maximise the number of disability-adjusted life-years (DALYs) averted. In general, the interventions that were found to be both cost-effective (and even cost-saving, in that the cost of prevented health care exceeds the upfront cost of the intervention) and had a substantial impact on health tended to be population-wide and often regulatory in nature. For example, taxes on alcohol, tobacco and unhealthy food, and a polypill (combining multiple cardiovascular drugs) were all cost-saving with big health impacts.[344]

The ACE-prevention study also pointed to wasted health-care resource in the treatment of cardiovascular disease.[344] Australian treatment practices at the time averted 380,000 DALYs over the lifetime of the population, at a total cost of $12 billion – cost-effective, but still costly. An alternative regime that applied a combination of community heart health programmes, cheaper drugs (e.g., diuretics and calcium channel blockers), dieticians and phytosterols in margarine would have achieved the same health gain for only $2 billion – now very cost-effective, and liberating $10 billion for use elsewhere.

The ACE studies demonstrate that we can achieve the same health gain for much less than we currently spend. Looked at another way, we could achieve greater health gain with the same resource applied in a different way. It sounds simple, and to some extent it is, but not always. We value things other than increased longevity as a society and as individuals. For example, we may turn a social blind-eye to high-salt foods, but want to spend lots of money helping people who develop strokes (of which some could have been prevented through no-cost regulation of the food industry to reduce salt in foods). Also, we may choose to say 'enough is enough' and put more effort into quality of life (be it disability support services or improving the physical environment), rather than focusing on quantity of life.

If we did want to put New Zealand once more at the top of the league tables in life expectancy, it could be done by more aggressive and extensive prevention, and by withdrawing funding from cost-ineffective treatments and spending on interventions in health care that have a more robust evidence base. (Then wait 5 to 30 years.) The biggest challenges will be agreeing on trade-offs; accommodating other social values; and managing the influence of industry (e.g., the food industry), health-care providers and other lobby groups. But technically, we know a lot about what needs to be done to achieve major increases in life expectancy in the next 20 years without huge cost. Here are some examples: drastically reducing the sale of tobacco products (by regulation or taxation); halving salt in the food chain; reformulating energy-dense, nutrient-poor foods; simple and informative nutritional labels on food (e.g., so-called traffic-light labels with red, amber and green colouring); banning or taxing heavily sugar-sweetened beverages; promoting active transport (e.g., by congestion charging in cities, pay-as-you-drive insurance and registration levies, and simple roadway changes that favour pedestrians and cyclists over motorised traffic); and prioritising within the menu of health-care treatments those that are cost-effective in terms of life-years saved. Importantly, many of these high-value, population-wide interventions would reduce inequalities in health.[496; 497]

Improve wider determinants of health

Future advances in life expectancy will depend on improvements in the underlying determinants of health, including real incomes, education, workplace safety, urban design, air pollution, nutritional quality and accessibility. It is possible to make gains from redistribution of access to resources without necessarily growing the pie. For example, the beneficial impact on health of an extra $100 a month is greater for someone in poverty than for someone who is already wealthy.[244; 498; 499] For someone in poverty, an extra $100 a month is more likely to go to basic, health-sustaining expenditures such as housing, heating and a decent diet. Given the widening income inequalities seen in New Zealand (and many other countries) since the 1970s and 1980s, there is ample 'mathematical' ability to narrow income distributions again. However, globalisation and the concentration of wealth in fewer hands through the global free market make it challenging for governments to redistribute income.

Social policy

Unless there is a rapid and substantial increase in fertility rates, or the number of young immigrants is greatly increased, longer lifespans mean a larger proportion of the population in the 'old' and 'very old' categories. Here we confront an anachronism, the notion of a static dependency ratio, conventionally defined as the ratio of 0–14-year-olds plus 65+-year-olds, to the 'working age' 15-to-64-year-olds. Social policy analysis often starts from this premise. But the reality is that the average health, mobility and vitality of a 65-year-old today is vastly improved compared to circumstances in the middle of the twentieth century.

What are the expected years of life remaining if you actually reach the age of 65, now and into the future? According to Statistics New Zealand's 'period' life tables for 2011, life expectancy at age 65 is 21.6 years for non-Māori females, 19.1 for non-Māori males, and 16.9 and 15.3 years for Māori females and males. But these figures assume that death rates observed in 2011 will apply into the future. Between 1956 and 2011 the death rate at age 75 fell by about 1.5 per cent per annum, and we believe this trend will continue. Let's assume the 1.5 per cent per year downward trend continues for the next 40 years, for men and women in all ethnic groups. If this is so, the actual or 'cohort' life expectancies of persons reaching age 65 are considerably greater than the Statistics New Zealand projections (Figure 56, overleaf).

This is good news if you are about to turn 65 – longevity has never been better! A non-Māori female who turned 65 years of age in 2011 probably had about 24 years of life ahead of her (i.e., she is expected to live to 89 years of age, considerably more than the 84 years suggested from period life tables).

How will the country pay for these extra years of life? The age of entitlement to government superannuation may need to increase if we want to keep super universal, *and* keep it tied to the average wage. Otherwise it seems likely that New Zealand will shunt even more of its benefit spend in the direction of older citizens, who are already relatively well supported. By far and away the biggest ticket item in the social welfare budget is superannuation – about $7–8 billion per annum, or 60 per cent of all benefits paid out by the Ministry of Social Development. This fraction gets little political attention compared with – say – the unemployment benefit, and will increase further unless the rules of entitlement are changed. There are good reasons to re-balance our social investment across the age span. For instance, rates of child poverty in New Zealand are high compared with other OECD countries, and we are, all of us, the poorer on account of the long tail of under-achievement at school.

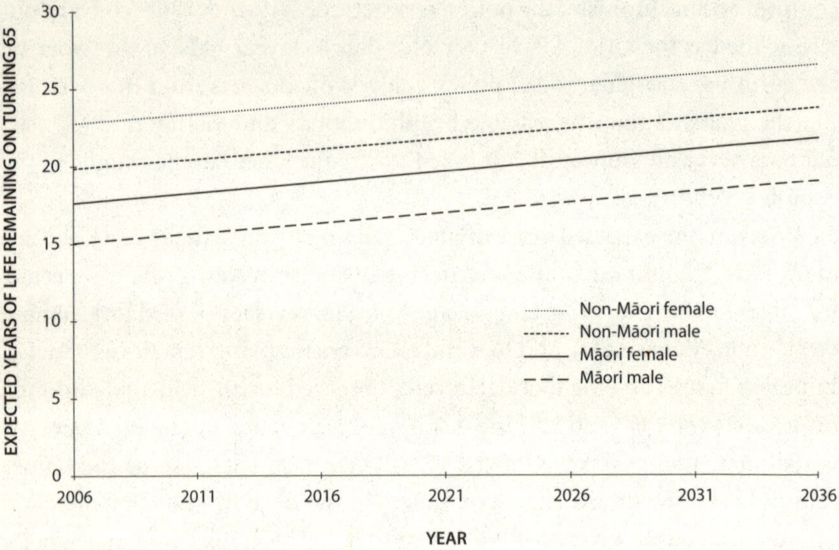

Figure 56: Estimated cohort life expectancy by calendar year at which someone turns 65
Source: Based on Statistics New Zealand life tables for 2011.

The graph also shows inequalities by ethnicity. Māori on turning 65 are likely to enjoy about five fewer years of life than non-Māori. As a society we want to close this gap, and maybe we will see it reduce in the next 20–40 years through faster mortality rate reductions for Māori consistent with what has happened at younger ages in the twentieth century. Regardless, there is a sizeable gap now and into the near future. How do we address this gap? One suggestion is to have different ages of entitlement by ethnicity. But what about people with chronic disease, and those in arduous and risky occupations? And low-income people? How would graded access to superannuation be defined, implemented, monitored? In our view, introducing different ages of entitlement for different groups in the population would be unworkable, and health inequities must be tackled in other policy.

In order to increase the age of entitlement fairly, there is another change that should be made at the same time – this is adjusting the invalid's benefit so that it is the same amount as the superannuation benefit. As argued by Gareth Morgan and Susan Guthrie in their book *The Big Kahuna*,[500] it makes no sense, and it is quite unfair that such differences exist. The Big Kahuna, a single living wage for every New Zealander, may be some way off, but equalising the superannuation benefit and the invalid's benefit is a sensible starting point. It would help to settle the concern that disease and disability will prevent some working beyond the age of 65, a particular issue for less advantaged groups in society. The New Zealand Retirement Commissioner has made a similar argument, that there should be an increase in the age of entitlement provided there is targeted-based-on-ability-to-work early eligibility for super.[501]

Conclusion

... Tanemahuta's forests of jade green
rivers, lakes, underground springs
a green belt around this nation's hips
kissed all over by Moana's blue lips.
From Te Wai Pounamu to Te Ika a Maui
greenstone to fishtail, lucky, lucky country.

— SELINA TUSITALA MARSH, FROM 'NEW ZEALAND, THE LUCKY COUNTRY'

World-wide, the advance in 'best practice' life expectancy in the last 150 years has been unwavering, and indicates that the force of mortality in the healthiest populations is reducing in a remarkably regular fashion. Many countries, including New Zealand, have tracked close to the 'best practice' trend line, with pauses, interruptions and setbacks from time to time, but no permanent reversals. Improvement in countries that are (temporarily) left behind appears to accelerate when the life expectancy curve bends upwards again. Like stretching a rubber band, the further the deviation from the long-term trend, the more rapid the recovery. Others have a more chequered history. Countries in Eastern Europe, sub-Saharan Africa and the Middle East, for instance, have suffered, or are presently immersed in, long periods of high mortality. But there are two high-level themes that emerge from our history: overall, a radical improvement in survival (more than doubling global average life expectancy in a hundred years); and convergence (in the same period, 1900–2000, the distance between the best and worst performers has reduced).

There are explanations as to why particular health problems in particular populations may have improved at a given point in time, for example, with the passing of the tobacco epidemic or the decline in vaccine-preventable diseases. But none of these explanations is big enough to account satisfactorily for the full picture. Perhaps we need to think of mortality decline as a field phenomenon – something that happens in many places simultaneously, that began small (England in the eighteenth century, arguably) but is now widely seeded and exerts a similar force whatever the setting.

An optimist would say: this phenomenon is inclusive. All populations, whether they are rich or poor, techno-quick or dawdling in the digital slow lane, democratically ruled or under the thumb of despots, all are eventually tugged along. And it is directional: for 150 years the tide has been running in, pushing life expectancy further and further up the shore. Knowledgeable people frequently say 'it will go no higher', and stick flags in the sand to mark the turning point. They hardly turn their backs and the flags are under water. What can we call this? Modernity?

Another view pays more attention to outliers than to averages, and asks: what about those who have not (yet) benefited from mortality decline? Zimbabwe, Afghanistan, Ukraine, Nauru – these are examples of populations following different trajectories, and a comprehensive explanation of life expectancy must account for differences.

We have not attempted a world-wide account. But one model that fits with observations of mortality decline both in New Zealand and elsewhere is stocks and flows, as proposed by Murray and Chen,[18] and described in an earlier chapter. There has been, long term, an accumulation of health credits – biological (e.g., stature), social (such as normative attitudes to unhealthy behaviours) and political (acceptance of the principle, if not the detail, of comprehensive health care, for instance). These are the stocks, the basis of the improvement in mortality from decade to decade. As well there are short-term runs of energy and resource, the flows (such as the arrival of a virulent strain of influenza, or take-up of a potent medical technology like blood transfusion) that detract from or add to population health. Flows generally provide the explanation for acute changes in health status; the gathering of stocks determines where health currently stands. This is rather like the difference between explaining the amplitude of waves on the surface of the lake, and understanding what determines the depth of the lake.

We have mentioned already Stephen Pinker's views on the decline in violence,[46] and believe there are parallels with mortality more generally. With minor interruptions, Pinker argues, there has been a cog-wheel advance of expectations, knowledge and technology that builds on what has gone before, is difficult to turn back and is contagious. The new norms are spread by contact, and because contact, real and virtual, is now almost immediate, is repetitive and, increasingly, is global, ways of behaving and ways of organising societies are converging.

In the introduction we sketched out four ways of thinking about mortality decline. These were: through our knowledge of the biology of ageing; a focus on technology and other products of human ingenuity; an analysis of the social determinants of health; and a systems view drawing on the principles of ecology. All these ways of thinking provide valuable insights, which are often, but not always, complementary.

The 'cog-wheel advance' idea that we ascribe to Pinker, for example, draws on the creativity of human problem-solving and the force of social institutions (e.g., those that enable trade and mass education). The decline of mortality from violence and other causes depends also on certain social norms (such as greater respect for the interests and values of women) being embedded in the world-view of new generations. From this angle, the future looks rosy. Why should there be any ceiling on cleverness and good governance? It is ecology that reminds us that human ingenuity and social determinism operate within a closed system, and on this basis it would be unwise to assume that old ways of doing things can continue.

What prompted us to write this book was the observation that the New Zealand non-Māori population had the lowest mortality in the world for roughly 70 years. We have rehearsed already the most likely reasons, which include: exclusion (and exploitation) of Māori; the wealth of natural resources locally; health-selection of migrants; lack of the crowd- and industry-related pressures that stalled Europe's mortality decline; a relatively even distribution of land and opportunity amongst non-Māori; early initiatives to extend education and promote the position of women; and economic good fortune when New Zealand became grocer to the British Empire.

Reasons for New Zealand being overtaken after 1940 include loss of the impetus provided by 'healthy migration', a change in the prevalent causes of death, dietary disadvantage in the new age of chronic diseases, lack of health service sophistication to match other highly developed countries, an epidemic of road traffic crashes, and a more comprehensive accounting for the national population (including Māori).

Could New Zealand be number one again? It may be that mortality league tables mean much less in a globalised age when international influences and rapid diffusions tend to dominate. However, New Zealand does retain important advantages. The country benefits still from abundant fresh water, a temperate climate and productive grasslands (one New Zealand company, Fonterra, is responsible for almost a third of the world's dairy exports). Although the population has quadrupled since the late nineteenth century, New Zealand remains relatively uncrowded. Again this is relative, in the age of jet travel and global pollution, but New Zealand is still, in many respects, a long way from trouble. In global terms, New Zealand's population is highly educated, its public administration is remarkably free from corruption, and the health system is efficient and innovative: as a consequence the country is well placed to make the most of its chances.

What would it take for New Zealand to increase life expectancy and at least to match countries like Japan (present-day longest-lived women) and Iceland (longest-lived men)?[502] We suggest taking some pages out of Japan's book. That country made remarkable advances on the basis of an educated, egalitarian state with few health inequalities, strong public health programmes targeted at the prevalent causes of ill-health and premature mortality (such as high blood pressure), and accessible health care.

In the future, with the growing influence of medicine on mortality, Japan may be constrained by its high-volume, low-cost health system. New Zealand likewise will find it tough to fund all new services of proven benefit, and if extended longevity and quality of life are accepted as important social goals, then it is likely the share of the national budget that goes to the health sector will have to increase. In public health, there are plenty of opportunities to do better with problems that are common and well understood. We have calculated the gains that would/will be made if/when New Zealand goes smoke-free. Other hurdles to be cleared on the way to catching Japan and Iceland include an unbalanced food environment (one that promotes high-energy, low-nutrient options), and human settlements designed to entrench sedentary living.

In Japan, inequalities in wealth and health have widened since the collapse of the asset bubble in the early 1990s,[503] but are still less than in New Zealand.[24] What would happen if we reduced differences in social and ethnic mortality to Japan-like proportions, or better? It would be challenging to achieve, but if New Zealand could flatten the socio-economic gradient to the extent that mortality rates of the most deprived quintile of the population were only 15 per cent higher than those in the least deprived quintile, then life expectancy at birth would be boosted by two to three years. This would lift New Zealand clear of all other OECD countries, Japan included (and put us roughly two years ahead of Australian average life expectancy).

We have followed the history of life expectancy from earliest *Homo sapiens* to the beginning of the twenty-first century. The average lifespan is a rough measure of human welfare, inadequate as a measure on its own, but surely, we have argued, a necessary component of the full package. All our lives have been radically transformed by dwindling mortality even if this thought seldom crosses most people's minds: it is human nature to take current expectations for granted.

There are many explanations for what has happened, but none alone account satisfactorily for the regularity of the phenomenon. The non-Māori population of New Zealand benefited from the early fall in mortality, and indeed was so far ahead of the rest of the world in the middle of the nineteenth century that it took everyone else 80 years to catch up. The experience of Māori in New Zealand was different, and illustrates another important point in the book – in mortality studies, as in the rest of life, there is no such thing as a free lunch. Improvements in life expectancy, in this country and everywhere else, have been achieved by diversion of resources and energy, and the full costs of the transfer are often overlooked.

In the short term, the future for further improvements in life expectancy looks bright – there is no sign that we are close to the biological limits on longevity. However, the social consequences of an extremely aged population will be challenging. The environmental costs of the high-energy economy that propelled lifespans upwards and onwards have escalated, and these now include serious threats to global systems. Sustaining the astounding decline in human mortality will require efficient health care, determined public health programmes, the wisdom of Solomon in social policy and greater respect for the planet on which the future of our species depends.

REFERENCES

1. Kunitz, Stephen J. *The Health of Populations: General Theories and Particular Realities*. New York: Oxford University Press, 2007.
2. Statistics New Zealand. 'A History of Survival in New Zealand: Cohort Life Tables 1876–2004.' Wellington: Statistics New Zealand, 2007.
3. Durie, Mason. 'Understanding Health and Illness: Research at the Interface between Science and Indigenous Knowledge.' *International Journal of Epidemiology* 33, no. 5 (2004): 1138–43.
4. Cutler, David M., Angus S. Deaton, and Adriana Lleras-Muney. 'The Determinants of Mortality.' *Journal of Economic Perspectives* 20, no. 3 (2006): 97–120.
5. Helliwell, J. F., R. Layard, and J. Sachs, eds. *World Happiness Report 2013*. New York: UN Sustainable Development Solutions Network, 2013.
6. Caldwell, J. C., P. H. Reddy, and P. Caldwell. 'The Social Component of Mortality Decline: An Investigation in South India Employing Alternative Methodologies.' *Population Studies* 37, no. 2 (1983): 185–205.
7. Wang, Haidong, Laura Dwyer-Lindgren, Katherine T. Lofgren, Julie Knoll Rajaratnam, Jacob R. Marcus, Alison Levin-Rector, Carly E. Levitz, Alan D. Lopez, and Christopher J. L. Murray. 'Age-Specific and Sex-Specific Mortality in 187 Countries, 1970–2010: A Systematic Analysis for the Global Burden of Disease Study 2010.' *The Lancet* 380, no. 9859 (15 December 2012): 2071–94.
8. Mesle, F., and J. Vallin. 'Historical Trends in Mortality.' In *International Handbook of Adult Mortality*, edited by R. G. Rogers and E. M. Crimmins. London: Springer, 2011.
9. Wood, Tony. 'Russia Vanishes.' *London Review of Books* (6 December 2012): 39–41.
10. Waigandt, A., and M. Reichle. 'The Potential Effects of Accident Prevention on Population Longevity.' *Journal of Safety Research* 19 (1988): 1–44.
11. Weale, M. 'Economic Progress and Health Improvement.' *British Medical Journal* 339 (2009): b4575.
12. Murphy, Kevin M., and Robert H. Topel. 'The Value of Health and Longevity.' *NBER Working Paper Series* (13 July 2005).
13. Durie, Mason. *Whaiora: Maori Health Development*. Auckland: Oxford University Press, 1994.
14. Thomson, A. S. *The Story of New Zealand: Past and Present – Savage and Civilized*, vol. 2. London: John Murray, 1859.
15. Wilmshurst, Janet M., Atholl J. Anderson, Thomas F. G. Higham, and Trevor H. Worthy. 'Dating the Late Prehistoric Dispersal of Polynesians to New Zealand Using the Commensal Pacific Rat.' *Proceedings of the National Academy of Sciences* 105, no. 22 (3 July 2008): 7676–80.
16. Crosby, A. W. *Ecological Imperialism: The Biological Expansion of Europe, 900–1900*. Cambridge: Cambridge University Press, 1986.
17. Li, Y., D. S. Carroll, et al. 'On the Origin of Smallpox: Correlating Variola Phylogenics with Historical Smallpox Records.' *Proceedings of the National Academy of Sciences* 104, no. 40 (2007): 15787–92.

18. United Nations Development Programme. 'Human Development Report 2013. The Rise of the South: Human Progress in a Diverse World.' New York: United Nations Development Programme, 2013.
19. Murray, C., and L. Chen. 'In Search of a Contemporary Theory for Understanding Mortality Change.' *Social Science & Medicine* 36, no. 2 (1993): 143–55.
20. Riley, James C. *Low Income, Social Growth, and Good Health: A History of Twelve Countries.* Berkeley: University of California Press, 2008.
21. Powles, J. 'Commentary: Mediterranean Paradoxes Continue to Provoke.' *International Journal of Epidemiology* 30, no. 5 (October 2001): 1076–7.
22. Hajat, A., T. Blakely, S. Dayal, and S. Jatrana. 'Do New Zealand's Immigrants Have a Mortality Advantage? Evidence from the New Zealand Census-Mortality Study.' *Ethnicity & Health* 15, no. 5 (2010): 531–47.
23. Horiuchi, S. 'Major Causes of the Rapid Longevity Extension in Postwar Japan.' *Japanese Journal of Population* 9, no. 1 (2011): 162–71.
24. Di Cesare, Mariachiara, Young-Ho Khang, Perviz Asaria, Tony Blakely, Melanie J. Cowan, Farshad Farzadfar, Ramiro Guerrero, et al. 'Inequalities in Non-Communicable Diseases and Effective Responses.' *The Lancet* 381, no. 9866 (2013): 585–97.
25. Evans, R. G. 'Thomas McKeown, Meet Fidel Castro: Physicians, Population Health and the Cuban Paradox.' *Healthcare Policy* 3, no. 4 (2008): 21–32.
26. Willcox, D. C., B. J. Willcox, S. Yasura, and I. Ashitomi. 'Gender Gap in Healthspan and Life Expectancy in Okinawa: Health Behaviours.' *Asian Journal of Gerontology & Geriatrics* 7, no. 1 (2012).
27. Cournil, A., and T. B. Kirkwood. 'If You Would Live Long, Choose Your Parents Well.' *Trends in Genetics* 17, no. 5 (May 2001): 233–5.
28. Christensen, K., and J. W. Vaupel. 'Genetic Factors and Adult Mortality.' In *International Handbook of Adult Mortality*, edited by E. G. Rogers and Eileen M. Crimmins. New York: Springer, 2011: 399–410.
29. Stearns, S. C., ed. *Evolution in Health and Disease.* Oxford: Oxford University Press, 1999.
30. Kluger, Jeffrey. 'How America's Children Packed on the Pounds.' *Time* (12 June 2008).
31. de Grey, Aubrey D. N. J. 'Escape Velocity: Why the Prospect of Extreme Human Life Extension Matters Now.' *PLoS Biology* 2, no. 6 (15 July 2004): e187.
32. Olshansky, S. Jay, Douglas J. Passaro, Ronald C. Hershow, Jennifer Layden, Bruce A. Carnes, Jacob Brody, Leonard Hayflick, et al. 'A Potential Decline in Life Expectancy in the United States in the 21st Century.' *New England Journal of Medicine* 352, no. 11 (2005): 1138–45.
33. Ho, J. Y. 'Mortality under Age 50 Accounts for Much of the Fact that US Life Expectancy Lags that of Other High-Income Countries.' *Health Affairs* 32, no. 3 (4 April 2013): 459–67.
34. Caldwell, John C. 'Health Transition: The Cultural, Social and Behavioural Determinants of Health in the Third World.' *Social Science & Medicine* 36, no. 2 (1993): 125–35.
35. White, K. M. 'Longevity Advances in High-Income Countries 1955–96.' *Population and Development Review* 28, no. 1 (2002): 59–76.

36. Dubos, R. *Mirage of Health: Utopias, Progress and Biological Change.* New York: Harper & Row, 1959.
37. Diamond, J. *Collapse: How Societies Choose to Fail or Succeed.* New York: Viking, 2005.
38. Cohen, M. N. *Health and the Rise of Civilization.* New Haven: Yale University Press, 1989.
39. Gurven, Michael, and Hillard Kaplan. 'Longevity among Hunter-Gatherers: A Cross-Cultural Examination.' *Population and Development Review* 33, no. 2 (July 2007): 321–65.
40. Howell, N. *Demography of the Dobe !Kung.* New York: Academic Press, 1979.
41. Hoppa, R. D. 'Paleodemography: Demographic Aspects.' In *International Encyclopedia of Social & Behavioral Sciences.* Elsevier, 2001: 11005–9.
42. McCaa, R. 'Paleodemography of the Americas: From Ancient Times to Colonialism and Beyond.' In *The Backbone of History: Health and Nutrition in the Western Hemisphere*, edited by R. H. Steckel and J. C. Rose. Cambridge: Cambridge University Press, 2002: 94–126.
43. McMichael, A. J. *Human Frontiers, Environments and Disease: Past Patterns, Uncertain Futures.* Cambridge: Cambridge University Press, 2001.
44. Howell, N. 'Towards a Uniformitarian Theory of Human Paleodemography.' *Journal of Human Evolution* 5 (1976): 25–40.
45. Callaway, E. 'Ancient Warfare: Fighting for the Common Good.' *New Scientist* (4 June 2009).
46. Pinker, Steven. *The Better Angels of Our Nature: The Decline of Violence in History and Its Causes.* London: Allen Lane, 2011.
47. Scott, J. C. 'Crops, Towns, Government.' *London Review of Books* (21 November 2013): 13–15.
48. McNeill, W. H. *Plagues and Peoples.* Harmondsworth: Penguin, 1976.
49. Eaton, S. B., and M. J. Konner. 'Paleolithic Nutrition: A Consideration of Its Nature and Current Implications.' *New England Journal of Medicine* 312 (1985): 283–9.
50. Sahlins, M. *Stone Age Economics.* Chicago & New York: Aldine Atherton, 1972.
51. Powles, J. 'Diseases of Civilisation: Thinking About the Health Costs and Benefits of Material Progress since the Enlightenment.' Unpublished booklet. Department of Social and Preventive Medicine, Monash Medical School, Prahran, 1985 (www.phpc.cam.ac.uk/dr-john-powles/publications-for-dr-john-powles).
52. Dobson, A. 'People and Disease.' In *The Cambridge Encyclopedia of Human Evolution*, edited by S. Jones, R. Martin and D. Pilbeam. Cambridge: Cambridge University Press, 1992: 411–20.
53. Frier, B. 'Roman Life Expectancy: Ulpian's Evidence.' *Harvard Studies in Classical Philology* 86 (1982): 213–51.
54. Pilkington, N. 'Growing up Roman: Infant Mortality and Reproductive Development.' *Journal of Interdisciplinary History* xliv, no. 1 (Summer 2013): 1–35.
55. Angel, J. L. 'Health as a Crucial Factor in the Changes from Hunting to Developed Farming in the Eastern Mediterranean.' In *Paleopathology at the Origins of Agriculture*, edited by M. N. Cohen and G. J. Armelagos. New York: Academic Press, 1984: 51–73.
56. Black, F. L. 'Infectious Diseases in Primitive Societies.' *Science* 187 (1975): 515–18.

57. Steckel, R. H., and J. C. Rose. 'Patterns of Health in the Western Hemisphere.' In *The Backbone of History: Health and Nutrition in the the Western Hemisphere*, edited by R. H. Steckel and J. C. Rose. Cambridge: Cambridge University Press, 2004: 563–82.
58. Weisenfeld, S. L. 'Sickle-Cell Trait in Human Biological and Cultural Evolution.' *Science* 157 (1967): 1134–40.
59. Comas, I., M. Coscolla, T. Luo, S. Borrell, K. E. Holt, M. Kato-Maeda, J. Parkhill, et al. 'Out-of-Africa Migration and Neolithic Coexpansion of *Mycobacterium tuberculosis* with Modern Humans.' *Nature Genetics* 45, no. 10 (2013): 1176–82.
60. Brosch, R., S. V. Gordon, M. Marmiesse, P. Brodin, C. Buchrieser, K. Eiglmeier, T. Garnier, et al. 'A New Evolutionary Scenario for the *Mycobacterium tuberculosis* Complex.' *Proceedings of the National Academy of Sciences* 99, no. 6 (2002): 3684–9.
61. Rüsch-Gerdes, S., C. Locht, S. Brisse, and A. Meyer. 'Origin, Spread and Demography of the *Mycobacterium tuberculosis* Complex.' *PLoS Pathogens* 4, no. 9 (2008).
62. Kirch, P. V. *The Lapita Peoples*. Oxford: Blackwell Scientific, 1997.
63. McGlone, M. S., J. M. Wilmshurst, and H. M. Leach. 'An Ecological and Historical Review of Bracken (*Pteridium esculentum*) in New Zealand, and Its Cultural Significance.' *New Zealand Journal of Ecology* 29, no. 2 (2005): 165–84.
64. Gray, R. D., A. J. Drummond, and S. J. Greenhill. 'Language Phylogenies Reveal Expansion Pulses and Pauses in Pacific Settlement.' *Science* 323 (2009): 479–83.
65. Kirch, P. V. *The Evolution of the Polynesian Chiefdoms*. Cambridge: Cambridge University Press, 1989.
66. Anderson, A., et al. 'Prehistoric Maritime Migration in the Pacific Islands: An Hypothesis of Enso Forcing.' *The Holocene* 16, no. 1 (2006): 1–6.
67. Wilmshurst, J. M., et al. 'High-Precision Radiocarbon Dating Shows Recent and Rapid Initial Human Colonization of East Polynesia.' *Proceedings of the National Academy of Sciences* 108, no. 5 (2011): 1815–20.
68. McGlone, M. S., A. J. Anderson, et al. 'An Ecological Approach to the Polynesian Settlement of New Zealand.' In *The Origins of the First New Zealanders*, edited by D. G. Sutton. Auckland: Auckland University Press, 1994: 136–63.
69. Howe, K. R. *The Quest for Origins: Who First Discovered and Settled New Zealand and the Pacific Islands?* Auckland: Penguin, 2003.
70. Beaglehole, J. C. *The Exploration of the Pacific*. London: Adam and Charles Black, 1966.
71. Salmond, Anne. *Two Worlds: First Meetings between Maori and Europeans 1642–1772*. Auckland: Viking, 1991.
72. Floud, R., K. Wachter, and A. Gregory. *Height, Health and History: Nutritional Status in the United Kingdom, 1750–1980*. Cambridge: Cambridge University Press, 1990.
73. Fortuine, R. 'The Health of the Eskimos as Portrayed in the Earliest Written Accounts.' *Bulletin of the History of Medicine* 45 (1971): 97–114.
74. McLauchlan, Gordon. *Great Tales from New Zealand History*. Auckland: Penguin, 2005.
75. Davidson, J. *The Prehistory of New Zealand*. Auckland: Longman Paul, 1984.
76. Matisoo-Smith, E. 'More Than Just Old Bones: On the Contribution of Biological Anthropology to New Zealand Archaeology.' In *Change through Time: 50 Years*

of New Zealand Archaeology, edited by L. Furey and S. Holdaway. Auckland: New Zealand Archaeological Assocation, 2004: 235–50.

77. Philipps, M. A. L. 'An Estimation of Fertility in Prehistoric New Zealanders.' *New Zealand Journal of Archaeology* 2 (1980): 149–67.
78. Belich, J. *Making Peoples*. Auckland: Allen Lane, Penguin, 1996.
79. Brewis, A., M. A. Molloy, and D. G. Sutton. 'Modeling the Prehistoric Maori Population.' *American Journal of Physical Anthropology* 81 (1990): 343–56.
80. Houghton, Philip. *The First New Zealanders*. Auckland: Hodder and Stoughton, 1980.
81. Buckley, Hallie R., Nancy Tayles, Siân E. Halcrow, Kasey Robb, and Roger Fyfe. 'The People of Wairau Bar: A Re-Examination.' *Journal of Pacific Archaeology* 1, no. 1 (2010): 1–20.
82. Brewis, A. 'Assessing Infant Mortality in Prehistoric New Zealand: A Life Table Approach.' *New Zealand Journal of Archaeology* 10 (1988): 73–82.
83. Murray-McIntosh, Rosalind P., Brian J. Scrimshaw, Peter J. Hatfield, and David Penny. 'Testing Migration Patterns and Estimating Founding Population Size in Polynesia by Using Human mtDNA Sequences.' *Proceedings of the National Academy of Sciences* 95, no. 15 (1998): 9047–52.
84. Matisoo-Smith, E., R. M. Roberts, et al. 'Patterns of Prehistoric Human Mobility in Polynesia Indicated by mtDNA from the Pacific Rat.' *Proceedings of the National Academy of Sciences* 95, no. 25 (1998): 45–15150.
85. Sutton, D. G. 'Maori Demographic Change, 1769–1840: The Inner Workings of "A Picturesque but Illogical Simile".' *Journal of the Polynesian Society* 95, no. 3 (1985): 291–339.
86. Lange, R. *May the People Live: A History of Maori Health Development 1900–1920*. Auckland: Auckland University Press, 1999.
87. Buck, P. *The Coming of the Maori*. Wellington: Maori Purposes Fund Board and Whitcombe and Tombs, 1949.
88. Gluckman, L. *Tangiwai: A Medical History of 19th Century New Zealand*. Christchurch: Whitcoulls, 1976.
89. Duncan, S. R., S. Scott, and C. J. Duncan. 'Smallpox Epidemics in Cities in Britain.' *Journal of Interdisciplinary History* 25, no. 2 (1994): 255–71.
90. Murton, B. 'Australia and New Zealand.' In *The Cambridge World History of Food*, edited by K. Kiple and K. Ornelas. Cambridge: Cambridge University Press, 2000: 1339–50.
91. James, H. F., T. W. Stafford, D. W. Steadman, S. L. Olson, P. S. Martin, A. J. T. Jull, and P. C. McCoy. 'Radiocarbon Dates on Bones of Extinct Birds from Hawaii.' *Proceedings of the National Academy of Sciences* 84 (1987): 2350–54.
92. Hughes, R. *The Fatal Shore: A History of the Transportation of Convicts to Australia 1787–1868*. London: Collins, 1987.
93. Berentson, Q. *Moa: The Life and Death of New Zealand's Legendary Bird*. Nelson: Craig Potton Publishing, 2012.
94. Holdaway, R. N., and C. Jacomb. 'Rapid Extinction of the Moas (Aves: Dinornithiformes): Model, Test, and Implications.' *Science* 287, no. 5461 (24 April 2000): 2250–54.
95. Walker, R. *Ka Whawhai Tonu Matou: Struggle without End*. Auckland: Penguin, 2004.

96. Wright-St Clair, R. E. 'Early Accounts of Maori Diet and Health, 2.' *New Zealand Medical Journal* 70, no. 451 (December 1969): 415–9.
97. Steckel, Richard H. 'Biological Measures of the Standard of Living.' *Journal of Economic Perspectives* 22, no. 1 (Winter 2008): 129–52.
98. Beaglehole, J. C., ed. *The Journals of Captain James Cook on His Voyages of Discovery: The Voyage of the Endeavour 1768–1771.* Cambridge: Cambridge University Press, 1955.
99. Floud, R., Robert W. Fogel, Bernard Harris, and Sok Chul Hong. *The Changing Body: Health, Nutrition, and Human Development in the Western World since 1700.* Cambridge: Cambridge University Press, 2011.
100. Belgrave, Michael. 'Arthur Saunders Thomson.' *Te Ara – The Encyclopedia of New Zealand* (www.TeAra.govt.nz/en/biographies/1t95/thomson-arthur-saunders).
101. Thomson, A. S. 'Observations on the Stature, Bodily Weight, Magnitude of Chest, and Physical Strength of the New Zealand Race of Men.' *Journal of the Royal Geographical Society* XXIII (1851): 87–93.
102. Houghton, Philip. 'Selective Influences and Morphological Variation Amongst Pacific *Homo Sapiens*.' *Journal of Human Evolution* 21, no. 1 (1991): 49–59.
103. Houghton, Philip. *People of the Great Ocean: Aspects of the Human Biology of the Early Pacific.* Cambridge, 1996.
104. Chapple, S. 'Sex Inequality in the Maori Population in the Prehistoric, Proto-Historic and Early Historic Eras in a Trans-Polynesian Context.' *Journal of Pacific History* 40, no. 1 (2005): 1–21.
105. Pool, I. *The Seeds of Rangiatea: Contact, Colonisation and Maori Development, New Zealand 1769–circa 1900.* Under review.
106. Wrigley, E. A., and R. S. Schofield. *The Population History of England, 1541–1871.* London: Arnold, 1981.
107. Fogel, Robert W. 'Economic Growth, Population Theory, and Physiology: The Bearing of Long-Term Processes on the Making of Economic Policy.' *The American Economic Review* 84, no. 3 (1994): 369–89.
108. Perrenoud, A. 'The Attenuation of Mortality Crises and the Decline of Mortality.' In *The Decline of Mortality in Europe*, edited by R. S. Schofield, D. Reher and A. Bideau. Oxford: Clarendon Press, 1991: 18–37.
109. Zhang, David D., Harry F. Lee, Cong Wang, Baosheng Li, Qing Pei, Jane Zhang, and Yulun An. 'The Causality Analysis of Climate Change and Large-Scale Human Crisis.' *Proceedings of the National Academy of Sciences* 108, no. 42 (18 October 2011): 17296–301.
110. Lancaster, H. O. *Expectations of Life: A Study in the Demography, Statistics and History of World Mortality.* New York: Springer-Verlag, 1990.
111. Peller, S. 'Studies on Mortality since the Renaissance. E. Men's Reproductive Activity; F. Men's Mortality.' *Bulletin of the History of Medicine* 21 (1947): 51–101.
112. Schofield, R., D. Reher, and A. Bideau, eds. *The Decline of Mortality in Europe.* Oxford, UK: Oxford University Press, 1991.
113. Fogel, Robert W. *The Escape from Hunger and Premature Death, 1700–2100: Europe, America and the Third World.* Cambridge: Cambridge University Press, 2004.
114. Riley, James C. *Rising Life Expectancy: A Global History*. Cambridge: Cambridge University Press, 2001.

115. Rogers, E. G., and Eileen M. Crimmins, eds. *International Handbook of Adult Mortality*. New York: Springer, 2011.
116. Galloway, P. R. 'Basic Patterns in Annual Variations in Fertility, Nuptiality, Mortality, and Prices in Pre-Industrial Europe'. *Population Studies* 42, no. 2 (1988): 275–303.
117. Riley, J. C. *The Eighteenth-Century Campaign to Avoid Disease*. London: Macmillan, 1987.
118. Bruce-Chwatt, L., and J. de Zulueta. *The Rise and Fall of Malaria in Europe*. Oxford: Oxford University Press, 1980.
119. Riley, James C. 'Insects and the European Mortality Decline.' *American Historical Review* 91 (1986): 833–58.
120. Hill, Christopher. *The Pelican Economic History of Britain Volume 2: Reformation to Industrial Revolution*. Harmondsworth: Penguin, 1969.
121. Civil Aviation Authority of New Zealand. 'CAA to Recommend Standard Passenger Weight Increase.' Media release, 5 December 2003.
122. Ministry of Health. *The Health of New Zealand Adults 2011/12: Key Findings of the New Zealand Health Survey*. Wellington: Ministry of Health, 2012.
123. Komlos, J. 'Shrinking in a Growing Economy? The Mystery of Physical Stature During the Industrial Revolution.' *Journal of Economic History* 58, no. 3 (1998): 779–802.
124. Galloway, P. R. 'Long-Term Fluctuations in Climate and Population in the Preindustrial Era.' *Population and Development Review* 12, no. 1 (1986): 1–24.
125. Mercer, A. J. 'Smallpox and Epidemiological Demographic Change in Europe: The Role of Vaccination.' *Population Studies* 39, no. 2 (1985): 287–307.
126. Pool, D. I. *Te Iwi Maori: A New Zealand Population, Past, Present and Projected*. Auckland: Auckland University Press, 1991.
127. Vallin, P. 'Mortality in Europe 1720–1914.' In *The Decline of Mortality in Europe*, edited by R. S. Schofield, D. Reher and A. Bideau. Oxford: Clarendon Press, 1991: 38–67.
128. Orange, C. 'The Maori People and the British Crown (1769–1840).' In *The Oxford Illustrated History of New Zealand*, edited by K. Sinclair. Auckland: Oxford University Press, 1990: 21–48.
129. Shawcross, W. 'Ethnographic Economics and the Study of Population in Prehistoric New Zealand: Viewed through Archaeology.' *Mankind* 7, no. 4 (1970): 279–91.
130. Bannister, S. 'An Account of the Changes and Present Condition of the Population of New Zealand.' *Journal of the Statistical Society (London)* 1 (1838): 362–76.
131. Pool, D. I. *The Maori Population of New Zealand 1769–1971*. Auckland: Auckland University Press, 1977.
132. Wright, M. *Guns and Utu: A Short History of the Musket Wars*. Auckland: Penguin Books, 2011.
133. McLean, G. 'When Worlds Collide.' In *Frontiers of Dreams: The Story of New Zealand*, edited by B. Dalley and G. McLean. Auckland: Hodder Moa, 2005: 62–91.
134. Salmond, Anne. *Between Worlds: Early Exchanges between Maori and Europeans 1773–1815*. Auckland: Viking, 1997.
135. Walsh, Archdeacon. 'The Passing of the Maori: An Inquiry into the Principal Causes of the Decay of the Race.' *Transactions and Proceedings of the New Zealand Institute*, no. 40 (1907): art. XIII, 154–76.

136. King, Michael. *Moriori: A People Rediscovered*, revised edition. Auckland: Viking, 2000.
137. Dow, Derek A. *Safeguarding the Public Health: A History of the New Zealand Department of Health*. Wellington: Victoria University Press, 1995.
138. Aaby, Peter. 'Lessons for the Past: Third World Evidence and the Reinterpretation of Developed World Mortality Declines.' *Health Transition Review* 2, supplement (7 July 1992): 155–83.
139. Aaby, Peter. 'Patterns of Exposure and Severity of Measles Infection Copenhagen 1915–1925.' *Annals of Epidemiology* 2, no. 3 (June 1992): 257–62.
140. Gould, S. J. *The Mismeasure of Man*. New York: W. W. Norton & Company, 1981.
141. Garenne, M., and P. Aaby. 'Pattern of Exposure and Measles Mortality in Senegal.' *The Journal of Infectious Diseases* 161, no. 6 (July 1990): 1088–94.
142. Black, F. L. 'Why Did They Die?' *Science* 258 (11 December 1992): 1739–40.
143. Knapp, Michael, K. Ann Horsburgh, Stefan Prost, Jo-Ann Stanton, Hallie R. Buckley, Richard K. Walter, and Elizabeth A. Matisoo-Smith. 'Complete Mitochondrial DNA Genome Sequences from the First New Zealanders.' *Proceedings of the National Academy of Sciences* 109, no. 45 (25 October 2012): 18350–4.
144. Mamelund, S. E. 'Geography May Explain Adult Mortality from the 1918–20 Influenza Pandemic.' *Epidemics* 3 (2011): 46–60.
145. Burström, B., F. Diderichsen, and L. Smedman. 'Child Mortality in Stockholm During 1885–1910: The Impact of Household Size and Number of Children in the Family on the Risk of Death from Measles.' *American Journal of Epidemiology* 149, no. 12 (15 July 1999): 1134–41.
146. Owens, J. 'Missionary Medicine and Maori Health: The Record of the Wesleyan Mission to New Zealand before 1840.' *Journal of the Polynesian Society* 81, no. 4 (1972): 418–36.
147. Wood, P. *Dirt: Filth and Decay in a New World Arcadia*. Auckland: Auckland University Press, 2005.
148. Fenton, Francis D. *Observations on the State of the Aboriginal Inhabitants of New Zealand*. Auckland: Government Print, 1859.
149. Phillips, J., and T. Hearn. *Settlers: New Zealand Immigrants from England, Ireland and Scotland 1800–1945*. Auckland: Auckland University Press, 2008.
150. Orange, C. *The Treaty of Waitangi*. Wellington: Allen & Unwin, 1987.
151. Salesa, T. D. 'The Power of the Physician: Doctors and the "Dying Maori" in Early Colonial New Zealand.' *Health and History* 3, no. 1 (2001): 13–40.
152. Andrews, J. *No Other Home Than This: A History of European New Zealanders*. Nelson: Craig Potton Publishing, 2009.
153. King, Michael. *The Penguin History of New Zealand*. Auckland: Penguin Books, 2003.
154. Dow, Derek A. *Maori Health and Government Policy 1840–1940*. Wellington: Victoria University Press, 1999.
155. Moon, P. *The Edges of Empires: New Zealand in the Middle of the Nineteenth Century*. Auckland: David Ling Publishing, 2009.
156. Wohlers, J. F. K. 'On the Conversion and Civilization of the Maoris in the South of New Zealand.' *Transactions and Proceedings of the New Zealand Institute*, no. XIV (1881).

157. Belich, J. 'The Governors and the Maori (1840–1872).' In *The Oxford Illustrated History of New Zealand*, edited by K. Sinclair. Auckland: Oxford University Press, 1990: 75–98.
158. Ashby, W. *New Zealand, the Land of Health, Wealth and Prosperity*. London: 1889.
159. Oeppen, J., and J. Vaupel. 'Broken Limits to Life Expectancy.' *Science* 296 (2002): 1029–31.
160. Christensen, Kaare, Gabriele Doblhammer, Roland Rau, and James W. Vaupel. 'Ageing Populations: The Challenges Ahead.' *The Lancet* 374, no. 9696 (3 October 2009): 1196–208.
161. Newman, A. K. 'Is New Zealand a Healthy Country?' *Proceedings of the Royal Society of New Zealand* 15 (1882): 493–510.
162. Pool, I. 'Mortality Trends and Differentials.' *Country Monograph Series No. 12: Population of New Zealand*, edited by Population Division Economic and Social Commission for Asia and the Pacific. New York: United Nations, 1985: 209–42.
163. Pool, D. I. 'Is New Zealand a Healthy Country?' *New Zealand Population Review* 8, no. 2 (1982): 2–27.
164. Human Mortality Database (www.mortality.org).
165. Lessof, Elizabeth. 'Mortality in New Zealand and England and Wales.' *Population Studies* 3, no. 1 (1949): 76–99.
166. New Zealand Government. *Statistics of New Zealand for the Year 1857*. Auckland: WC Wilson, 1858.
167. New Zealand Government. *Statistics of the Colony of New Zealand for the Year 1881*. Wellington: Government Printer, 1882.
168. Statistics New Zealand. 'A History of Survival in New Zealand: Cohort Life Tables 1876–2004.' Wellington: Statistics New Zealand, 2006.
169. Pool, I., and J. Cheung. 'Why Were New Zealand Levels of Life Expectation So High at the Dawn of the Twentieth Century?' *Genus* 61, no. 2 (2005): 9–33.
170. Gibson, C. *Demographic History of New Zealand*. University of California at Berkeley, PhD thesis, 1972.
171. Razum, O., H. Zeeb, and S. Rohrmann. 'The "Healthy Migrant Effect" – Not Merely a Fallacy of Inaccurate Denominator Figures.' *International Journal of Epidemiology* 29, no. 1 (February 2000): 191–2.
172. Gadd, M., S. E. Johansson, J. Sundquist, and P. Wandell. 'Morbidity in Cardiovascular Diseases in Immigrants in Sweden.' *Journal of Internal Medicine* 254, no. 3 (2003): 236–43.
173. Albin, B., K. Hjelm, J. Ekberg, and S. Elmstahl. 'Mortality among 723,948 Foreign- and Native-Born Swedes 1970–1999.' *European Journal of Public Health* 15, no. 5 (2005): 511–17.
174. Harding, S., M. Rosato, and A. Teyhan. 'Trends for Coronary Heart Disease and Stroke Mortality among Migrants in England and Wales, 1979–2003: Slow Declines Notable for Some Groups.' *Heart* 94, no. 4 (2008): 463–70.
175. Rubalcava, Luis N., Graciela M. Teruel, Duncan Thomas, and Noreen Goldman. 'The Healthy Migrant Effect: New Findings from the Mexican Family Life Survey.' *American Journal of Public Health* 98, no. 1 (January 2008): 78–84.
176. Bryder, L. '"A Health Resort for Consumptives": Tuberculosis and Immigration to New Zealand, 1880–1914.' *Medical History* 40, no. 4 (1996): 453–71.

177. Robb, D. *Medical Odyssey*. Auckland: Collins, 1967.
178. Borrie, W. D. 'Immigration to New Zealand, 1854–1938.' Australian National University, 1991.
179. Belich, J. *Replenishing the Earth: The Settler Revolution and the Rise of the Anglo-World, 1783–1939*. Oxford: Oxford University Press, 2009.
180. Abraido-Lanza, A. F., B. P. Dohrenwend, D. S. Ng-Mak, and J. B. Turner. 'The Latino Mortality Paradox: A Test of the "Salmon Bias" and Healthy Migrant Hypotheses.' *American Journal of Public Health* 89, no. 10 (1999): 1543–48.
181. Government Statistician of Victoria. *Victorian Year-Book 1903*. The Government of Victoria, 1904.
182. McClean, Rosalind. '"How We Prepare Them in India": British Diasporic Imaginings and Migration to New Zealand'. *New Zealand Journal of History* 37, no. 2 (2003): 1–18.
183. Catton, E. *The Luminaries*. Wellington: Victoria University Press, 2013.
184. Strong, K., P. Trickett, and K. Bhatia. 'The Health of Overseas-Born Australians, 1994–1996.' *Australian Health Review* 21, no. 2 (1998): 124–33.
185. Bade, J. H. 'Germans.' In *Settler and Migrant Peoples of New Zealand*, edited by L. J. Phillips. Auckland: David Bateman, 2006.
186. Phillips, J. 'History of immigration.' *Te Ara – The Encyclopedia of New Zealand*, retrieved 3 July 2009 (www.TeAra.govt.nz/NewZealanders/NewZealandPeoples/HistoryOfImmigration/en).
187. Arnold, Rollo. 'Clayden, Arthur 1829–1899.' *Te Ara – The Encyclopedia of New Zealand*, retrieved 2007 (www.TeAra.govt.nz/en/biographies/2c19/clayden-arthur).
188. Friedlander, D., Jona Schellekens, E. Ben-Moshe, and Ariela Keysar. 'Socio-Economic Characteristics and Life Expectancies in Nineteenth-Century England: A District Analysis.' *Population Studies* 39, no. 1 (1985): 137–51.
189. Peacocke, Kathryn. 'Ranstead, William 1859–1944.' *Te Ara – The Encyclopedia of New Zealand* (www.TeAra.govt.nz/en/biographies/3r3/ranstead-william).
190. Taylor, R., M. Lewis, and J. Powles. 'The Australian Mortality Decline: All-Cause Mortality 1788–1990.' *Australian & New Zealand Journal of Public Health* 22, no. 1 (February 1998): 27–36.
191. Coghlan, T. A. *A Statistical Account of the Seven Colonies of Australasia, 1895–6*. Sydney: Government Printer, 1896.
192. Curtin, P. D. *Death by Migration: Europe's Encounter with the Tropical World in the Nineteenth Century*. Cambridge: Cambridge University Press, 1989.
193. Pickens, K. A. 'The Origins of the Population of Nineteenth Century Canterbury.' *New Zealand Geographer* 33 (1977): 69–75.
194. Barker, D. 'The Origins of the Developmental Origins Theory.' *Journal of Internal Medicine* 261 (2007): 412–17.
195. Preston, S. H., and M. R. Haines. *Fatal Years: Child Mortality in Late Nineteenth-century America*. Princeton: Princeton University Press, 1991.
196. Sceats, J. E. 'Family Formation in New Zealand: An Analysis of the Timing and Spacing of Pregnancies.' *New Zealand Population Review* 7, no. 3 (1981): 29–47.
197. Jones, E. F. 'Fertility Decline in Australia and New Zealand 1861–1936.' *Population Index* 37, no. 4 (1971): 301–338.

198. Pool, D. I. 'Changing Patterns of Sex Differentials in Survival: An Examination of Data for Maoris and Non-Maoris in New Zealand.' In *Sex Differentials in Mortality: Trends, Determinants and Consequences*, edited by A. D. Lopez and L. T. Ruzicka. Canberra: Department of Demography, Australian National University. Miscellaneous Series No. 4 (1983): 193–219.
199. Neels, K., Z. Theunynck, et al. 'Economic Recession and First Births in Europe: Recession-Induced Postponement and Recuperation of Fertility in 14 European Countries between 1970 and 2005.' *International Journal of Public Health* 58 (2013): 43–55.
200. Dalziel, R. '120 Years of Women's Suffrage.' *UniNews: The University of Auckland News for Staff* 43, no. 16 (2013).
201. Reves, R. 'Declining Fertility in England and Wales as a Major Cause of the Twentieth Century Decline in Mortality: The Role of Changing Family Size and Age Structure in Infectious Disease Mortality in Infancy.' *American Journal of Epidemiology* 122 (1985): 112–126.
202. Rutstein, S. O. 'Effects of Preceding Birth Intervals on Neonatal, Infant and Under-Five Years Mortality and Nutritional Status in Developing Countries: Evidence from the Demographic and Health Surveys.' *International Journal of Gynaecology and Obstetrics* 89 (suppl. 1) (2005): S7–S24.
203. Diamond, J. *Guns, Germs and Steel: The Fates of Human Societies*. New York: W. W. Norton, 1999.
204. Lewis, M. W. 'Environmental Determinism, Ellsworth Huntington and the Decline of Geography.' *Geocurrents* (2011): 1–2.
205. Burnett, J. 'Housing and the Decline in Mortality.' In *The Decline of Mortality in Europe*, edited by R. S. Schofield, D. Reher and A. Bideau. Oxford: Clarendon Press, 1991: 158–76.
206. Preston, S. H., and E. v. d. Walle. 'Urban French Mortality in the Nineteenth Century.' *Population Studies* 32, no. 2 (1978): 275–297.
207. Chadwick, E. *Report on the Sanitary Condition of the Labouring Population of Great Britain*. London: Her Majesty's Stationery Office, 1842; reprinted by Edinburgh University Press, 1965.
208. Rice, G. W. 'Public Health in Christchurch, 1875–1910: Mortality and Sanitation.' In *A Healthy Country: Essays on the Social History of Medicine in New Zealand*, edited by L. Bryder. Wellington: Bridget Williams Books, 1991: 85–108.
209. Clark, G., M. Huberman, et al. 'A British Food Puzzle, 1770–1850.' *Economic History Review* 48, no. 2 (1995): 215–37.
210. McMichael, A. J., J. W. Powles, et al. 'Food, Livestock Production, Energy, Climate Change, and Health.' *The Lancet* (2007).
211. Burton, D. *Two Hundred Years of New Zealand Food and Cookery*. Wellington: A. H. & A. W. Reed, 1982.
212. Goodyear, R. K. *'Sunshine and Fresh Air': An Oral History of Childhood and Family Life in Interwar New Zealand, with Some Comparisons to Interwar Britain*. Victoria University of Wellington, PhD thesis, 1998.
213. Inwood, K., L. Oxley, et al. 'Physical Stature in Nineteenth-Century New Zealand: A Preliminary Interpretation.' *Australian Economic History Review* 50, no. 3 (2010): 262–83.

214. New Zealand Division of Public Health Family Health Branch. *Physical Development of New Zealand School Children 1969*. Wellington: Department of Health, 1971.
215. Inwood, K., L. Oxley, et al. 'Physical Stature in Nineteenth-Century New Zealand: A Preliminary Interpretation.' *Australian Economic History Review* 50, no. 3 (2010): 262–83.
216. Simon Denny, personal communication, 20 June 2013.
217. Ferriman, A. 'BMJ Readers Choose the "Sanitary Revolution" as Greatest Medical Advance since 1840.' *British Medical Journal* 334, no. 7585 (2007): 111-a.
218. Condran, G., and E. Crimmins-Gardner. 'Public Health Measures and Mortality in U.S. Cities in the Late Nineteenth Century.' *Human Ecology* 6, no. 1 (1978): 27–54.
219. van Poppel, F., and C. van der Heijden. 'The Effects of Water Supply on Infant and Childhood Mortality: A Review of Historical Evidence.' *Health Transition Review* 7 (1997): 113–48.
220. Aiello, A. E., E. L. Larson, et al. 'Hidden Heroes of the Health Revolution. Sanitation and Personal Hygiene.' *American Journal of Infection Control* 36, no. 10 (suppl.) (2008): S128–51.
221. Mein Smith, P., and L. Frost. 'Suburbia and Infant Death in Later Nineteenth- and Early Twentieth-century Adelaide.' *Urban History* 21 (1994): 251–72.
222. Cohn, R. L. 'The Determinants of Individual Immigrant Mortality on Sailing Ships, 1836–1853.' *Explorations in Economic History* 24, no. 4 (1987): 371–91.
223. Haines, R., and R. Shlomowitz. 'Explaining the Modern Mortality Decline: What Can We Learn from Sea Voyages?' *Social History of Medicine* 11, no. 1 (1998): 15–48.
224. Szreter, S. 'The Importance of Social Intervention in Britain's Mortality Decline c. 1850–1914: A Re-Interpretation of the Role of Public Health.' *Social History of Medicine* 1, no. 1 (1988): 1–37.
225. Sherman, I. W. *The Power of Plagues*. Washington, DC: ASM Press, 2006.
226. Bryder, L. 'New Zealand's Infant Welfare Services and Maori, 1907–1960.' *Health & History* 3, no. 1 (2001): 65–86.
227. Bryder, L. *The Plunket Nurses as a New Zealand Icon*. UK Centre for the History of Nursing and Midwifery, 2002.
228. Bryder, L. '"Babies of the Empire": The Evolution of Infant Welfare Services in New Zealand and Britain in the First Half of the Twentieth Century.' In *The Practice of Reform in Health, Medicine and Science, 1500–2000*, edited by M. Pelling and S. Mandelbrote. Aldershot: Ashgate, 2005: 247–262.
229. Chapman, L. *In a Strange Garden: The Life and Times of Truby King*. Auckland: Penguin Books, 2003.
230. Mein Smith, P. 'Infant Welfare Services and Infant Mortality: A Historian's View.' *Australian Economic Review* 93 (1991): 21–34.
231. Beaver, M. W. 'Infant Mortality and Milk.' *Population Studies* 27, no. 2 (1973): 243–54.
232. McCalman, J., R. Morley, et al. 'A Health Transition: Birth Weights, Households and Survival in an Australian Working-class Population Sample Born 1857–1900.' *Social Science & Medicine* 66, no. 5 (2008): 1070–83.
233. Davies, P. D. O., and J. M. Grange. 'Factors Affecting Susceptibility and Resistance to Tuberculosis.' *Thorax* 56, suppl. II (2001): ii23–ii29.

234. Nnoaham, K. E., and A. Clarke. 'Low Serum Vitamin D Levels and Tuberculosis: A Systematic Review and Meta-analysis.' *International Journal of Epidemiology* 37, no. 1 (February 2008): 113–9.
235. Martineau, A. R., S. Nhamoyebonde, et al. 'Reciprocal Seasonal Variation in Vitamin D Status and Tuberculosis Notifications in Cape Town, South Africa.' *Proceedings of the National Academy of Sciences* 108, no. 47 (2011): 19013–17.
236. Martineau, A. R., F. U. Honecker, et al. 'Vitamin D in the Treatment of Pulmonary Tuberculosis.' *The Journal of Steroid Biochemistry and Molecular Biology* 103, no. 3–5 (2007): 793–8.
237. Seckmeyer, G., M. Glandorf, et al. 'Europe's Darker Atmosphere in the UV-B.' *Photochemical & Photobiological Sciences* 7, no. 8 (2008): 925.
238. Sjögren, I., and I. Sutherland. 'Studies of Tuberculosis in Relation to Infection in Cattle.' *Tubercle* 56, no. 2 (1975): 113–27.
239. de Lisle, G. W. 'Bovine Tuberculosis: The New Zealand Problem.' *Proceedings of the New Zealand Grassland Association* 55 (1993): 199–202.
240. Brenner, M. H. 'Commentary: Economic Growth is the Basis of Mortality Rate Decline in the 20th Century – Experience of the United States 1901–2000.' *International Journal of Epidemiology* 34, no. 6 (2005): 1214–21.
241. Greasley, D., and L. Oxley. 'The Pastoral Boom, the Rural Land Market and Long Swings in New Zealand Economic Growth, 1873–1939.' *Economic History Review* 62, no. 2 (2009): 324–49.
242. Whitwell, G., C. de Souza, and S. Nicholas. 'Height, Health and Economic Growth in Australia, 1860–1940.' In *Health and Welfare During Industrialization*, edited by R. H. Steckel and R. Flound. Chicago and London, 1997: 379–423.
243. Wilkinson, R., and K. Pickett. *The Spirit Level: Why Equality Is Better for Everyone*, second edition. Penguin Books, 2010.
244. Lynch, J., G. Davey Smith, S. Harper, M. Hillemeier, N. Ross, G. A. Kaplan, and M. Wolfson. 'Is Income Inequality a Determinant of Population Health? Part 1. A Systematic Review.' *Milbank Q* 82, no. 1 (2004): 5–99.
245. Sinclair, K., with additional material by R. Dalziel. *A History of New Zealand* revised edition. Auckland: Penguin Group, 2000.
246. Hamer, D. W. 'The Making of Urban New Zealand.' *Journal of Urban History* 22, no. 1 (1995): 6–39.
247. Hamer, D. A., ed. *The Webbs in New Zealand 1898*. Wellington: 1974.
248. Olssen, E., C. Griffen, and F. Jones. *An Accidental Utopia? Social Mobility and the Foundations of an Egalitarian Society, 1880–1940*. Dunedin: Otago University Press, 2011.
249. McKeown, T. *The Modern Rise of Population*. New York: Academic Press, 1976.
250. Preston, S. 'The Changing Relation between Mortality and Level of Economic Development.' *Population Studies* 29, no. 2 (1975): 231–48.
251. Omran, A. R. 'The Epidemiological Transition: A Theory of the Epidemiology of Population Change.' *The Milbank Memorial Fund Quarterly* 49, no. 4 (1971): 509–38.
252. Newman, A. K. 'A Study of the Causes Leading to the Extinction of the Maori.' *Transactions and Proceedings of the New Zealand Institute*, no. LXXV (1881).
253. Binney, Judith. *Stories without End: Essays 1975–2010*. Wellington: Bridget Williams Books, 2010.

254. Pope, J. H. *Health for the Maori: A Manual for Use in Native Schools*. Wellington: 1884.
255. Pool, I., and K. C. Chan. 'Differential Declines in Tuberculosis Mortality.' Paper presented at the Proceedings, General Conference, International Union for the Scientific Study of Population, London, 1969.
256. Belich, J. *Paradise Reforged: A History of the New Zealanders from the 1880s to the Year 2000*. Auckland: Penguin Press, 2001.
257. Sorrenson, M. P. K. 'Land Purchase Methods and Their Effect of Maori Population, 1865–1901.' *Journal of the Polynesian Society* 65, no. 3 (1956): 183–99.
258. Kunitz, S. J. *Disease and Social Diversity: The European Impact on the Health of Non-Europeans*. New York: Oxford University Press, 1994.
259. Maclean, F. S. *Challenge for Health: A History of Public Health in New Zealand*. Wellington: Government Printer, 1964.
260. Rice, G. W. 'Maori Mortality in the 1918 Influenza Pandemic.' *New Zealand Population Review* 9 (1983): 44–61.
261. Rice, G. *Black November: The 1918 Influenza Pandemic in New Zealand*. Wellington: Allen & Unwin, 1988.
262. Wilson, N., L. T. Barnard, et al. 'Differential Mortality Rates by Ethnicity in 3 Influenza Pandemics Over a Century, New Zealand.' *Emerging Infectious Diseases* 18, no. 1 (2012): 71–7.
263. Bryder, L. '"If Preventable, Why Not Prevented?": New Zealand Response to Tuberculosis, 1901–1940.' In *A Healthy Country: Essays on the Social History of Medicine in New Zealand*, edited by L. Bryder. Wellington: Bridget Williams Books, 1991: 109–27.
264. Turbott, H. B. *Tuberculosis in the Maori, East Coast, New Zealand*. Wellington: Government Printer, 1935.
265. O'Malley, Vincent. *The Meeting Place: Māori and Pākehā Encounters, 1642–1840*. Auckland: Auckland University Press, 2013.
266. Tahu Kukutai, personal communication, November 2013.
267. Durie, Mason. *Mauri Ora: The Dynamics of Maori Health*. Auckland: Oxford University Press, 2001.
268. Pool, D. I. 'Post-War Trends in Maori Population Growth.' *Population Studies* 21, no. 2 (1967): 87–98.
269. Morikawa, J. *Whaling in Japan: Power, Politics and Diplomacy*. Columbia University Press, 2009.
270. Ikeda, Nayu, Eiko Saito, Naoki Kondo, Manami Inoue, Shunya Ikeda, Toshihiko Satoh, Koji Wada, et al. 'What Has Made the Population of Japan Healthy?' *The Lancet* 378, no. 9796 (2011): 1094–105.
271. Tobias, M., K. Sexton, S. Mann, and N. Sharpe. 'How Low Can It Go? Projecting Ischaemic Heart Disease Mortality in New Zealand to 2015.' *New Zealand Medical Journal* 119, no. 1232 (2006): U1932.
272. Lancaster, H. O., and J. W. Donovan. 'A Study in New Zealand Mortality. 1. Population Data.' *New Zealand Medical Journal* 65, no. 412 (December 1966): 946–53.
273. Lancaster, H. O., and J. W. Donovan. 'A Study in New Zealand Mortality. 2. Mortality Data.' *New Zealand Medical Journal* 66, no. 424 (November 1967): 769–77.

274. Donovan, J. W. 'A Study in New Zealand Mortality. 5. Tuberculosis.' *New Zealand Medical Journal* 70, no. 447 (August 1969): 94–103.
275. Beaglehole, R., D. R. Hay, F. H. Foster, and D. N. Sharpe. 'Trends in Coronary Heart Disease Mortality and Associated Risk Factors in New Zealand.' *New Zealand Medical Journal* 93, no. 685 (10 June 1981): 371–5.
276. Beaglehole, R. 'Coronary Heart Disease in New Zealand Maoris: An Epidemiological Study.' University of Otago, Doctor of Medicine thesis, 1977.
277. Jackson, R. T., and R. Beaglehole. 'Trends in Dietary Fat and Cigarette Smoking and the Decline in Coronary Heart Disease in New Zealand.' *International Journal of Epidemiology* 16, no. 3 (1 September 1987): 377–82.
278. Tobias, Martin, Richard Taylor, Li-Chia Yeh, Ken Huang, Stewart Mann, and Norman Sharpe. 'Did It Fall or Was It Pushed? The Contribution of Trends in Established Risk Factors to the Decline in Premature Coronary Heart Disease Mortality in New Zealand.' *Australian & New Zealand Journal of Public Health* 32, no. 2 (April 2008): 117–25.
279. Capewell, S., R. Beaglehole, M. Seddon, and J. McMurray. 'Explanation for the Decline in Coronary Heart Disease Mortality Rates in Auckland, New Zealand, between 1982 and 1993.' *Circulation* 102, no. 13 (2000): 1511–6.
280. Bonita, R., and R. Beaglehole. 'Trends in Cerebrovascular Disease Mortality in New Zealand.' *New Zealand Medical Journal* 95, no. 710 (23 June 1982): 411–4.
281. Metcalf, Patricia, Robert K. Scragg, David Schaaf, Lorna Dyall, Peter Black, and Rod Jackson. 'Trends in Major Cardiovascular Risk Factors in Auckland, New Zealand: 1982 to 2002–2003.' *New Zealand Medical Journal* 119, no. 1245 (2006): U2308.
282. Prior, I. A. 'Cardiovascular Epidemiology in New Zealand and the Pacific.' *New Zealand Medical Journal* 80, no. 524 (25 September 1974): 245–52.
283. Prior, I. A. M., A. Hooper, J. Huntsman, J. M. Stanhope, and C. Salmond. 'The Tokelau Island Migrant Study.' *Population Structure and Human Variation* 2 (1977): 165–86.
284. Patrick, R. C., I. A. Prior, J. C. Smith, and A. H. Smith. 'Relationship between Blood Pressure and Modernity among Ponapeans.' *International Journal of Epidemiology* 12, no. 1 (March 1983): 36–44.
285. Salmond, C. E., J. G. Joseph, I. A. Prior, D. G. Stanley, and A. F. Wessen. 'Longitudinal Analysis of the Relationship between Blood Pressure and Migration: The Tokelau Island Migrant Study.' *American Journal of Epidemiology* 122, no. 2 (August 1985): 291–301.
286. Salmond, C. E., I. A. Prior, and A. F. Wessen. 'Blood Pressure Patterns and Migration: A 14-Year Cohort Study of Adult Tokelauans.' *American Journal of Epidemiology* 130, no. 1 (July 1989): 37–52.
287. Wessen, A. F., A. Hooper, J. Huntsman, I. A. M. Prior, and C. E. Salmond. *Migration and Health in a Small Society*. Oxford: Clarendon Press, 1992.
288. Beaglehole, R., R. Bonita, and A. Stewart. 'Cardiovascular Disease Mortality Trends in the Western Pacific, 1968–1984.' *New Zealand Medical Journal* 101, no. 849 (13 July 1988): 441–3.
289. O'Donoghue, B., P. Howden-Chapman, and A. Woodward. 'Why Do Australians Live Longer Than New Zealanders?' *Health Education & Behavior* 27, no. 3 (1 July 2000): 307–16.

290. Woodward, A., C. Mathers, and M. Tobias. 'Migrants, Money and Margarine: Possible Explanations for Australia New Zealand Mortality Differences.' In *The Social Origins of Health and Well-Being*, edited by R. Eckersley, J. Dixon and R. Douglas. Cambridge: Cambridge University Press, 2001: 114–28.
291. Steel, F. 'A Source of Our Wealth, Yet Adverse to Our Health? Butter and the Diet–Heart Link in New Zealand to c. 1990.' *Social History of Medicine* 18, no. 3 (2005): 475–93.
292. Donovan, J. W. 'Cancer Mortality in New Zealand. 1. General.' *New Zealand Medical Journal* 72, no. 458 (July 1970): 9–12; '2. Digestive System.' *New Zealand Medical Journal* 72, no. 459 (August 1970): 104–10; and '4. Other Primary Sites.' *New Zealand Medical Journal* 75, no. 478 (March 1972): 144–8.
293. Ministry of Health. 'Cancer: New Registrations and Deaths 2010.' Wellington: Ministry of Health, 2013.
294. Aune, D., D. S. M. Chan, R. Lau, R. Vieira, D. C. Greenwood, E. Kampman, and T. Norat. 'Dietary Fibre, Whole Grains, and Risk of Colorectal Cancer: Systematic Review and Dose-Response Meta-Analysis of Prospective Studies.' *British Medical Journal* 343, no. d6617 (2011).
295. Potter, J., and D. Hunter. 'Colorectal Cancer.' In *Textbook of Cancer Epidemiology*, edited by H. O. Adami, D. Hunter and D. Trichopoulos. New York: Oxford University Press, 2008.
296. Cox, B., and J. Little. 'Reduced Risk of Colorectal Cancer among Recent Generations in New Zealand.' *British Journal of Cancer* 66, no. 2 (August 1992): 386–90.
297. Cox, B., and M. J. Sneyd. 'School Milk and Risk of Colorectal Cancer: A National Case-Control Study.' *American Journal of Epidemiology* 173, no. 4 (15 February 2011): 394–403.
298. Blakely, T., J. J. Barendregt, R. H. Foster, S. Hill, J. Atkinson, D. Sarfati, and R. Edwards. 'The Association of Active Smoking with Multiple Cancers: National Census-Cancer Registry Cohorts with Quantitative Bias Analysis.' *Cancer Causes Control* 24 (12 April 2013): 1243–55.
299. Office of the Surgeon General. 'How Tobacco Smoke Causes Disease: The Biology and Behavioral Basis for Smoking-Attributable Disease: A Report of the Surgeon General.' Rockville, MD: Department of Health and Human Services, Public Health Service, Office of Surgeon General, 2010.
300. King, D. R., A. H. Smith, and D. M. Salter. 'Mortality Attributable to Smoking in New Zealand.' *New Zealand Medical Journal* 96, no. 728 (23 March 1983): 195–9.
301. Carter, K. N., T. Blakely, and M. Soeberg. 'Trends in Survival and Life Expectancy by Ethnicity, Income and Smoking: 1980s to 2000s.' *New Zealand Medical Journal* 123, no. 1320 (13 August 2010): 1–13.
302. Murray, Christopher J. L. 'Why Is Japanese Life Expectancy So High?' *The Lancet* 378, no. 9797 (2011): 1124–5.
303. Hunt, Darren, Tony Blakely, Alistair Woodward, and Nick Wilson. 'The Smoking-Mortality Association Varies over Time and by Ethnicity in New Zealand.' *International Journal of Epidemiology* 34 (19 July 2005): 1020–28.
304. Blakely, Tony, Jackie Fawcett, Darren Hunt, and Nick Wilson. 'What is the Contribution of Smoking and Socioeconomic Position to Ethnic Inequalities in Mortality in New Zealand?' *The Lancet* 368, no. 9529 (2006): 44–52.

305. Wilson, Nick, Tony Blakely, and Martin Tobias. 'What Potential Has Tobacco Control for Reducing Health Inequalities? The New Zealand Situation.' *International Journal for Equity in Health* 5, no. 1 (2006): 14; and 'Correction: What Potential Has Tobacco Control for Reducing Health Inequalities? The New Zealand Situation.' *International Journal for Equity in Health* 5, no. 1 (2006): 16.
306. Johnston, Susie C. 'Lighting Up: The Social History of Smoking in New Zealand c. 1920 to 1962.' Victoria University of Wellington, 2009.
307. Statistics New Zealand. 'New Zealand Official Yearbook.' Wellington: Statistics New Zealand, 1901.
308. Laugesen, M. 'Tobacco Statistics 1991: Trends in Tobacco Consumption and Smoking Prevalence in New Zealand.' Wellington: Cancer Society, 1992.
309. Ruhm, Christopher J. 'Are Recessions Good for Your Health?' In *Working Paper 5570*. Cambridge, MA: National Bureau of Economic Research, 1996.
310. Blakely, T., and M. McCleod. 'Will the Financial Crisis Get Under the Skin and Affect Our Health? Learning from the Past, Predicting the Future.' *New Zealand Medical Journal* 122, no. 1307 (2009).
311. Stuckler, David, Sanjay Basu, Marc Suhrcke, Adam Coutts, and Martin McKee. 'The Public Health Effect of Economic Crises and Alternative Policy Responses in Europe: An Empirical Analysis.' *The Lancet* 374, no. 9686 (31 July 2009): 315–23.
312. Stuckler, D., and Sanjay Basu. *The Body Economic: Why Austerity Kills*. Basic Books, 2013.
313. Laugesen, M. 'Tobacco Statistics 2000.' Wellington: Cancer Society, 2000.
314. Easton, B. 'Smoking in New Zealand: A Census Investigation.' *Australian Journal of Public Health* 19, no. 2 (April 1995): 125–9.
315. Lopez, A. D., N. E. Collishaw, and T. Piha. 'A Descriptive Model of the Cigarette Epidemic in Developed Countries.' *Tobacco Control* 3, no. 3 (1 September 1994): 242–7.
316. Sorrenson, M. P. K. 'The Maori People and the City of Auckland.' *Te Ao Hou* 7, no. 3 (1959): 8–13.
317. Reid, P., and R. Pouwhare. *Te Taonga Mai Tawhiti (The Gift from a Distant Place)*. Auckland: Nino Taniwha, 1991.
318. Commission on Social Determinants of Health. 'Closing the Gap in a Generation: Health Equity through Action on the Social Determinants of Health.' Geneva: The World Health Organization, 2008.
319. Tukuitonga, C. F., A. Stewart, and R. Beaglehole. 'Coronary Heart Disease among Pacific Island People in New Zealand.' *New Zealand Medical Journal* 103, no. 898 (26 September 1990): 448–9.
320. McKeown, T. *Medicine in Modern Society*. London: George Allen & Unwin, 1965.
321. Blakely, Tony, Martin Tobias, and June Atkinson. 'Inequalities in Mortality During and after Restructuring of the New Zealand Economy: Repeated Cohort Studies.' *British Medical Journal* 336 (24 January 2008): 371–5.
322. Ajwani, S., T. Blakely, B. Robson, J. Atkinson, and C. Kiro. 'Unlocking the Numerator-Denominator Bias III: Adjustment Ratios by Ethnicity for 1981–1999 Mortality Data. The New Zealand Census-Mortality Study.' *New Zealand Medical Journal* 116, no. 1175 (2004): 6.

323. Blakely, T., J. Atkinson, and J. Fawcett. 'Ethnic Counts on Mortality and Census Data (Mostly) Agree for 2001–2004: New Zealand Census-Mortality Study Update.' *New Zealand Medical Journal* 121, no. 1281 (5 September 2008): 58–62.
324. Beaglehole, R., C. E. Salmond, and I. A. Prior. 'Prevalence of Coronary Heart Disease in Samples of New Zealand Maoris and Pakehas.' *New Zealand Medical Journal* 82, no. 546 (27 August 1975): 119–22.
325. Beaglehole, R., I. Prior, C. Salmond, and E. Eyles. 'Coronary Heart Disease in Maoris: Incidence and Case Mortality.' *New Zealand Medical Journal* 88, no. 618 (23 August 1978): 138–41.
326. Blakely, T., M. Tobias, J. Atkinson, L.-C. Yeh, and K. Huang. 'Tracking Disparity: Trends in Ethnic and Socioeconomic Inequalities in Mortality, 1981–2004.' Wellington: Ministry of Health, 2007.
327. Tobias, Martin, Tony Blakely, Don Matheson, Kumanan Rasanathan, and June Atkinson. 'Changing Trends in Indigenous Inequalities in Mortality: Lessons from New Zealand.' *International Journal of Epidemiology* 38, no. 6.
328. Russell, D., W. Parnell, and N. Wilson. 'NZ Food: NZ People. Key Results of the 1997 National Nutrition Survey.' Wellington: 1999.
329. University of Otago and Ministry of Health. 'A Focus on Nutrition: Key Findings of the 2008/09 New Zealand Adult Nutrition Survey.' Wellington: Ministry of Health, 2011.
330. Peter Herbison, personal communication, October 2011.
331. McLean, R. M., S. Williams, J. I. Mann, J. C. Miller, and W. R. Parnell. 'Blood Pressure and Hypertension in New Zealand: Results from the 2008/09 Adult Nutrition Survey.' *New Zealand Medical Journal* 126, no. 1372 (2013).
332. International Agency for Research on Cancer. 'Tobacco Smoke and Involuntary Smoking.' *IARC Monographs on the Evaluation of Carcinogenic Risks to Humans* 83 (2004): 1–1438.
333. Office of the Surgeon General. 'The Health Consequences of Smoking: A Report of the Surgeon General.' Washington, DC: Department of Health and Human Services, Centers for Disease Control and Prevention, National Center for Chronic Disease Prevention and Health Promotion, Office on Smoking and Health, 2004.
334. Gandini, S., E. Botteri, S. Iodice, M. Boniol, A. B. Lowenfels, P. Maisonneuve, and P. Boyle. 'Tobacco Smoking and Cancer: A Meta-Analysis.' *International Journal of Cancer* 122, no. 1 (2008): 155–64.
335. Ministry of Health. 'Cancer Incidence Projections: 1999–2003 Update.' Wellington: Ministry of Health, 2008.
336. Ministry of Health. 'Tobacco Trends 2008: A Brief Update of Tobacco Use in New Zealand.' Wellington: Ministry of Health, 2009.
337. Blakely, Tony, Caroline Shaw, June Atkinson, Ruth Cunningham, and Diana Sarfati. 'Social Inequalities or Inequities in Cancer Incidence? Repeated Census-Cancer Cohort Studies, New Zealand 1981–1986 to 2001–2004.' *Cancer Causes and Control* 22, no. 9 (2011): 1307–18.
338. Hunink, M. G., L. Goldman, A. N. Tosteson, M. A. Mittleman, P. A. Goldman, L. W. Williams, J. Tsevat, and M. C. Weinstein. 'The Recent Decline in Mortality

from Coronary Heart Disease, 1980–1990. The Effect of Secular Trends in Risk Factors and Treatment.' *JAMA: The Journal of the American Medical Association* 277, no. 7 (1997): 535–42.

339. Unal, Belgin, Julia Alison Critchley, and Simon Capewell. 'Modelling the Decline in Coronary Heart Disease Deaths in England and Wales, 1981–2000: Comparing Contributions from Primary Prevention and Secondary Prevention.' *British Medical Journal* (17 August 2005): bmj.38561.633345.8F
340. Law Commission. 'Alcohol in Our Lives: Curbing the Harm. A Report on the Review of the Regulatory Framework for the Sale and Supply of Liquor.' Wellington: Law Commission, 2010.
341. Scragg, R. 'A Quantification of Alcohol-Related Mortality in New Zealand.' *Australian and New Zealand Journal of Medicine* 25 (1995): 5–11.
342. Connor, J., R. Kydd, Kevin Shield, and Jürgen T. Rehm. 'Alcohol-Attributable Burden of Disease and Injury in New Zealand: 2004 and 2007.' Dunedin: University of Otago, 2013.
343. Cobiac, L., T. Vos, C. Doran, and A. Wallace. 'Cost-Effectiveness of Interventions to Prevent Alcohol-Related Disease and Injury in Australia.' *Addiction* 104, no. 10 (2009): 1646–55.
344. Vos, T., R. Carter, et al. 'Assessing Cost-Effectiveness in the Prevention (ACE-Prevention): Final Report.' Brisbane and Melbourne: University of Queensland and Deakin University, 2010.
345. Powles, J. 'Greek Migrants in Australia.' In *Migrants, Minorities and Health: Historical and Contemporary Studies*, edited by L. Marks and M. Worboys. London: Routledge, 1997: 210–27.
346. Haig, R. 'Working across the Ditch – New Zealanders Working in Australia.' Wellington: Department of Labour, 2010.
347. Statistics New Zealand. 'What Is the Extent of Crowding in New Zealand? An Analysis of Crowding in New Zealand Households 1986–2001.' Wellington: Statistics New Zealand, 2003.
348. Baker, M., R. Goodyear, L. Telfar Barnard, and P. Howden-Chapman. 'The Distribution of Household Crowding in New Zealand: An Analysis Based on 1991 to 2006 Census Data.' Wellington: He Kainga Oranga, Housing and Health Research Programme, University of Otago, 2012.
349. Baker, M. G., L. T. Barnard, A. Kvalsvig, A. Verrall, J. Zhang, M. Keall, N. Wilson, T. Wall, and P. Howden-Chapman. 'Increasing Incidence of Serious Infectious Diseases and Inequalities in New Zealand: A National Epidemiological Study.' *The Lancet* 379, no. 9821 (24 March 2012): 1112–9.
350. Baker, M., A. McNicholas, N. Garrett, N. Jones, J. Stewart, V. Koberstein, and D. Lennon. 'Household Crowding a Major Risk Factor for Epidemic Meningococcal Disease in Auckland Children.' *Pediatric Infectious Disease Journal* 19 (2000): 983–90.
351. Lim, Stephen S., Theo Vos, Abraham D. Flaxman, Goodarz Danaei, Kenji Shibuya, Heather Adair-Rohani, Markus Amann, et al. 'A Comparative Risk Assessment of Burden of Disease and Injury Attributable to 67 Risk Factors and Risk Factor Clusters in 21 Regions, 1990–2010: A Systematic Analysis for the Global Burden of Disease Study 2010.' *The Lancet* 380, no. 9859 (2012): 2224–60.

352. Ministry for the Environment. 'Environment New Zealand 2007.' Wellington: Ministry for the Environment, 2007.
353. Kuschel, G., J. Metcalfe, E. Wilton, J. Guria, S. Hales, K. Rolfe, and A. Woodward. 'Updated Health and Air Pollution in New Zealand Study.' Auckland: Emission Impossible, 2012.
354. Ministry of Transport. 'Road Deaths and Reported Injury Casualties 1921 to 2012.' Wellington: New Zealand Ministry of Transport, 2013.
355. Australian Transport Council, and Australian Transport Safety Bureau. *National Road Safety Strategy, 2011–2020*. Canberra: ATSB, Australian Federal Department of Infrastructure and Transport, 2011.
356. Ministry of Transport. 'The New Zealand Vehicle Fleet.' In *Annual Fleet Statistics 2012*. Ministry of Transport, 2013.
357. Advisory Committee to the Surgeon General of the Public Health Service. 'Smoking and Health: Report of the Advisory Committee to the Surgeon General of the Public Health Service.' DHEW publication no. (PHS) 64–1103. Washington, DC: Public Health Service, 1964.
358. Young, Leanne, and Boyd Swinburn. 'Impact of the Pick the Tick Food Information Programme on the Salt Content of Food in New Zealand.' *Health Promotion International* 17, no. 1 (1 March 2002): 13–19.
359. Hart, J. T. 'The Inverse Care Law.' *The Lancet* 1, no. 7696 (1971): 405–12.
360. Victora, C. G., J. P. Vaughan, F. C. Barros, A. C. Silva, and E. Tomasi. 'Explaining Trends in Inequities: Evidence from Brazilian Child Health Studies.' *The Lancet* 356 (2000): 1093–8.
361. Veronesi, U., P. Boyle, A. Goldhirsch, and G. Viale. 'Breast Cancer.' *The Lancet* 365 (2005): 1727–41.
362. Hankinson, S., R. Tamimi, and D. Hunter. 'Breast Cancer.' In *Textbook of Cancer Epidemiology*, second edition, edited by H. O. Adami, D. Hunter and D. Trichopoulos. New York: Oxford University Press, 2008.
363. Jeffreys, M., V. Stevanovic, M. Tobias, C. Lewis, L. Ellison-Loschmann, N. Pearce, and T. Blakely. 'Ethnic Inequalities in Cancer Survival in New Zealand: Linkage Study.' *American Journal of Public Health* 95, no. 5 (May 2005): 834–7.
364. Jeffreys, M., D. Sarfati, V. Stevanovic, M. Tobias, C. Lewis, N. Pearce, and T. Blakely. 'Socioeconomic Inequalities in Cancer Survival in New Zealand: The Role of Extent of Disease at Diagnosis.' *Cancer Epidemiology, Biomarkers and Prevention* 18, no. 3 (March 2009): 915–21.
365. Soeberg, M., T. Blakely, D. Sarfati, M. Tobias, R. Costilla, K. Carter, and J. Atkinson. 'Cancertrends: Trends in Cancer Survival by Ethnic and Socioeconomic Group, New Zealand 1991–2004.' Wellington: University of Otago and Ministry of Health, 2012.
366. Commission on Social Determinants of Health. 'Achieving Health Equity: From Root Causes to Fair Outcomes. Interim Statement.' Geneva: The World Health Organization, 2007.
367. Commission on Social Determinants of Health. 'Closing the Gap in a Generation: Health Equity Through Action on the Social Determinants of Health.' Geneva: The World Health Organization, 2008.
368. Cheyne, C., M. O'Brien, and M. Belgrave. *Social Policy in Aotearoa New Zealand:*

A Critical Introduction. Auckland: Oxford University Press, 1997.

369. Boston, J., P. Dalziel, and S. St John. *Redesigning the Welfare State in New Zealand: Problems, Policies and Prospects*, vol. 1. Auckland: Oxford University Press, 1999.
370. Statistics New Zealand. *New Zealand Now: Incomes*. Wellington: Statistics New Zealand, 1999.
371. Howden-Chapman, P., and M. Tobias, eds. *Social Inequalities in Health: New Zealand 1999*. Wellington: Ministry of Health, 2000.
372. Te Puni Kokiri. 'Progress Towards Closing the Social and Economic Gaps between Maori and Non-Maori. A Report to the Minister of Maori Affairs.' Wellington: Te Puni Kokiri, Ministry of Maori Development, 2000.
373. Mowbray, M. 'Distributions and Disparity: New Zealand Household Incomes.' Wellington: Ministry of Social Policy, 2001.
374. Förster, M., and M. M. d'Ercole. 'Income Distribution and Poverty in OECD Countries in the Second Half of the 1990s.' In *OECD Social, Employment And Migration Working Papers*, edited by OECD. Paris: OECD, 2005.
375. Ministry of Social Policy. *The Social Report: Te Purongo Oranga Tangata 2009*. Wellington: Ministry of Social Policy, 2009.
376. Perry, B. 'Household Incomes in New Zealand: Trends in Indicators of Inequality and Hardship 1982 to 2004.' Wellington: Ministry of Social Development, 2007.
377. Fletcher, M., and M. Dwyer. 'A Fair Go for All Children: Actions to Address Child Poverty in New Zealand.' Wellington: Office of the Children's Commission, 2008.
378. Khang, Young-Ho, John W. Lynch, and George A. Kaplan. 'Impact of Economic Crisis on Cause-Specific Mortality in South Korea.' *International Journal of Epidemiology* 34, no. 6 (1 December 2005): 1291–301.
379. Leon, D. A., L. Chenet, V. M. Shkolnikov, J. Shaprio, G. Rakhmanova, S. Vassin, and M. McKee. 'Huge Variation in Russian Mortality Rates 1984–94: Artefact, Alcohol, or What?' *The Lancet* 350 (1997): 383–8.
380. Shkolnikov, V., M. McKee, and D. A. Leon. 'Changes in Life Expectancy in Russia in the Mid-1990s.' *The Lancet* 357, no. 9260 (2001): 917–21.
381. Men, Tamara, Paul Brennan, Paolo Boffetta, and David Zaridze. 'Russian Mortality Trends for 1991–2001: Analysis by Cause and Region.' *British Medical Journal* 327, no. 7421 (25 October 2003): 964–70.
382. Lundin, A., I. Lundberg, L. Hallsten, J. Ottosson, and T. Hemmingsson. 'Unemployment and Mortality: A Longitudinal Prospective Study on Selection and Causation in 49321 Swedish Middle-Aged Men.' *Journal of Epidemiology and Community Health* 64, no. 1 (January 2010): 22–28.
383. Blakely, T., S. Collings, and J. Atkinson. 'Unemployment and Suicide: New Zealand Evidence for a Causal Association.' *Journal of Epidemiology & Community Health* 57 (2003): 594–600.
384. Keefe, Vera, Papaarangi Reid, Clint Ormsby, Bridget Robson, Gordon Purdie, Joanne Baxter, and Ngati Kahungunu Iwi Incorporated. 'Serious Health Events Following Involuntary Job Loss in New Zealand Meat Processing Workers.' *International Journal of Epidemiology* 31, no. 6 (1 December 2002): 1155–61.
385. Karsten, I. P., and K. Moser. 'Unemployment Impairs Mental Health: Meta-Analyses.' *Journal of Vocational Behaviour* 74 (2009): 264–82.
386. Fawcett, J., T. Blakely, and A. Kunst. 'Are Mortality Differences and Trends by

Education Any Better or Worse in New Zealand? A Comparison Study with Norway, Sweden and Finland, 1980–90s.' *European Journal of Epidemiology* 20, no. 8 (2005): 683–9.

387. Statistics New Zealand. 'National Population Estimates: December 2010 quarter.' Statistics New Zealand, 2011.
388. Rau, R., E. Soroko, D. Jasilionis, and J. W. Vaupel. 'Continued Reductions in Mortality at Advanced Ages.' *Population and Development Review* 34, no. 4 (2008): 747–68.
389. Wang, Haidong, and Samuel H. Preston. 'Forecasting United States Mortality Using Cohort Smoking Histories.' *Proceedings of the National Academy of Sciences* 106, no. 2 (2009): 393–8.
390. Statistics New Zealand. 'National Population Projections: 2011(Base)–2061.' In *Hot off the Press*. Wellington: Statistics New Zealand, 2012.
391. Goldstein, Joshua R., and Kenneth W. Wachter. 'Relationships between Period and Cohort Life Expectancy: Gaps and Lags.' *Population Studies* 60, no. 3 (November 2006): 257–69.
392. Shkolnikov, V. M., D. A. Jdanov, et al. 'Steep Increase in Best-Practice Cohort Life Expectancy.' *Population and Development Review* 37, no. 3 (2011): 419–34.
393. Office for National Statistics. 'What Are the Chances of Living to Age 100?' (29 August 2012): 1–10.
394. Reither, E. N., R. M. Haser, and Y. Yang. 'Do Birth Cohorts Matter? Age-Period-Cohort Analyses of the Obesity Epidemic in the United States.' *Social Science & Medicine* 69 (2009): 1439–48.
395. Ministry of Health. 'Tracking the Obesity Epidemic.' *Public Health Intelligence Occasional Bulletin No. 24*. Wellington: 2004.
396. Allman-Farinelli, M. A., T. Chey, A. E. Bauman, T. Gill, and W. P. T. James. 'Age, Period and Birth Cohort Effects on Prevalence of Overweight and Obesity in Australian Adults from 1990 to 2000.' *European Journal of Clinical Nutrition* 62, no. 7 (2008): 898–907.
397. Capewell, Simon, and Martin O'Flaherty. 'What Explains Declining Coronary Mortality? Lessons and Warnings.' *Heart* 94, no. 9 (1 September 2008): 1105–8.
398. Critchley, J., J. Liu, D. Zhao, W. Wei, S. Capewell, Julia Critchley, Jing Liu, et al. 'Explaining the Increase in Coronary Heart Disease Mortality in Beijing between 1984 and 1999.' *Circulation* 110, no. 10 (7 September 2004): 1236–44.
399. Rose, Geoffrey. 'Sick Individuals and Sick Populations.' *International Journal of Epidemiology* 14, no. 1 (1985): 32–8.
400. Farooqi, I. S., and S. O'Rahilly. 'Genetic Factors in Human Obesity.' *Obesity Reviews* 8, no. s1 (2007): 37–40.
401. Young, Lisa R., and Marion Nestle. 'Expanding Portion Sizes in the US Marketplace: Implications for Nutrition Counseling.' *Journal of the American Dietetic Association* 103, no. 2 (February 2003): 231–4.
402. Bleich, Sara N., David Cutler, Christopher Murray, and Alyce Adams. 'Why Is the Developed World Obese?' *Annual Review of Public Health* 29, no. 1 (2008): 273–95.
403. Bray, George A., Samara Joy Nielsen, and Barry M. Popkin. 'Consumption of High-Fructose Corn Syrup in Beverages May Play a Role in the Epidemic of Obesity.' *American Journal of Clinical Nutrition* 79, no. 4 (2004): 537–43.

404. Barker, D. J. 'The Fetal and Infant Origins of Adult Disease.' *British Medical Journal* 301, no. 6761 (17 November 1990): 1111.
405. Rosenberg, M. 'Birth Weights in Three Norwegian Cities, 1860–1984. Secular Trends and Influencing Factors.' *Annals of Human Biology* 15, no. 4 (July 1988): 275–88.
406. Childress, J. F., R. R. Faden, R. D. Gaare, L. O. Gostin, J. Kahn, R. J. Bonnie, N. E. Kass, et al. 'Public Health Ethics: Mapping the Terrain.' *Journal of Law, Medicine & Ethics* 30, no. 2 (2002): 170–8.
407. Public Health Leadership Society. 'Principles of the Ethical Practice of Public Health.' USA, 2002.
408. Lord Krebs, K., J. Unwin, et al. 'Public Health: Ethical Issues.' London: Nuffield Council on Bioethics, 2007.
409. Tannahill, A. 'Beyond Evidence – to Ethics: A Decision-Making Framework for Health Promotion, Public Health and Health Improvement.' *Health Promotion International* 23, no. 4 (December 2008): 380–90.
410. Have, Marieke ten, I. D. De Beaufort, J. P. Mackenbach, and A. van der Heide. 'An Overview of Ethical Frameworks in Public Health: Can They Be Supportive in the Evaluation of Programs to Prevent Overweight?' *BMC Public Health* 10 (2010): 638.
411. Drummond, M. F., M. J. Sculpher, G. W. Torrance, B. J. O'Brien, and G. L. Stoddart. *Methods for the Economic Evaluation of Health Care Programmes*, third edition. London: Oxford University Press, 2005.
412. Williams, A. 'Intergenerational Equity: An Exploration of the "Fair Innings" Argument.' *Health Economics* 6, no. 2 (April 1997): 117–32.
413. Roland, Rau, Soroko Eugeny, Jasilionis Domantas, and W. Vaupel James. 'Continued Reductions in Mortality at Advanced Ages.' *Population and Development Review* 34, no. 4 (2008): 747–68.
414. Rossi, I. A., V. Rousson, and F. Paccaud. 'The Contribution of Rectangularization to the Secular Increase of Life Expectancy: An Empirical Study.' *International Journal of Epidemiology* 42, no. 1 (21 December 2012): 250–8.
415. Kirkwood, Thomas B. L. 'A Systematic Look at an Old Problem.' *Nature* 451, no. 7179 (7 February 2008): 644–7.
416. Zhang, Guo, Juxue Li, Sudarshana Purkayastha, Yizhe Tang, Hai Zhang, Ye Yin, Bo Li, Gang Liu, and Dongsheng Cai. 'Hypothalamic Programming of Systemic Ageing Involving Ikk-B, Nf-Kb and Gnrh.' *Nature* 497, no. 7448 (2013): 211–16.
417. Shanley, Daryl P., and Thomas B. L. Kirkwood. 'Caloric Restriction Does Not Enhance Longevity in All Species and Is Unlikely to Do So in Humans.' *Biogerontology* 7, no. 3 (June 2006): 165–8.
418. Anderson, R., M., and R. Weindruch. 'The Caloric Restriction Paradigm: Implications for Healthy Human Aging.' *American Journal of Human Biology* 24, no. 2 (2012): 101–6.
419. Colman, R. J., R. M. Anderson, et al. 'Caloric Restriction Delays Disease Onset and Mortality in Rhesus Monkeys.' *Science* 325, no. 5937 (2009): 201–4.
420. Caplan, Arthur L. 'Death as an Unnatural Process. Why Is It Wrong to Seek a Cure for Aging?' *EMBO Reports* 6, suppl. 1 (July 2005): S72–5.
421. Kirkwood, Thomas B. L. 'Genes That Shape the Course of Ageing.' *Trends in Endocrinology & Metabolism* 14, no. 8 (October 2003): 345–7.

422. Hjelmborg, J. vB. 'Genetic Influences on Human Lifespan and Longevity.' *Human Genetics* 119 (2006): 312–21.
423. Horiuchi, Shiro, and J. R. Wilmoth. 'Deceleration in the Age Pattern of Mortality at Older Ages.' *Demography* 35 (1998): 391–412.
424. Kirkwood, Thomas B. L. 'Time of Our Lives. What Controls the Length of Life?' *EMBO Reports* 6 Spec No (July 2005): S4–8.
425. Falus, Andras, Istvan Marton, Erika Borbenyi, Adam Tahy, Pal Karadi, Janos Aradi, Adrienne Stauder, and Maria Kopp. 'A Challenging Epigenetic Message: Telomerase Activity Is Associated with Complex Changes in Lifestyle.' *Cell Biology International* 35, no. 11 (2011): 1079–83.
426. Epel, Elissa. 'How "Reversible" Is Telomeric Aging?' *Cancer Prevention Research* 5, no. 10 (2012): 1163–8.
427. von Zglinicki, Thomas. 'Will Your Telomeres Tell Your Future?' *British Medical Journal* 344 (2012): e1727.
428. Armanios, Mary. 'Telomeres and Age-Related Disease: How Telomere Biology Informs Clinical Paradigms.' *Journal of Clinical Investigation* 123, no. 3 (2013): 996–1002.
429. Hovatta, Iiris, Vanessa D. F. de Mello, Laura Kananen, Jaana Lindstrom, Johan G. Eriksson, Pirjo Ilanne-Parikka, Sirkka Keinanen-Kiukaanniemi, et al. 'Leukocyte Telomere Length in the Finnish Diabetes Prevention Study.' *PLoS ONE* (electronic resource) 7, no. 4 (2012): e34948.
430. Amsellem, Valerie, Guillaume Gary-Bobo, Elisabeth Marcos, Bernard Maitre, Vicky Chaar, Pierre Validire, Jean-Baptiste Stern, et al. 'Telomere Dysfunction Causes Sustained Inflammation in Chronic Obstructive Pulmonary Disease.' *American Journal of Respiratory & Critical Care Medicine* 184, no. 12 (2011): 1358–66.
431. Hochstrasser, Tanja, Josef Marksteiner, and Christian Humpel. 'Telomere Length Is Age-Dependent and Reduced in Monocytes of Alzheimer Patients.' *Experimental Gerontology* 47, no. 2 (2012): 160–3.
432. Honig, Lawrence S., Min Suk Kang, Nicole Schupf, Joseph H. Lee, and Richard Mayeux. 'Association of Shorter Leukocyte Telomere Repeat Length with Dementia and Mortality.' *Archives of Neurology* 69, no. 10 (2012): 1332–9.
433. Cohen, Sheldon, Denise Janicki-Deverts, Ronald B. Turner, Margaretha L. Casselbrant, Ha-Sheng Li-Korotky, Elissa S. Epel, and William J. Doyle. 'Association between Telomere Length and Experimentally Induced Upper Respiratory Viral Infection in Healthy Adults.' *JAMA: The Journal of the American Medical Association* 309, no. 7 (2013): 699–705.
434. Steptoe, Andrew, Mark Hamer, Lee Butcher, Jue Lin, Lena Brydon, Mika Kivimaki, Michael Marmot, Elizabeth Blackburn, and Jorge D. Erusalimsky. 'Educational Attainment but not Measures of Current Socioeconomic Circumstances are Associated with Leukocyte Telomere Length in Healthy Older Men and Women.' *Brain, Behavior, & Immunity* 25, no. 7 (2011): 1292–8.
435. Batty, G. D., Y. Wang, S. W. Brouilette, P. Shiels, C. Packard, J. Moore, N. J. Samani, and I. Ford. 'Socioeconomic Status and Telomere Length: The West of Scotland Coronary Prevention Study.' *Journal of Epidemiology and Community Health* 63, no. 10 (2009): 839–41.

436. Needham, Belinda L., Nancy Adler, Steven Gregorich, David Rehkopf, Jue Lin, Elizabeth H. Blackburn, and Elissa S. Epel. 'Socioeconomic Status, Health Behavior, and Leukocyte Telomere Length in the National Health and Nutrition Examination Survey, 1999–2002.' *Social Science & Medicine* 85, no. C (1 June 2013): 1–8.
437. Kirkwood, T. 'Evolution of Aging.' *Nature* 270 (1977): 301–4.
438. Bonneux, L., Jan J. Barendregt, and P. J. Van der Maas. 'The Expiry Date of Man: A Synthesis of Evolutonary Biology and Public Health.' *Journal of Epidemiology and Community Health* 52 (1998): 619–23.
439. Mitteldorf, J. 'Female Fertility and Longevity.' *Age (Dordr)* 32, no. 1 (March 2010): 79–84.
440. Flannery, T. *The Future Eaters.* Chatswood, NSW: Reed Books, 1994.
441. Goklany, Indur M. 'Humanity Unbound. How Fossil Fuels Saved Humanity from Nature and Nature from Humanity.' *Cato Institute Policy Analysis*, no. 715 (20 December 2012): 1–36.
442. McMichael, A. J., and J. W. Powles. 'Human Numbers, Environment, Sustainability, and Health. [See Comment].' *British Medical Journal* 319, no. 7215 (9 October 1999): 977–80.
443. Steckel, Richard H. 'Heights and Human Welfare: Recent Developments and New Directions.' *Explorations in Economic History* 46, no. 1 (2009): 1–23.
444. Gleick, P. H. 'The Changing Water Paradigm: A Look at Twenty-First Century Water Resources Development.' *Water International* 25, no. 1 (2000): 127–38.
445. Postel, S. N., G. C. Daily, and P. R. Ehrlich. 'Human Appropriation of Renewable Fresh Water.' *Science* 271 (1996): 785–8.
446. Mackenbach, Johan, Lany Slobbe, Caspar Looman, Agnes van der Heide, Johan Polder, and Joop Garssen. 'Sharp Upturn of Life Expectancy in the Netherlands: Effect of More Health Care for the Elderly?' *European Journal of Epidemiology* 26 (2011): 903–14.
447. Peters, Glen P., Robbie M. Andrew, Tom Boden, Josep G. Canadell, Philippe Ciais, Corinne Le Quéré, Gregg Marland, Michael R. Raupach, and Charlie Wilson. 'The Challenge to Keep Global Warming Below 2°C.' *Nature Climate Change* 3, no. 1 (2 December 2012): 4–6.
448. Kump, Lee R. 'The Last Great Global Warming.' *Scientific American* 305, no. 1 (July 2011): 56–61.
449. Battisti, D. 'Historical Warnings of Future Food Insecurity with Unprecedented Seasonal Heat.' *Science* 323, no. 5911 (2009): 240.
450. Dunne, John P., Ronald J. Stouffer, and Jasmin G. John. 'Reductions in Labour Capacity from Heat Stress under Climate Warming.' *Nature Climate Change* 3, no. 4 (24 March 2013): 1–4.
451. Hsiang, Solomon M., Kyle C. Meng, and Mark A. Cane. 'Civil Conflicts Are Associated with the Global Climate.' *Nature* 476, no. 7361 (16 August 2011): 438–41.
452. Franco, Manuel, Pedro Ordunez, Benjamin Caballero, Jose A. Tapia Granados, Mariana Lazo, Jose Luis Bernal, Eliseo Guallar, and Richard S. Cooper. 'Impact of Energy Intake, Physical Activity, and Population-Wide Weight Loss on Cardiovascular Disease and Diabetes Mortality in Cuba, 1980 2005.' *American Journal of Epidemiology* 166, no. 12 (2007): 1374–80.
453. Pope, C. Arden, 3rd, Majid Ezzati, and Douglas W. Dockery. 'Fine-Particulate

Air Pollution and Life Expectancy in the United States.' *New England Journal of Medicine* 360, no. 4 (2009): 376–86.

454. Haines, Andy, Kirk R. Smith, Dennis Anderson, Paul R. Epstein, Anthony J. McMichael, Ian Roberts, Paul Wilkinson, James Woodcock, and Jeremy Woods. 'Policies for Accelerating Access to Clean Energy, Improving Health, Advancing Development, and Mitigating Climate Change.' *The Lancet* 370, no. 9594 (6 October 2007): 1264–81.
455. Rogelj, Joeri, William Hare, Jason Lowe, Detlef P. van Vuuren, Keywan Riahi, Ben Matthews, Tatsuya Hanaoka, Kejun Jiang, and Malte Meinshausen. 'Emission Pathways Consistent with a 2 Degrees C Global Temperature Limit.' *Nature Climate Change* 1, no. 11 (23 October 2011): 413–18.
456. Fries, J. 'Aging, Natural Death, and the Compression of Morbidity.' *New England Journal of Medicine* 303 (1980): 130–5.
457. Crimmins, E. M. 'Mortality and Health in Human Life Spans.' *Experimental Gerontology* 36, no. 4–6 (2001): 885–97.
458. Manton, K. G. 'Recent Declines in Chronic Disability in the Elderly U.S. Population: Risk Factors and Future Dynamics.' *Annual Review of Public Health* 29 (2008): 91–113.
459. Statistics New Zealand, and Ministry of Health. 'Longer Life, Better Health? Trends in Health Expectancy in New Zealand, 1996–2006.' Wellington: Statistics New Zealand, 2009.
460. Robine, Jean-Marie, and Fred Paccaud. 'Nonagenarians and Centenarians in Switzerland, 1860–2001: A Demographic Analysis.' *Journal of Epidemiology & Community Health* 59, no. 1 (January 2005): 31–7.
461. Graham, P., T. Blakely, P. Davis, A. Sporle, and N. Pearce. 'Compression, Expansion, or Dynamic Equilibrium? The Evolution of Health Expectancy in New Zealand.' *Journal of Epidemiology & Community Health* 58, no. 8 (2004): 659–66.
462. Schoeni, Robert F., Jersey Liang, Joan Bennett, Hidehiro Sugisawa, Taro Fukaya, and Erika Kobayashi. 'Trends in Old-Age Functioning and Disability in Japan, 1993–2002.' *Population Studies: A Journal of Demography* 60, no. 1 (2006): 39–53.
463. Crimmins, Eileen M., and Hiram Beltrán-Sánchez. 'Mortality and Morbidity Trends: Is There Compression of Morbidity?' *The Journals of Gerontology* 66B, no. 1 (2011): 75.
464. Jagger, C., and J.-M. Robine. 'Healthy Life Expectancy.' In *International Handbook of Adult Mortality,* edited by EG Rogers and EM Crimmins, 2011.
465. Christensen, Kaare, M. McGue, I. Petersen, B. Jeune, and J. Vaupel. 'Exceptional Longevity Does Not Result in Excessive Levels of Disability.' *Proceedings of the National Academy of Sciences* 105 (2008): 13274–9.
466. Kinsella, K. G. 'Future Longevity – Demographic Concerns and Consequences.' *Journal of the American Geriatrics Society* 53 (2005): S299-S303.
467. Boyd, M., M. Connolly, N. Kerse, S. Foster, M. Randow, and C. Chelimo, et al. 'Changes in Aged Care Residents' Characteristics and Dependency in Auckland 1988 to 2008.' Auckland: University of Auckland, 2009.
468. Tobias, M., L. C. Yeh, and E. Johnson. 'Burden of Alzheimer's Disease: Population-Based Estimates and Projections for New Zealand, 2006–2031.' *Australian & New Zealand Journal of Psychiatry* 42, no. 9 (September 2008): 828–36.

469. Christensen, K., M. Thinggaard, A. Oksuzyan, T. Steenstrup, K. Andersen-Ranberg, B. Jeune, M. McGue, and J. W. Vaupel. 'Physical and Cognitive Functioning of People Older Than 90 Years: A Comparison of Two Danish Cohorts Born 10 Years Apart.' *The Lancet* 382, no. 9903 (2013): 1507–13.
470. Schrijvers, Elisabeth M. C., Benjamin F. J. Verhaaren, Peter J. Koudstaal, Albert Hofman, M. Arfan Ikram, and Monique M. B. Breteler. 'Is Dementia Incidence Declining? Trends in Dementia Incidence since 1990 in the Rotterdam Study.' *Neurology* 78, no. 19 (2012): 1456–63.
471. Olshansky, S. Jay, and L. Hayflick. 'Public Policies Intended to Influence Adult Mortality.' In *International Handbook of Adult Mortality*, edited by E. G. Rogers and Eileen M. Crimmins. New York: Springer, 2011: 571–81.
472. Murray, Christopher J. L., Theo Vos, Rafael Lozano, Mohsen Naghavi, Abraham D. Flaxman, Catherine Michaud, Majid Ezzati, et al. 'Disability-Adjusted Life Years (Dalys) for 291 Diseases and Injuries in 21 Regions, 1990–2010: A Systematic Analysis for the Global Burden of Disease Study 2010.' *The Lancet* 380, no. 9859 (2012): 2197–223.
473. Salomon, Joshua A., Theo Vos, Daniel R. Hogan, Michael Gagnon, Mohsen Naghavi, Ali Mokdad, Nazma Begum, et al. 'Common Values in Assessing Health Outcomes from Disease and Injury: Disability Weights Measurement Study for the Global Burden of Disease Study 2010.' *The Lancet* 380, no. 9859 (2012): 2129–43.
474. Ministry of Health. 'Health Loss in New Zealand: A Report from the New Zealand Burden of Diseases, Injuries and Risk Factors Study, 2006–2016.' Wellington: Ministry of Health, 2013.
475. Doll, R., R. Peto, J. Boreham, and I. Sutherland. 'Mortality in Relation to Smoking: 50 Years' Observations on Male British Doctors.' *British Medical Journal* 328, no. 7455 (26 June 2004): 1519.
476. Blakely, Tony, George Thomson, Nick Wilson, Richard Edwards, and Heather Gifford. 'The Maori Affairs Select Committee Inquiry and the Road to a Smokefree Aotearoa.' *New Zealand Medical Journal* 123, no. 1326 (2010): 7–18.
477. New Zealand Parliament. 'Inquiry into the Tobacco Industry in Aotearoa and the Consequences of Tobacco Use for Māori, Report of the Māori Affairs Committee.' Wellington: New Zealand Parliament, 2010.
478. Blakely, T., K. Carter, N. Wilson, R. Edwards, A. Woodward, G. Thomson, and D. Sarfati. 'If Nobody Smoked Tobacco in New Zealand from 2020 Onwards, What Effect Would This Have on Ethnic Inequalities in Life Expectancy?' *New Zealand Medical Journal* 123, no. 1320 (2010): 26–36.
479. Turley, M., M. Tobias, et al. 'Non-Fatal Disease Burden Associated with Excess Body Mass Index and Waist Circumferencei New Zealand Adults.' *Australian & New Zealand Journal of Public Health* 30, no. 3 (2006): 231–7.
480. Renehan, A. G., M. Tyson, et al. 'Body-Mass Index and incidence of Cancer: A Systematic Review and Meta-Analysis of Prospective Observational Studies.' *The Lancet* 371, no. 9612 (2008): 569–78.
481. Prospective Studies Collaboration. 'Body-Mass Index and Cause-Specific Mortality in 900 000 Adults: Collaborative Analyses of 57 Prospective Studies.' *The Lancet* 373, no. 9669 (2009): 1083–96.
482. Peeters, A., J. J. Barendregt, et al. 'Obesity in Adulthood and its Consequences

for Life Expectancy: A Life-Table Analysis.' *Annals of Internal Medicine* 138, no. 1 (2003): 24.

483. Panel on Understanding Divergent Trends in Longevity in High-Income Countries. *Explaining Divergent Levels of Mortality in High-Income Countries.* National Research Council, 2011: 1–194.
484. Mehta, N. K., and V. W. Chang. 'Secular Declines in the Association between Obesity and Mortality in the United States.' *Population and Development Review* 37, no. 3 (2011): 435–51.
485. Flegal K. M., B. K. Kit, H. Orpana, and B. I. Graubard. 'Association of All-Cause Mortality with Overweight and Obesity Using Standard Body Mass Index Categories: A Systematic Review and Meta-Analysis.' *JAMA: The Journal of the American Medical Association* 309, no. 1 (2013): 71–82.
486. Gregg, E. W., Y. J. Cheng, et al. 'Secular Trends in Cardiovascular Disease Risk Factors According to Body Mass Index in US Adults.' *JAMA: The Journal of the American Medical Association* 293, no. 15 (2005): 1868–74.
487. Stewart, S. T., D. M. Cutler, et al. 'Forecasting the Effects of Obesity and Smoking on U.S. Life Expectancy.' *New England Journal of Medicine* 361, no. 23 (2009): 2252–60.
488. Preston, S. H., A. Stokes, et al. 'Projecting the Effect of Changes in Smoking and Obesity on Future Life Expectancy in the United States.' The National Bureau of Economic Research, 2012.
489. van Baal, P. H., R. T. Hoogenveen, et al. 'Estimating Health-Adjusted Life Expectancy Conditional on Risk Factors: Results for Smoking and Obesity.' *Population Health Metrics* 4 (2006): 14.
490. Klijs, B., J. P. Mackenbach, et al. 'Obesity, Smoking, Alcohol Consumption and Years Lived with Disability: A Sullivan Life Table Approach.' *BMC Public Health* 11 (2011): 378.
491. Laatikainen, T., J. Critchley, et al. 'Explaining the Decline in Coronary Heart Disease Mortality in Finland between 1982 and 1997.' *American Journal of Epidemiology* 162, no. 8 (2005): 764–73.
492. Capewell, S., D. K. Hayes, et al. 'Life-Years Gained Among US Adults From Modern Treatments and Changes in the Prevalence of 6 Coronary Heart Disease Risk Factors Between 1980 and 2000.' *American Journal of Epidemiology* 170, no. 2 (2009): 229–36.
493. Aspelund, T., V. Gudnason, et al. 'Analysing the Large Decline in Coronary Heart Disease Mortality in the Icelandic Population Aged 25–74 between the Years 1981 and 2006.' *PLoS ONE* 5, no. 11 (2010): e13957.
494. PHARMAC Pharmaceutical Management Agency. 'Pharmaceutical Management Agency Annual Report: For the Year Ended 30 June 2012.' Wellington: PHARMAC Pharmaceutical Management Agency, 2012.
495. Yi Lee, Y., J. L. Veerman, et al. 'The Cost-Effectiveness of Laparoscopic Adjustable Gastric Banding in the Morbidly Obese Adult Population of Australia.' *PLoS ONE* 8, no. 5 (2013): e64965.
496. Thomas, S., D. Fayter, et al. 'Population Tobacco Control Interventions and Their Effects on Social Inequalities in Smoking: Systematic Review.' *Tobacco Control* 17, no. 4 (2008): 230–37.
497. Capewell, S., and H. Graham. 'Will Cardiovascular Disease Prevention Widen

Health Inequalities?' *PLoS Medicine* 7, no. 8 (2010): e1000320.

498. Subramanian, S. V., and I. Kawachi. 'Income Inequality and Health: What Have We Learned So Far?' *Epidemiologic Reviews* 26 (2004): 78–91.
499. Blakely, T., and N. Wilson. 'Shifting Dollars, Saving Lives: What Might Happen to Mortality Rates, and Socio-Economic Inequalities in Mortality Rates, if Income was Redistributed?' *Social Science & Medicine* 62, no. 8 (2006): 2024–34.
500. Morgan, G., and S. Guthrie. *The Big Kahuna: Turning Tax and Welfare in New Zealand on its Head*. New Zealand: Public Interest Publishing, 2011.
501. Retirement Commissioner. *Review of Retirement Income Policy*. Wellington: Office of the Retirement Commissioner, 2010.
502. Salomon, J. A., H. Wang, et al. 'Healthy Life Expectancy for 187 Countries, 1990–2010: A Systematic Analysis for the Global Burden Disease Study 2010.' *The Lancet* 380, no. 9859 (2012): 2144–62.
503. Suzuki, E., S. Kashima, et al. 'Social And Geographic Inequalities in Premature Adult Mortality In Japan: A Multilevel Observational Study From 1970 to 2005.' *BMJ Open* 2, no. 2 (2012): e000425–e000425.
504. Cobiac, L., T. Ikeda, N. Nghiem, T. Blakely, and N. Wilson. 'Modelling the Implications of Regular Increases in Tobacco Taxes as a Tobacco Endgame Strategy.' *Tobacco Control*, in press (2014).

INDEX

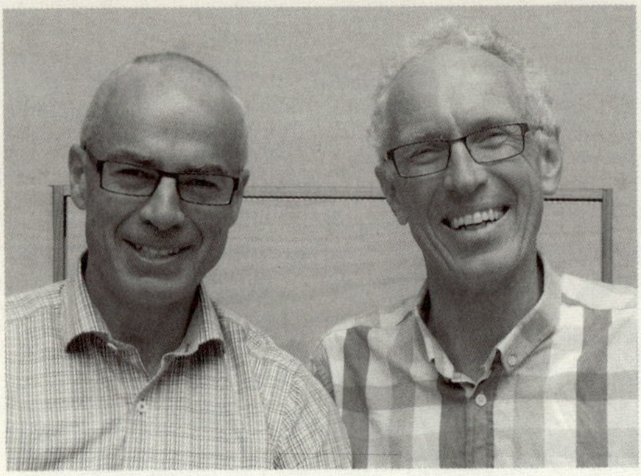

Alistair Woodward is Professor of Epidemiology and Biostatistics at the University of Auckland and was head of the School of Population Health from 2004 to 2013. His first degree was in medicine and he undertook his postgraduate training in public health in the United Kingdom. Woodward has a PhD in epidemiology from the University of Adelaide. Prior to taking up a post at the University of Auckland, he was professor of Public Health at the University of Otago, Wellington. His research interests include tobacco, radio-frequency radiation and health, transport and injury, and climate change. He has worked for the World Health Organization throughout the Pacific, and led the writing of the health chapter in the fifth assessment report of the Intergovernmental Panel on Climate Change. Since 2009 Woodward has been an editor of the *Australian and New Zealand Journal of Public Health.*

Tony Blakely is an epidemiologist at the University of Otago. His extensive research portfolio includes initiating the New Zealand Census-Mortality Study, a pioneering study linking the national censuses with mortality data to allow research on ethnic and socio-economic inequalities and the contribution of smoking to mortality. He has also led the parallel study, CancerTrends, that links census and cancer registration data to allow for cancer incidence and survival studies. Blakely directs a Health Inequalities Research Programme that is built around these two studies and includes both the health component of a panel study of 20,000 adults followed up for eight years and a series of neighbourhoods and health research projects. Since 2010, he has directed the HRC-funded Burden of Disease Epidemiology, Equity and Cost Effectiveness Programme. This ambitious programme reviews the health impact and cost effectiveness of a range of preventative and cancer control interventions. Cutting across all Blakely's research is a strong focus and interest in epidemiological and quantitative research methodologies; he teaches short courses in social epidemiology and epidemiological methods. He has published more than 150 peer-reviewed journal articles.